Men's Health®

TOTAL-BODY
Health & Fitness Guide
2013

RODALE.

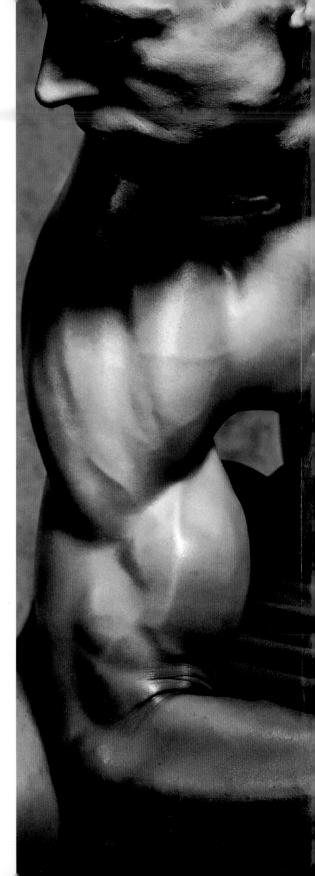

© 2013 by Rodale Inc.

Printed in the United States of America

Rodale Inc. makes every effort to use acid-free ∞, recycled paper ♲.

Library of Congress Cataloging-in-Publication Data is on file with the publisher.

ISBN: 978–1–60961–928–2

2   4   6   8   10   9   7   5   3   1   hardcover

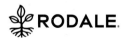 **RODALE.**

We inspire and enable people to improve their lives and the world around them.
For more of our products visit **rodalestore.com** or call 800-848-4735.

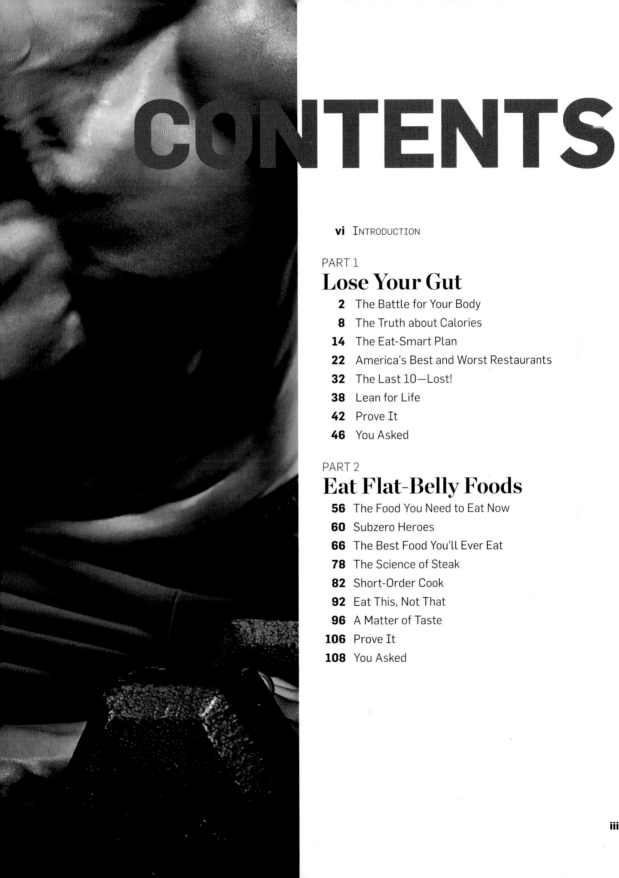

CONTENTS

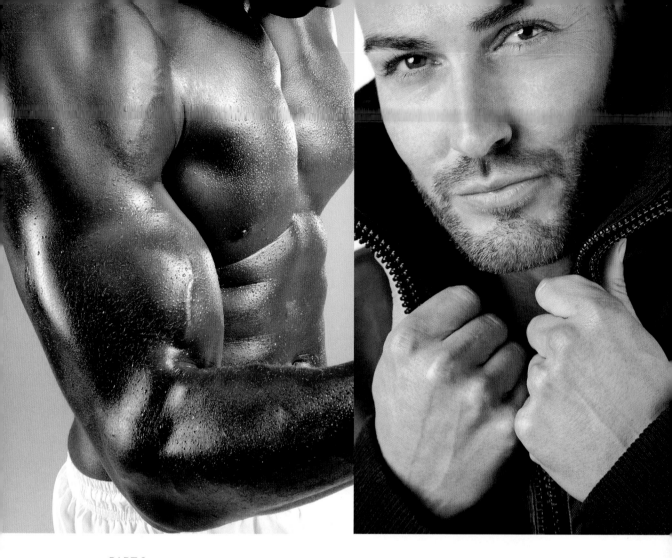

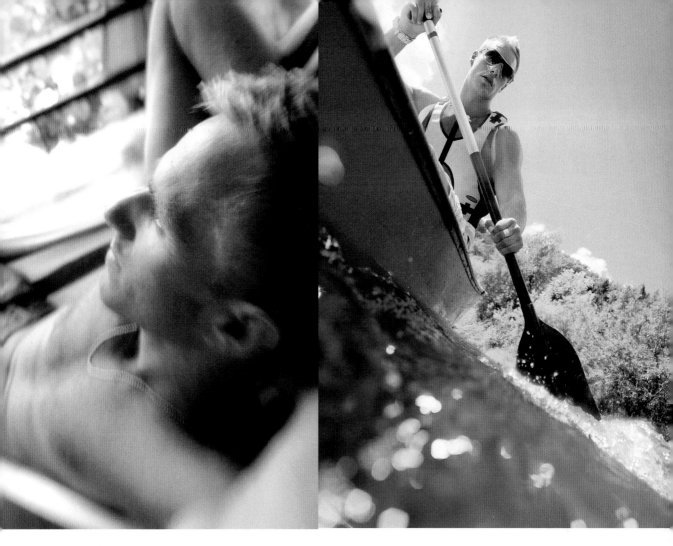

INTRODUCTION

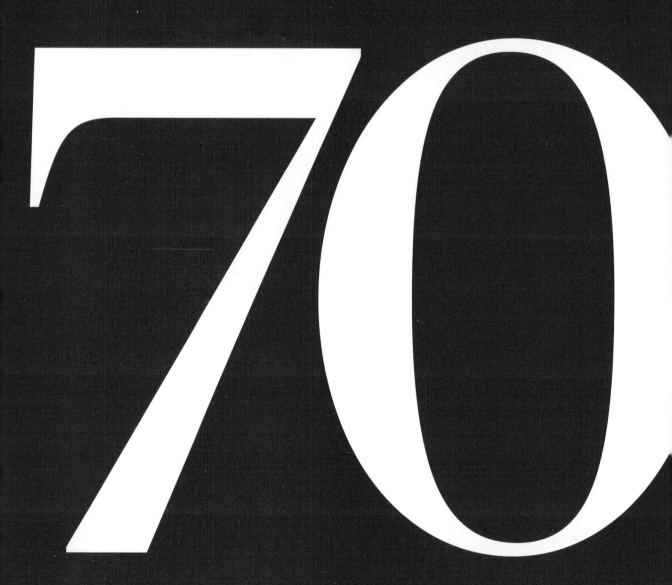

70

That's the percentage of men who are overweight and obese. Hand in hand with that sobering stat is 37: That's the percentage of men who are sedentary. If you are a member of either of those two groups—or worse yet of *both* of those two groups—this book will help you boost your fitness as well as your overall health. With the tips in the *Men's Health Total-Body Health & Fitness Guide 2013,* you can take your life to the next level. You'll lose weight, eat better, muscle up, stay well, look great, and play every game—better.

In Part I, you'll take the first step and Lose Your Gut. Discover the "Rules of the Ripped," target visceral fat with our belly-busting workout, and for once and for all learn the "Truth about Calories."

Life is short; learn how to fill it with great foods in Part 2, Eat Flat-Belly Foods. Here you'll read about the "Food You Need to Eat Now," cook "The Best Food You'll Ever Eat," and manage to not undo all of your healthy eating when you eat at restaurants by knowing how to "Eat This, Not That."

In Part 3, you'll save time and get strong in Muscle Up Fast. First take our simple self-test. Then build strong shoulders, chest, abs, buns, and even those small, easily forgotten muscles—for big results, big gains.

You'll Look Better Instantly after reading Part 4. With some simple style strategies, you'll find out how to combine timeless essentials with timely trends. You'll save money and streamline your life with the most effective grooming products. And you'll learn "What Every Woman Wants."

In part 5, you'll find out how to Live Longer, Live Better. Discover how to have "Your Healthiest Year Ever." Plus you'll learn how you can prevent allergies, cancer—even heart disease.

Last, in part 6, you can Improve Your Game. Heed these tips to smash your personal records. Balance your body to take both your workout and game to the next level. And learn how to play everything better.

We hope that this book will inspire you to change your body—to change your life—by moving more. You'll add more years to your life, and more life to your years. Here's to your better health!

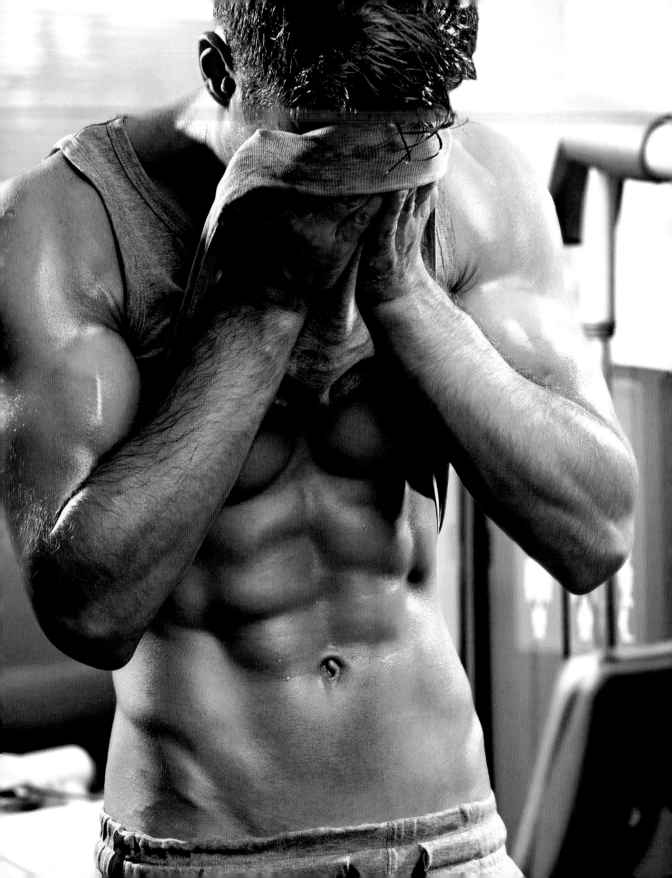

Lose Your Gut

The Battle for Your Body

Fat and Muscle are at war. Make sure the good guy wins.

The battle goes on whether you're awake or asleep, on the couch or on the treadmill. On one side, the good guy: Muscle. Muscle is like the doorman at your own personal nightclub. It's his job to make you look good, attract the cute girls, and keep out the riffraff. The riffraff, in this case, is a man called Fat.

2

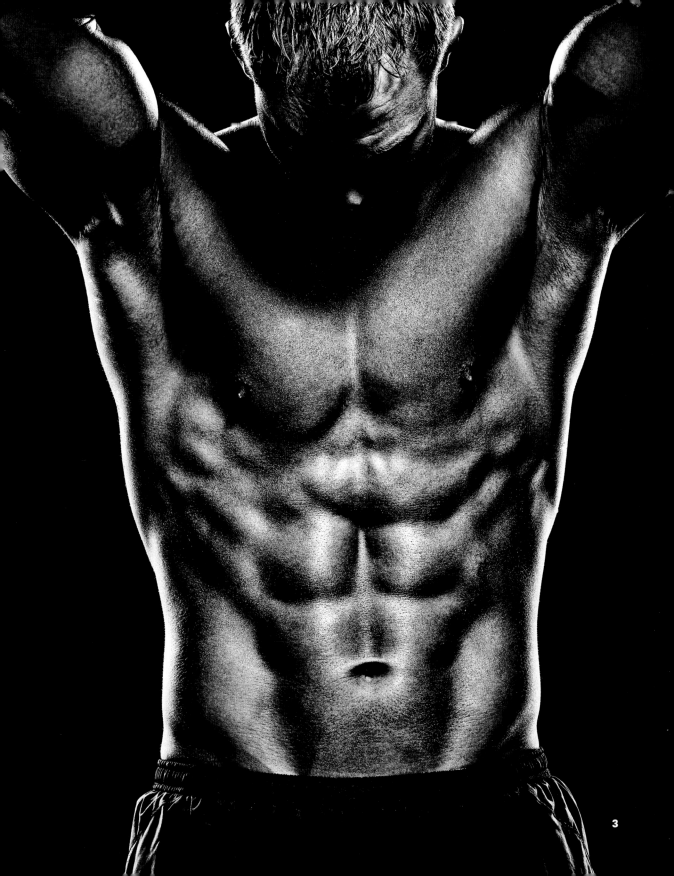

Fat hates Muscle, and the feeling is mutual. Fat wants to kill your metabolism with all his fat, lazy friends, who will just sit around bumming free drinks, eating all the peanuts at the bar, and scaring the women away. Fat also wants to run Muscle out of town.

You know which side you're rooting for: Muscle burns Fat for energy, which is why building and maintaining muscle is the key to losing flab and sculpting a lean, toned body. Muscle boosts metabolism, helping you burn calories day and night. Muscle heightens your testosterone level,

Visceral fat fights fitness by releasing compounds that degrade muscle quality.

keeping aging at bay and your sex drive revving. Muscle helps protect you from heart disease, back pain, arthritis, and depression. Help Muscle win the war against Fat, and you'll triumph over much more than your waistline. The key: firing up your metabolism.

Just what is metabolism? Simply put, it's all the various chemical reactions that happen inside your body 24-7 to keep you alive. Think of your metabolism as your caloric bouncer, ready to throw Fat out of Club You.

Your metabolism isn't an instant-makeover machine, but you can order it to keep an eye out for big fat party crashers and throw them back onto the street. Learn the following surprising truths, and you'll help Muscle conquer its flabby nemesis—once and for all.

Burning calories in the gym is (almost) a waste of time.

Sure, burning calories is great. But the energy you expend in the gym isn't as big a deal as those LED readouts on the treadmill might make it seem. In fact, we all have three distinct types of "burns" that make up our metabolism. Here they are.

Burn #1: Basal (resting) metabolism: 60 to 75 percent. Your basal metabolic rate, or BMR, accounts for 60 to 75 percent of your overall metabolism. Surprisingly, it represents the calories you burn doing nothing at all. It's fueled by your heart beating, your lungs working to breathe, and even your cells dividing.

Burn #2: Digestive metabolism: 10 percent. This burn results from the thermic effect of food, or TEF. Simply digesting food—converting carbohydrates to sugar and protein to amino acids—typically burns 10 percent of your daily calories. You burn more calories digesting protein than you do digesting carbohydrates and fat—about 25 calories for every 100 consumed, versus zero to 10 for carbs and fat.

Burn #3: Exercise and movement metabolism: 15 to 30 percent. This part of your metabolism includes your gym workouts and other physical activities, such as jogging or playing softball (called "exercise-activity thermogenesis," or EAT). It also includes your countless incidental movements throughout the day, such as turning the pages of this book (called "non-exercise activity thermogenesis," or NEAT).

So why is it so hard to lose weight just by exercising? Why do you see so many overweight people in the gym? The answer is simple. Exercise and movement account for only 15 to 30 percent of your fat burn. Up to 85 percent of your calorie burn in a given day has nothing to do with moving your body.

But that doesn't mean you should skip the gym! You just need to know how to make exercise work for you. The fact is, exercise can play an important role in preparing Muscle to conquer its greatest threat—Fat, of course.

Truth #2

The fatter you get, the fatter you'll get.

Fat doesn't just show up at your door one day, rent a room, and live quietly alone with a couple of cats. Fat loves company. The more fat you open the door to, the harder you'll find it to stop even more fat from inviting itself in. Here's why.

Your BMR—basal (resting) metabolic rate—accounts for the majority of the calories that you burn every day. It's

Rules of the Ripped

Hunger tells your body to store fat. So eat smart to fuel new muscle and stoke your metabolism. Here's how.

RULE #1 Eat protein with every meal and every snack.

At any given moment, even at rest, your body is breaking down and building up muscle, says Jeff S. Volek, PhD, RD, an exercise and nutrition researcher at the University of Connecticut. Every time you eat at least 10 to 15 grams of protein, you trigger a burst of muscle-building protein synthesis. And when you eat at least 30 grams, that period of synthesis lasts for about 3 hours, and that means even more muscle growth.

YOUR PLAN: Eat at least 30 grams of protein at all three meals, taking it in from meats, seafood, cheese, eggs, and milk. For each snack, eat at least 10 to 15 grams of protein, such as two hard-boiled eggs.

RULE #2 Never eat the world's worst breakfast.

What's the world's worst breakfast? No breakfast at all. When you wake up in the morning, your body is fuel deprived. It needs food to kick-start your metabolism.

"When you shift calories to the morning, you lose weight and keep it off," says David Grotto, RD, author of *101 Optimal Life Foods*. In fact, regularly skipping breakfast increases your risk of obesity by 450 percent.

YOUR PLAN: Eat a considerable portion of your calories—30 to 35 percent of your total intake—in the morning. The very best breakfasts match proteins and whole grains with produce and healthy fats. For example, try fried eggs on whole-grain toast and a protein-and-fruit smoothie.

RULE #3 Eat before and after exercise.

Here's great news for any man who loves to eat: You probably need to eat more. Eating before training speeds muscle growth, Dutch and British researchers report. Downing protein before and after weight training also helps blunt the fat-storing effects of cortisol, according to researchers at Syracuse University. What's more, pre- and postworkout protein also helps your body produce more stem cells, which aid in recovery and muscle growth, Finnish scientists have discovered.

YOUR PLAN: Eat a snack composed of carbohydrates and protein 30 minutes or so before your workout, and eat one of your protein-rich meals immediately after exercise. Remember, lost time is lost muscle.

determined by a number of factors: your bon, age, and height; your genes (most likely); and your body's ratio of fat to muscle. The problem is, fat slows your calorie burn. Fat is lazy on a metabolic level: It burns barely any calories at all. For your body to support a pound of fat, it needs to burn about 2 calories a day. Muscle, on the other hand, is metabolically very active. At rest, 1 pound of skeletal muscle burns three times as many calories every day just to sustain itself, and the more calories you burn, the more body fat you tend to lose. That's why Fat hates Muscle—because Muscle is constantly burning it off.

So Fat actually fights back, trying to erode Muscle. The main fat culprit is a nasty type called visceral fat, which resides behind your abdominal muscles

Target Visceral Fat with This Belly-Busting Workout

Here's how to flatten your gut in less than 30 minutes, 3 days a week.

CARDIO WORKOUT

Use this interval method. It's short and intense, so it'll save you time. And unlike traditional steady-state aerobic exercise, it'll keep your body burning fat at a higher rate for hours after you've finished.

You can perform this workout on the road or on a treadmill, but if you're packing more than an extra 20 pounds, opt for an exercise bike to reduce the stress on your knees.

1. *Start out at an easy pace (about 40 percent of your best effort) and keep it up for 90 seconds.*

2. *Sprint at the fastest pace you can maintain for 1 minute.*

3. *Rest for 1 minute.*

4. *Sprint at the fastest pace you can maintain for 30 seconds.*

5. *Rest for 30 seconds.*

6. *Sprint as fast as you can for 1 minute.*

CARDIO WORKOUT LENGTH:
5½ minutes
(including warmup)

WEIGHT WORKOUT

We're giving you two upper-body exercises, two lower-body exercises, and one core (abs and lower back) exercise. Do them as a circuit: That is, perform one after the other with no rest in between.

Working your muscles in this way will allow you to progress in less time, eliminating any excuses, says Todd Durkin, CSCS, author of *The IMPACT! Body Plan*. After all, this workout doesn't require tons of equipment, but it still provides the fast results you want.

Do 10 to 20 repetitions of each exercise; complete three circuits, resting for 2 minutes between them.

WEIGHT WORKOUT LENGTH: 15 to 20 minutes

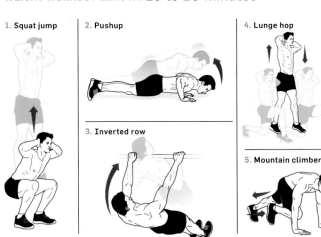

1. Squat jump
2. Pushup
3. Inverted row
4. Lunge hop
5. Mountain climber

and surrounds your internal organs (the viscera). And visceral fat works its mischief by releasing a variety of substances collectively called adipokines. Adipokines include compounds that raise your risks of high blood pressure, diabetes, arterial inflammation, and high blood sugar.

Visceral fat also messes with an important hormone called adiponectin, which regulates metabolism. The more visceral fat you have, the less adiponectin your body releases and the slower your metabolism is. So fat literally begets more fat. In fact, a study in the *Journal of Applied Physiology* showed that the biologically active molecules that are released from visceral fat can actually degrade muscle quality—which, again, leads to more fat.

The solution? Bigger muscles. In addition to boosting your metabolic rate, muscle mass plays a key role in preventing more common (but no less deadly) conditions such as cardiovascular disease and diabetes. A survey of scientific literature published in the journal *Circulation* linked the loss of muscle mass to insulin resistance (the main marker of type 2 diabetes), elevated blood lipid levels, and increased body fat, especially visceral fat.

Truth #3

Weight training is the ultimate fat fighter.

While muscle burns calories, bigger muscle burns more calories. That's because the physical work you need to do to build and maintain added muscle can have a dramatic effect on your overall metabolism. Research shows that a single weight-training session can spike your calorie burn for up to 39 hours after you lift. (And remember, this doesn't include the calories you burn while you're actually exercising. Think of those as a bonus.)

And the long-term calorie burn you enjoy from building muscle does more than just eliminate extra weight. It specifically targets fat! A study conducted by Jeff S. Volek, PhD, RD, an exercise and nutrition researcher at the University of Connecticut, showed that people who built muscle lost almost 40 percent more fat on restricted-calorie diets than non-exercisers and aerobic exercisers.

Here's another reason weight training is the ultimate fat fighter: The more muscle you have, the better your body uses the nutrients you consume, and the less likely it is to store your food (even junk food) as fat. See, your muscles store energy (read: calories) in the form of glycogen. When you exercise, your muscles call on that glycogen for fuel. After you exercise, your fat-storing hormones are subdued because your body wants to use incoming carbs to restore the glycogen depleted during your workout. So the carbs you eat after exercise are stored in your muscles, not in your spare tire.

But it gets better: If you complete a high-intensity workout (like the one on page 6), your body will burn calories at an advanced rate for hours afterward, and it'll be desperate for energy to keep your heart beating. Because the food you're eating is being stored in your muscles, your body has to hunt for something else to burn. Guess what that is? Fat. Score another one for Team Muscle.

The Truth about Calories

It's a basic unit tied to a tricky concept. But learn these secrets, and you'll start dropping pounds.

You can't go anywhere without being confronted by calories. Restaurants now print calorie counts on menus. You go to the supermarket and there they are, stamped on every box and bottle. You hop on the treadmill and watch your "calories burned" click upward.

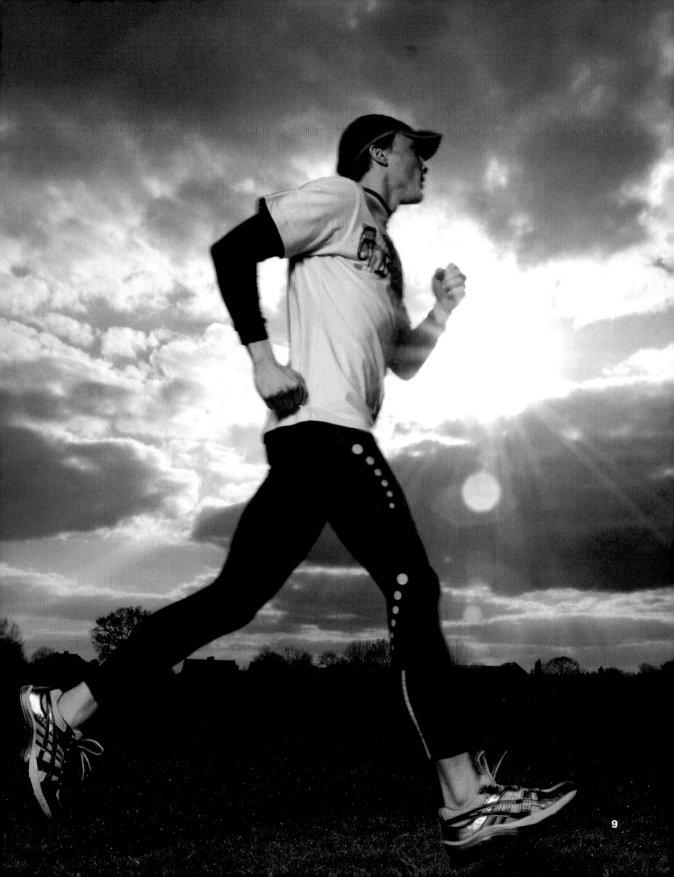

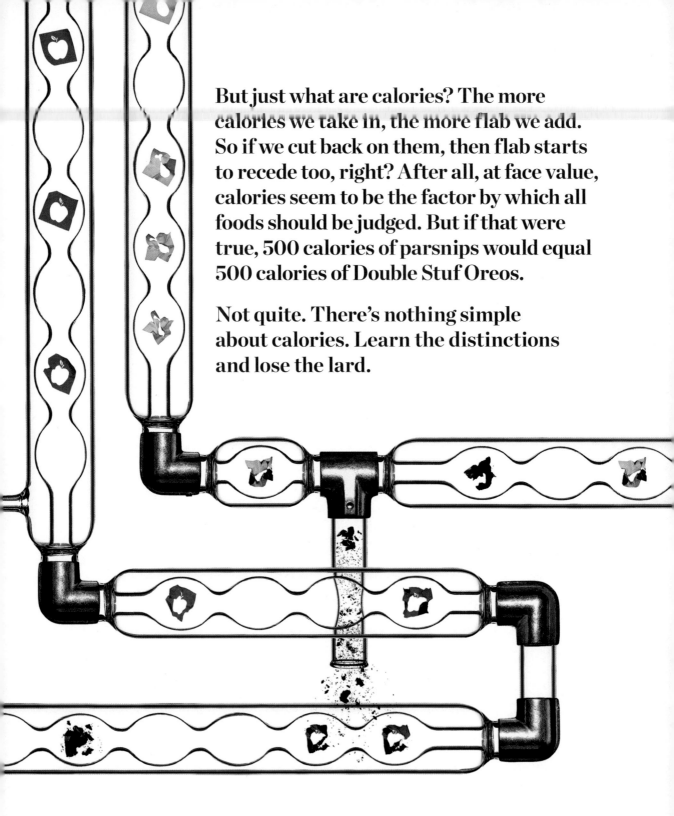

But just what are calories? The more calories we take in, the more flab we add. So if we cut back on them, then flab starts to recede too, right? After all, at face value, calories seem to be the factor by which all foods should be judged. But if that were true, 500 calories of parsnips would equal 500 calories of Double Stuf Oreos.

Not quite. There's nothing simple about calories. Learn the distinctions and lose the lard.

Calories Fuel Our Bodies?

ACTUALLY, THEY DON'T.

A calorie is simply a unit of measurement for heat. In the early 19th century, it was used to explain the theory of heat conservation and steam engines. The term entered the food world around 1890, when the U.S. Department of Agriculture appropriated it for a report on nutrition. Specifically, a calorie was defined as the unit of heat required to raise 1 gram of water 1 degree Celsius.

To apply this concept to foods like sandwiches, scientists used to set food on fire (really!) and then gauge how well the flaming sample warmed a water bath.

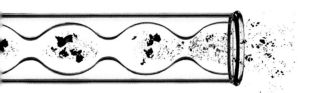

The warmer the water, the more calories the food contained. (Today, a food's calorie count is estimated from its carbohydrate, protein, and fat content.)

In the calorie's leap to nutrition, its definition evolved. The calorie we now see cited on nutrition labels is the amount of heat required to raise 1 kilogram of water by 1 degree Celsius.

Here's the problem: Your body isn't a steam engine. Instead of heat, it runs on chemical energy, fueled by the oxidation of carbohydrates, fat, and protein that occurs in your cells' mitochondria.

"You could say mitochondria are like small power plants," says Maciej Buchowski, PhD, a research professor of medicine at Vanderbilt University medical center. "Instead of one central plant, you have several billion, so it's more efficient."

YOUR MOVE

Track carbohydrates, fats, and protein—not just calories—when you're evaluating foods.

All Calories Are Created Equal?

NOT EXACTLY.

Our fuel comes from three sources: protein, carbohydrates, and fat. "They're handled by the body differently," says Alan Aragon, MS, a *Men's Health* nutrition advisor. So that old "calories in, calories out" formula can be misleading, he says. "Carbohydrates, protein, and fat have different effects on the equation."

Here's an example: For every 100 carbohydrate calories you consume, your body expends 5 to 10 in digestion. With fats, you expend slightly less (although thin people seem to break down more fat than heavy people do). The calorie-burn champion is protein: For every 100 protein calories you consume, your body needs 20 to 30 for digestion, Buchowski says. Carbohydrates and fat give up their calories easily: They're built to supply quick energy. In effect, carbs and fat yield more usable energy than protein does.

YOUR MOVE

If you want to lose weight, make protein a priority at every meal.

A Calorie Ingested Is a Calorie Digested?

IT'S NOT THAT SIMPLE.

Just because the food is swallowed doesn't mean it will be digested. It passes through your stomach and then reaches your small intestine, which slurps up all the nutrients it can through its spongy walls. But 5 to 10 percent of calories slide through unabsorbed. Fat digestion is relatively efficient: Fat easily enters your intestinal walls. As for protein, animal sources are more digestible than plant sources, so a top sirloin's protein will be better absorbed than tofu's.

Different carbs are processed at different rates too: Glucose and starch are rapidly absorbed, while fiber dawdles in the digestive tract. In fact, the insoluble fiber in some complex carbs, such as that in vegetables and whole grains, tends to block the absorption of other calories.

"With a very high-fiber diet, say 60 grams a day, you might lose as much as 20 percent of the calories you consume," says Wanda Howell, PhD, RD, a professor of nutritional sciences at the University of Arizona.

So a useful measure of calories is difficult. A lab technician might find that a piece of rock candy and a piece of broccoli have the same number of calories. But in action, the broccoli's fiber ensures that the vegetable contributes less energy. A study in the *Journal of Nutrition* found that a high-fiber diet leaves roughly twice as many calories undigested as a low-fiber diet does. And fewer calories means less flab.

YOUR MOVE

Aim to consume at least 35 to 40 grams of fiber every day.

Track the Burn

Here's one strategy for dropping pounds: Motivate yourself with gear that can help you monitor the calories you scorch, in and out of the gym.

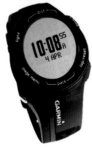

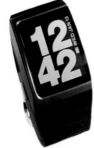

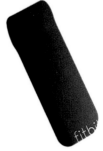

FOR THE SOCIAL-MEDIA ADDICT: Nike+ SportWatch GPS, $170, nike.com. Pair this watch with Nike+ sneakers to share goals, results, and challenges with other online users.

FOR THE CROSS-TRAINER: Garmin Forerunner 210, $250, garmin.com. This device includes a GPS and a heart-rate monitor to record distance and intensity on hikes, runs, and rides.

FOR THE ALL-DAY TRACKER: Fitbit Ultra, $100, fitbit.com. The tiny Fitbit slips easily in your pocket to track your calorie burn all day and then syncs wirelessly to your computer.

Exercise Burns Most of Our Calories?

NOT EVEN CLOSE.

As we talked about in the previous chapter, even the most fanatical fitness nuts burn no more than 30 percent of their daily calories at the gym. Most of your calories burn at a constant simmer, fueling the automated processes that keep you alive, says Warren Willey, DO, author of *Better Than Steroids*.

Some 60 to 75 percent of our total caloric expenditure goes toward normal bodily functions. This includes replacing old tissue, transporting oxygen, mending minor shaving wounds, and so on. For men, these processes require about 11 calories per pound of body weight a day, so a 200-pound man will incinerate 2,200 calories a day—even if he sits in front of the TV all day.

And then there are the calories you lose to NEAT, or non-exercise activity thermogenesis. NEAT consists of the countless daily motions you make outside the gym—the calories you burn while making breakfast, playing Nerf football in the office, or chasing the bus. Brandon Alderman, PhD, director of the exercise psychophysiology lab at Rutgers University, says emerging evidence suggests that "a conscious effort to spend more time on your feet might net a greater calorie burn than 30 minutes of daily exercise."

YOUR MOVE

Take frequent breaks from your desk (and couch) to move your body and burn bonus calories.

Low-Calorie Foods Help You Lose Weight?

NOT ALWAYS!

Processed low-calorie foods can be weak allies in the weight-loss war. Take sugar-free foods. Omitting sugar is perhaps the easiest way to cut calories. But food manufacturers generally replace those sugars with calorie-free sweeteners, such as sucralose or aspartame. And artificial sweeteners can backfire. One University of Texas study found that consuming as few as three diet sodas a week increases a person's risk of obesity by more than 40 percent. In a 2008 Purdue University study, rats that ate artificially sweetened yogurt took in more calories at subsequent meals, resulting in more flab. The theory is that the promise of sugar—without the caloric payoff—might actually lead to overeating.

"Too many people are counting calories instead of focusing on the content of food," says Alderman. "This just misses the boat."

YOUR MOVE

Avoid artificial sweeteners and load up your plate with the bona fide low-calorie saviors: fruits and vegetables.

The Eat-Smart Plan

Ditch the diet, lose the weight!
You don't have to go on a diet to lose
those extra pounds. Just eat smart—
and use our foolproof checklists.

Rise before the sun, jog before breakfast, and eat three home-cooked meals interspersed with protein- and fiber-rich snacks. Hit the gym every day and renounce beer, Chinese takeout, and any food that's breaded, battered, fried, or sweetened.

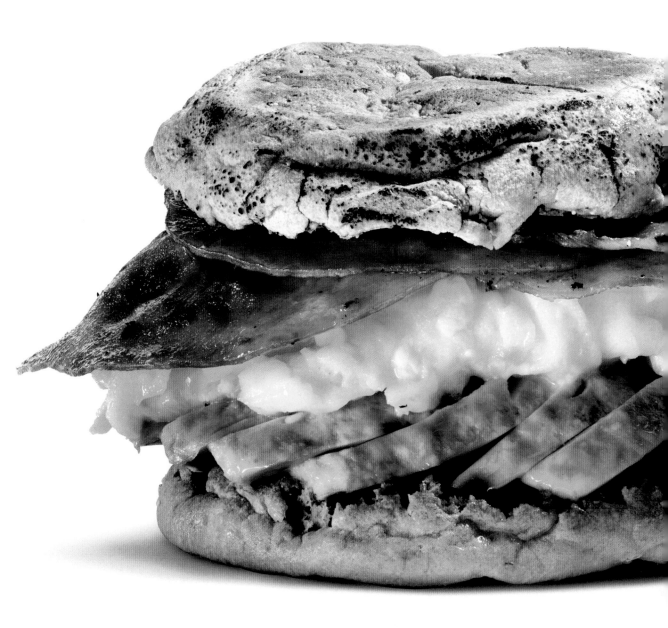

That's it: your blueprint for superlative health. If that sounds doable, you can stop reading now.

Still with us? Good. You're human. And you're busy. Chances are you've occasionally ordered greasy takeout while crunching a deadline, or scarfed down a candy bar as you rushed to a meeting. Real life interferes with diets—and maybe that's why a UCLA analysis of eight studies found that about 40 percent of dieters regain lost weight or even exceed their prediet weight after four or more years. It's tough to stick to a diet that doesn't adapt to your life.

Here's another problem with diets: They're usually built on self-denial, and people (most people, at least) aren't masochists.

"Anytime you withhold something enjoyable from somebody, whether it's television or affection or pizza, they'll resist it for only so long," says Brian Wansink, PhD, the author of *Mindless Eating*. "Those are deprivation diets. Effective in the short run, but not sustainable."

So we came up with an anti-diet. Our plan is flexible enough to fit your schedule and realistic enough to keep you from feeling deprived. We've started you off with a day of nutrient-dense eating. From there, use the checklists to guide your choices. Turns out you don't have to be superhuman to shrink your belly.

Word to the wise:
Concerned about high sodium levels?
They're hard to avoid in restaurant food,
so if you're trying to control your intake,
stick to the "At Home" options.

BREAKFAST

Too busy for breakfast? That's dangerous thinking. A University of Massachusetts medical school study found that people who regularly skipped breakfast had a risk of obesity that was 4¹/₂ times greater than those who routinely ate a morning meal. And when University of Minnesota researchers followed a group of high school students for 5 years, they found that the body mass indexes (BMIs) of students who always skipped breakfast were about 30 percent higher than those of students who ate every morning.

But don't eat just anything. In a study in the *Journal of the American College of Nutrition*, people who ate egg-based breakfasts consumed about 20 percent fewer calories during the day than those whose breakfasts were based on bread alone. The protein in those eggs might increase satiety and delay hunger pangs.

So how in the name of Jimmy Dean should you eat those eggs? Pair them with whole-grain bread and a lean protein such as ham for a smart sandwich that will fuel your race to the office.

BREAKFAST CHECKLIST

- ■ Can at least half the foods in this meal be described as protein sources?

- ■ Does this meal make up about a quarter of my day's calories? That's 550 for a 2,200-calorie diet, a reasonable goal for an average-height 30-year-old man who's moderately active and looking to lose weight.

- ■ If there's bread, a muffin, or cereal, is it made from whole grains?

AT HOME

Thomas' Light Multi-Grain English Muffin: Protein is crucial for satiety, but so is fiber. This Thomas' English muffin contains more fiber than a half cup of garbanzo beans.

Hormel Natural Choice Smoked Deli Ham (2 slices): This line of deli meats has no preservatives or added nitrites or nitrates.

Eggs (2 large): Scramble them in a small skillet.

Avocado (½): Avocado offers all the creaminess of cheese but has fewer than half the calories per gram.

Milk (1 cup, 1%)

FROM A RESTAURANT: PANERA BREAD

Breakfast Power Sandwich: Panera's egg sandwich boasts a fiber count that's rare among fast-food breakfast sandwiches. But the benefit doesn't end there: It has about as much protein as a 4-ounce pork tenderloin.

Apple: The apple doubles the fiber load of the meal and delivers plenty of quercetin and catechins, antioxidants that might help reduce your risk of cardiovascular disease, cancer, asthma, and diabetes.

Cappuccino (8.5 ounces): Why not brewed coffee? Because a cappuccino gives you a dose of dairy along with your caffeine fix.

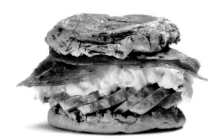

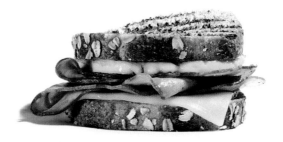

MEAL TOTAL: 575 calories, 32 grams protein, 49 grams carbohydrates, 31 grams fat, 14.5 grams fiber, 731 milligrams sodium

MEAL TOTAL: 540 calories, 31 grams protein, 63 grams carbohydrates, 18.5 grams fat, 8 grams fiber, 915 milligrams sodium

MIDMORNING SNACK

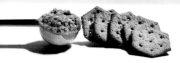

Smucker's Natural Chunky Peanut Butter (2 tablespoons): Smucker's Natural has no added oils, sweeteners, or fillers, and it boasts plenty of fiber and healthy fats. **+ Wheat Thins Fiber Selects 5-Grain Crackers** (5 crackers)

SNACK TOTAL: 246 calories, 8 grams protein, 14.5 grams carbohydrates, 17.5 grams fat, 4 grams fiber, 175 milligrams sodium

LUNCH

Lunch is a meal you're likely to buy rather than make, and the countless unhealthy options outside the home mean it's easy to pack in too many calories. But if you eat too few calories—or the wrong kind—you risk battling hunger pangs before dinner, priming you for overindulgence.

   To hit target calorie counts and sustain your energy all afternoon, you want a meal with a healthy dose of complex carbs, not refined ones. That's because complex carbs digest more slowly, helping you power past your 3 p.m. slump. And to ward off afternoon hunger pangs, make sure you include plenty of protein, which has been shown to increase satiety. Finally, pack in extra nutrients by picking a lunch that includes at least a serving or two of produce. One easy, tasty solution: chili. It delivers complex carbs (beans and vegetables), produce (tomatoes, onions, and peppers), and a hefty shot of protein—all in a single bowl.

LUNCH CHECKLIST

- ■ Am I eating this meal within 2 hours of my last snack?
- ■ Is there at least one source of protein and one source of fiber?
- ■ Can I identify the produce in this meal?

AT HOME

Amy's Organic Black Bean Chili (1 cup): This canned chili is more than just organic—it's also relatively low in sodium, high in protein, and totally jacked with fiber.

Sargento Mild Cheddar Cheese Cubes (30 grams, about 7 pieces): Shredded cheese is messy and hard to measure. Cubes are simple; just count them up and drop them into your bowl.

Fage Total 2% Plain Greek Yogurt (7 ounces): Greek yogurt is as luscious as sour cream but has more protein and fewer calories. Add a dollop to the chili and enjoy the rest with your orange.

Orange (1)

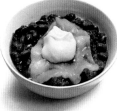

MEAL TOTAL: 532 calories, 41 grams protein, 55.5 grams carbohydrates, 17 grams fat, 16 grams fiber, 935 milligrams sodium

FROM A RESTAURANT: WENDY'S

Chili (small): Burger King and McDonald's both make decent burgers, but only Wendy's offers this hearty alternative to fries.

Double Stack: Pairing your chili with a burger adds another helping of protein. This burger's smaller bun helps lower the calorie count, while double the beef patties packs in the protein.

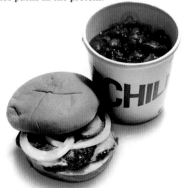

MEAL TOTAL: 580 calories, 41 grams protein, 48 grams carbohydrates, 25 grams fat, 7 grams fiber, 1,630 milligrams sodium

MIDAFTERNOON SNACK

Larabar Pecan Pie (1 bar): The typical snack bar is bloated with furtive sweeteners and heavily processed soy products, but this bar is honest food, simple and nutritious. Its sugar comes from natural dates, and outside that, you'll find only two ingredients: pecans and almonds.

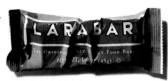

SNACK TOTAL: 220 calories, 3 grams protein, 24 grams carbohydrates, 14 grams fat, 4 grams fiber, 0 milligrams sodium

DINNER

<table>
<tr><td>

The average man eats about 900 calories at dinner. The problem? Dinner ought to be the smallest meal of the day. Loading up on energy before you head off on your day's errands makes sense, but doing that before you fall asleep in front of *The Colbert Report* doesn't. The goal is to keep your belly full during waking hours only.

So stop thinking of dinner as an end-of-day binge and start thinking of it as an opportunity to nab the last few nutrients you need for an optimal day of eating. Ideally, your dinner should be about half of what you're probably eating now—no more than about 450 calories. That's roughly 20 percent fewer calories than you took in at breakfast or lunch, and that's plenty if you've stuck to the plan so far. After two big meals and two hearty snacks, your appetite should be moderate and your cravings under control. Besides, you still have dessert to top it all off!

</td><td>

DINNER CHECKLIST

■ Am I eating this meal at least 2 hours before I go to sleep?

■ Can I identify at least one source of protein and one source of fiber?

■ Can I point to the produce in this meal?

■ Is this the smallest of my three main meals of the day?

</td></tr>
</table>

AT HOME

Kashi Stone-Fired Thin Crust Margherita Pizza (⅓ pizza)

Baby spinach (3 cups): Spinach boasts ample vitamin K and vitamin A, plus folic acid. A recent Swedish study found that a compound in spinach could also boost the efficiency of cells' mitochondria, in turn helping oxygen consumption during exercise.

Chopped walnuts (2 tablespoons): With the addition of walnuts, you transform a drab bed of dressed leaves into a legitimate salad. Plus, gram for gram, walnuts pack in even more omega-3 fats than salmon does.

Newman's Own Lite Balsamic Vinaigrette Dressing (2 tablespoons)

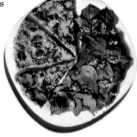

MEAL TOTAL: 422 calories, 18.5 grams protein, 36.5 grams carbohydrates, 23 grams fat, 7 grams fiber, 1,091 milligrams sodium

FROM A RESTAURANT: DOMINO'S PIZZA

Thin Crust Ham, Mushroom, Green Pepper, and Onion Pizza (¼ large pie): A combo of lean meat, three kinds of vegetables, and a thin crust keeps the calorie count low but your satisfaction high.

Garden Fresh Salad (½ salad): This side salad provides a couple of extra grams of fiber (the better to fill your belly), plus more than a third of your day's recommended intake of vitamin C and 120 percent of your vitamin A.

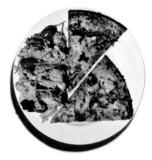

MEAL TOTAL: 490 calories, 20 grams protein, 43 grams carbohydrates, 22.5 grams fat, 4 grams fiber, 980 milligrams sodium

DESSERT

Sensible choices during the day leave you plenty of caloric space for dessert, and the anticipation of a reward will help keep you motivated.

Newman-O's Mint Creme Filled Chocolate Cookies (2): Newman-O's takes the gold trophy for cookie credibility with a recipe that features simple, mostly organic ingredients. Think Oreo or Famous Amos can make a claim like that? Not a chance. Add a small glass of milk for dunking and you earn a glucose-stabilizing shot of complete protein.
DESSERT TOTAL: 130 calories, 4.5 grams fat, 10 grams sugars

OR

Green & Black's Organic Dark 70% Bar (⅓ of a 3.5 ounce bar): Time to swear off milk chocolate. The dark stuff contains far more epicatechin, an antioxidant that may relax blood vessels. With 70 percent cocoa, this organic bar is perfect—dark enough to provide cocoa's benefits but sweet enough to be indulgent.
DESSERT TOTAL: 182 calories, 14 grams fat, 10 grams sugars

OR

Kashi TLC Soft-Baked Ripe Strawberry (1 bar, 35 grams): You wouldn't guess it, but the soft-baked shell is made with whole grains and the bar contains 3 grams of hunger-fighting fiber.
DESSERT TOTAL: 130 calories, 3 grams fat, 9 grams sugars

DESSERT CHECKLIST

- Have I met my other nutritional goals for the day so I can afford an indulgence?

- Am I eating this within 2 hours of dinner to help blunt a potential blood-sugar spike?

- Can I point to at least one beneficial ingredient, such as fruit, antioxidants, or dairy?

- Is this dessert smaller than a snack—about 200 calories or less?

For More Info . . .

For other ways to drop pounds in the real world, pick up a copy of *Eat This, Not That! No-Diet Diet*, by *Men's Health* Editor-in-Chief David Zinczenko with Matt Goulding, available in stores and at eatthisnotthatdiet.com.

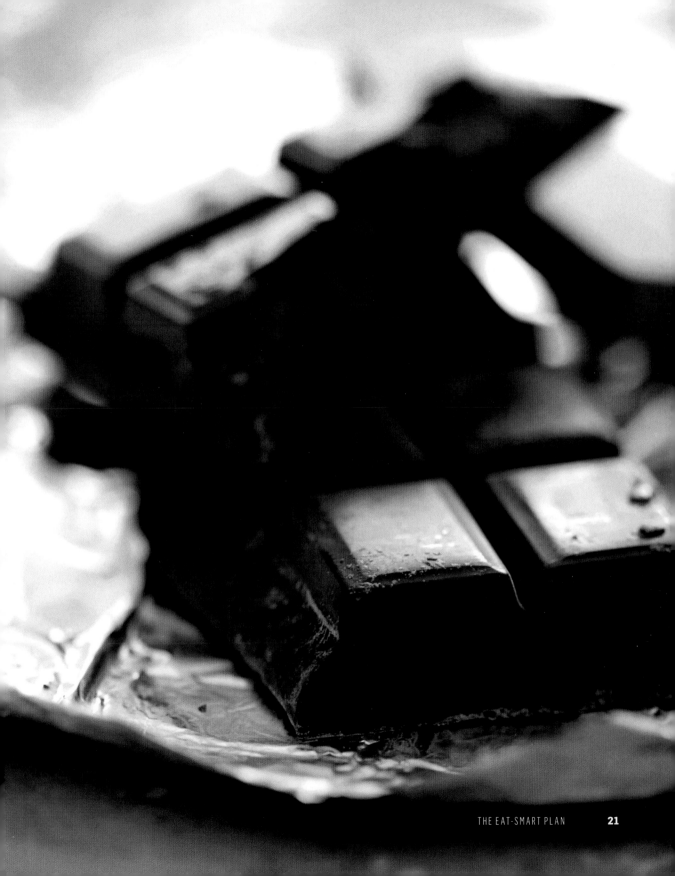

America's
Worst

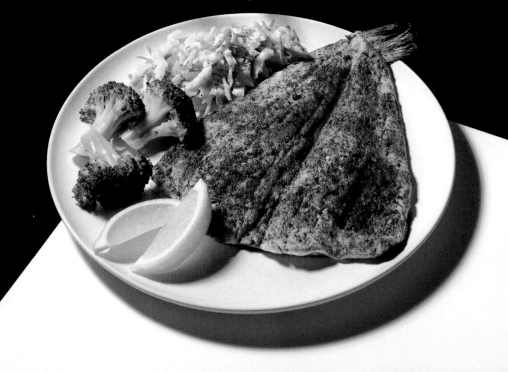

Best and Restaurants

We're fighting a battle for our waistlines.
Here's the lowdown on our allies—and our enemies.

Walking into a restaurant these days is like stepping onto a nutritional minefield. Safe passage is elusive, and dangers abound on all sides: sandwiches made with fried chicken instead of bread, pasta that packs over 1,500 calories in a single bowl. The edible enemies that hide in the shadows, masquerading as wholesome dishes, are even worse. The danger of a misstep? An exploding waistline.

The fact is, most restaurants are dangerous to your health. Every meal we eat out adds an average of 134 calories to our daily intake. And if you eat out as often as the average American man does (at least three times a week), those calories could tack on at least 6 pounds of mass every single year. Let's be clear: That's flab—not muscle. And if you eat out more, you gain more.

So what's the solution? We're not going to give up restaurants anytime soon. In 2010, 47.9 percent of the money the average American spent on food went toward dining out—that's about nine times what we spent in 1975. We're also not interested in spending our hard-earned cash on bland diet fare. A 2009 consumer research report found that even though most of us want to see healthier items on menus, only 20 percent of us actually order food based on nutritional considerations—probably because few of the options billed as "healthy" are as appealing as the other choices. Restaurants need to offer alternatives that are not only good for you but also tasty enough to rival the calorie bombs ticking alongside them.

And that's where this list comes in. We're naming the best restaurant chains, the ones that make scoring a healthy meal a deliciously easy task. We're also exposing the worst ones, where finding a decent entrée is an achievement worthy of a bloodhound. Follow our lead, and you'll enjoy the tastiest lean meals from America's biggest restaurants—and save your waistline and taste buds from mutually assured destruction.

SEAFOOD PLACE

BEST:
RED LOBSTER

Red Lobster ranks highest in the seafood category, and our nutritional analysis also taps Red Lobster as the best all-around sit-down restaurant. And it's not just the Lobster's abundant variety of heart-healthy seafood that helps it edge out the other seafood chains, like Bubba Gump's and Captain D's. Red Lobster relies primarily on simple cooking techniques, such as broiling, blackening, and wood-fire grilling, to accentuate the fresh flavor. One caveat: Unless you order from the Fresh Fish Menu, expect a heavy dose of sodium. Sorry, can't win 'em all.

Top pick: Blackened Rainbow Trout with fresh broccoli and coleslaw: Rainbow trout is a sustainable fish with low contamination levels. Wood-fired or broiled both work fine, but ask for it blackened. You'll enjoy a robust coat of smoky spice without extra calories.

MEAL TOTAL: 610 calories, 34 grams fat, 830 milligrams sodium

WORST:
LONG JOHN SILVER'S

It's fitting that this seafood chain was named after a nefarious pirate. Long John is perhaps the biggest villain in the restaurant industry. Why? Because of the restaurant's preferred method of cooking seafood: boiling nearly everything in a hot bath of partially hydrogenated soybean oil. That means any heart-health benefit you might receive from the seafood is negated by a boatload of nasty trans fats. Order a Fish Combo Basket, and you've just dropped a 12.5-gram trans fat mortar shell right into the depths of your belly.

Survival strategy: If it's fried, you don't want it. You can head off the relentless trans fat assault (and save on calories) by ordering from the Freshside Grille menu, which pairs grilled seafood—salmon, tilapia, or shrimp scampi—with rice and vegetables.

SANDWICH SHOP

BEST:
SUBWAY

Here's some good news: The leanest sandwiches in America come from the chain that's easiest to find. More than 25,100 Subway shops are spread out across the nation, which means your ride to work is about 59 percent more likely to swing you past a Subway than a McDonald's. Walk into any Subway, and you'll find at least ten 6-inch subs that come in at under 400 calories—and that includes the cheese toll. Plus, you can embellish your sub with as much produce as you like. You won't find heirloom tomatoes or fresh-picked arugula, but by fast-food standards, the Subway counter is a veritable farmers' market.

Top pick: Roast Beef and Swiss on 9-Grain Wheat (6-inch): No other sandwich on the menu—not even the oven-roasted chicken—manages to pack 30 grams of protein into so few calories. Just don't ruin it with mayonnaise; Subway's soybean-oil spread will cost you 110 calories per tablespoon. Instead, opt for mustard or marinara sauce to give your sandwich a kick.

MEAL TOTAL: 360 calories, 9 grams fat, 890 milligrams sodium

WORST:
QUIZNOS

In this case, Q stands for queasy. That's how the Quiznos menu—bloated with mayonnaise-spiked salads, oily dressings, briny bacon, and other waistline-threatening accoutrements—makes us feel. Sixty-five percent of the regular-size sandwiches carry more than 500 calories along with unhealthy overages of sodium. And the chain's tuna melt is quite likely the worst in the country: A large contains 1,260 calories. Even the regular-size version packs 870 calories, as many as you'd take in from two McDonald's Quarter Pounders with cheese. These submarines will sink your diet.

Survival strategy: Stick to the chain's Roadhouse Steak Sammies, which is a line of modestly sized flatbread sandwiches. Two Sammies make for a decent lunch of about 500 calories. If that's not enough to fill you up, order a bowl of chili or chicken noodle soup on the side.

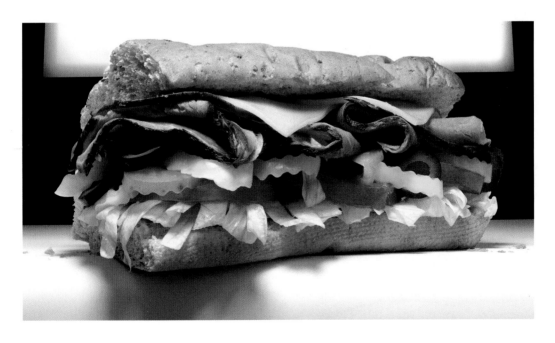

CHICKEN CHAIN

BEST:
CHICK-FIL-A

Chick-fil-A manages to pull off one feat that no other fast-food chain can match: Not a single entrée on the menu—not the Spicy Chicken Deluxe nor the Sausage Breakfast Burrito—packs more than 600 calories. In fact, only three entrées breach 500, which is an accomplishment bolstered by the fact that Chick-fil-A's grilled chicken sandwiches taste just as good, if not better, than the fried versions. The cast of sides also scores points because many of them, like the fruit cup and the carrot-and-raisin salad, don't visit the deep fryer on their way to your plate. Even the chicken salad and the coleslaw, while heavy on mayonnaise, make decent upgrades from fries.

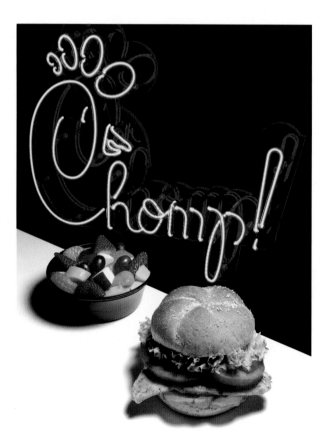

Top pick: Chargrilled Chicken Sandwich with a large fruit cup: Protein accounts for more than a third of the calories in this sandwich, and when you eat it with a side of fruit, you've satisfied 16 percent of your day's fiber needs—and filled your stomach. Bottom line: You won't find a better meal at any fast-food joint in the country.

MEAL TOTAL: 400 calories, 3.5 grams fat, 1,120 milligrams sodium

WORST:
CHURCH'S CHICKEN

Shockingly, Church's is one of the few remaining fast-food purveyors still pumping partially hydrogenated oil into its fryers, a fact that's even more unsettling when you consider the chain's specialty—fried chicken. In case you forgot, partially hydrogenated oil is the primary source of trans fat in the American diet, so anything submerged in the stuff becomes an instant hazard to your health. If you eat just one spicy fried chicken thigh, you've taken in more than double your trans fat limit for the day. It gets worse if you build a full meal around the chain's chicken. A half dozen boneless barbecue wings with a large side of fries deliver a full 15 grams of trans fat—about $7\frac{1}{2}$ times the recommended level. But wait—there's more bad news. Those six wings and fries also serve up 1,155 calories, 50 grams of fat, and a whopping 3,000 milligrams of sodium.

Survival strategy: Choose wisely and you might just make it out alive. Go for the Spicy Chicken Sandwich, which carries a reasonable 456 calories. Coincidentally, it's also among the few items on the menu that's not polluted with artery-clogging trans fat. Make it your go-to entrée, and for a side dish, choose a regular-size portion from the following nonfried options at Church's: mashed potatoes and gravy, corn on the cob, Cajun rice, or coleslaw. That will keep your meal hovering right around 600 calories if you skip the soda.

For More Info . . .

For more belly-saving tips, go to eatthisnotthatdiet. com and pick up a copy of the fully updated 2013 edition of *Eat This, Not That!* by *MH* Editor-in-Chief David Zinczenko with Matt Goulding.

ITALIAN RESTAURANT

BEST:
ROMANO'S MACARONI GRILL

Check out this story of restaurant redemption: Macaroni Grill used to be one of the most fattening sit-down chains in America. But things took a sharp turn for the better when the company recruited a new CEO in 2008. What followed was a multiphase plan to improve the nutritional quality of the entrées, and the chain has since become the caloric conscience of the red-sauce restaurants. In December 2008, a basic Fettuccine Alfredo at Macaroni Grill had 1,220 calories—the same amount you'll find in the Fettuccine Alfredo at Olive Garden today. Now Macaroni Grill's Fettuccine Alfredo has a mere 770 calories. That's a 37 percent drop! The chain also trimmed its Seafood Linguine from 1,230 calories to 650, its Lobster Ravioli from 1,350 to 710, and its Chicken Marsala from 1,180 to 810. Everything became, well, reasonable—exactly as it should be. The food tastes great too, so it's well worth the sauce stains on your shirt.

Top pick: Spaghetti Bolognese: "Bolognese" means meat sauce, and at Macaroni Grill, ordering it on your pasta instead of choosing spaghetti and meatballs with

tomato sauce will save you 260 calories and 16 grams of fat. Want something lighter still? Try the meatless Capellini Pomodoro, a tomato-based pasta with angel-hair noodles, which weighs in at only 490 calories.

MEAL TOTAL: 710 calories, 30 grams fat, 1,470 milligrams sodium

WORST:
OLIVE GARDEN

Sure, Italian food can be rich and starchy, but a true Italian doesn't let that stop him from looking svelte in his Dolce & Gabbana suit. The U.S. obesity rate is more than three times that of Italy. And why is that? Perhaps because of restaurants like Olive Garden, which combine the richness of Italian food with oversize American portions. Fully half of the dinner options on the Classic Pastas menu exceed 1,000 calories. Bottomless portions of carb-heavy breadsticks and dressing-soaked salads don't help.

Survival strategy: Come here for lunch, when the portions are smaller, and skip the bread and the salad. Two great options under 450 calories: Venetian Apricot Chicken and Linguine alla Marinara.

PIZZA PARLOR

BEST:
DOMINO'S

The pizza industry's ingredient-sourcing policies aren't worthy of praise, but when it comes to nutritional considerations, Domino's reigns supreme. Its plain pie ranks among the leanest available, and it boasts far more vegetable-topping varieties than the competition. Plus, unlike Papa John's, Domino's offers a thin-crust option for all its pizza sizes, and its pepperoni and sausage toppings are lower in fat than Pizza Hut's.

Top pick: Philly Cheese Steak Pizza thin crust (2 slices, based on a large pie): Want the leanest possible pie? Just skip the toppings and toss the cheese on the floor. But what's the point? You might as well gnaw on the pizza box. The Domino's Philly pie features plenty of lean beef, and the mushrooms, onions, and peppers provide a nice hit of fiber-rich vegetation.

MEAL TOTAL: 460 calories, 27 grams fat, 940 milligrams sodium

WORST:
CALIFORNIA PIZZA KITCHEN

While CPK's pies all have a relatively thin crust, their awkward sizing makes it difficult to eat a healthy portion. A 10-inch pie isn't enough for two people, and ordering one for yourself means a 1,000-calorie meal. Turning to other items on the menu, like the dozens of salad and pasta options, usually makes things worse. You might think you're doing yourself a favor by ordering the Waldorf Chicken Salad with Dijon Balsamic Vinaigrette, but you're actually padding your belly with 1,485 calories. The healthy-sounding Asparagus and Spinach Spaghettini with Grilled Chicken Breast is just as bad, with 1,340 calories.

Survival strategy: Split a pizza and a dish from the Small Cravings menu. Sharing the Four Seasons pie and the Asparagus and Arugula Salad makes for a meal that's around 563 calories.

BREAKFAST DINER

BEST:
BOB EVANS

Even though the breakfast at Bob Evans is fattier and brinier than anything you'd make at home, it still beats out the other chains. To net a decent meal, you still need strategy, and it goes like this: Forget the premade burritos, the greasy sausage scrambles, and the stuffed French toast. Instead, construct your own healthy meal from basic breakfast elements.

Top pick: 2 scrambled eggs, home fries, and a fruit dish: Choose eggs for belly-filling protein, and always pair them with a side of fruit. Have home fries instead of hash browns, and you'll save 161 calories, 2 grams of fat, and 414 milligrams of sodium. If you build a reasonable breakfast foundation, you can even afford to add on turkey sausage, bacon, or a parfait.

MEAL TOTAL: 390 calories, 16 grams fat, 1,163 milligrams sodium

WORST:
IHOP

Here's the short stack of IHOP foibles: Nearly every combo encourages you to order bacon or sausage, every regular order of pancakes comes crowned with a scoop of butter big enough to plug the mouth of an ice-cream cone, and nearly every omelet is packed with meat and cheese and often garnished with rich toppings like sour cream or hollandaise sauce. The fat assault is so severe that your omelet can contain as many as 82 grams of it—just 10 fewer than you'll find in a stick of butter. Just call it the International House of Pudge.

Survival strategy: Turn to the "Simple & Fit" selections, which come in at under 600 calories. Try the whole-wheat French toast topped with fresh banana—just take it easy with the syrup.

12 Months of Restaurant Survival Strategies Adopt one every time the

JANUARY:
AVOID THE COMBO MEALS.

A recent survey of New York City restaurants revealed that combo meals account for 31 percent of all burger-chain purchases, and the average calorie toll exceeds 1,200 per meal. Defend yourself by ignoring the preset combos and building your own meal with a couple of nutritious items instead.

FEBRUARY:
ORDER SMALL CUPS.

A Duke University study found that when people order drinks at fast-food joints, they tend to pick the medium size regardless of the volume of the cup. That means restaurants can

control how much you drink by deciding how big to make their "medium." Keep portions under control by sticking with the small soda. (You'll get at least 8 ounces, which is plenty.)

MARCH:
EAT MORE PLANTS.

Most restaurants offer a vegetable side other than fries. Order it. A University of Florida study that tracked the diets of two groups of young adults—an overweight and a normal-weight group—showed that both groups ate about the same number of calories. So why the difference in body weight? The thinner participants ate more calories from vegetables.

APRIL:
DRINK UP.

If your stomach is growling as you enter a restaurant, reach for the water first. In a Virginia Tech study, two groups ate low-calorie diets, but only one group also drank 2 cups of water before each meal. Over 12 weeks, the water drinkers lost nearly 5 pounds more than the control group. The reason? Water, like food, fills the stomach, blunting appetite.

MAY:
BAN THE HANDOUTS.

What do tortilla chips, dinner rolls, and breadsticks have in common? All of them are made from cheap refined carbohydrates, loaded into baskets, and doled out free

of charge to patrons. Take the bait and you'll end up with a few hundred worthless calories tacked onto your meal. The better option? Tell the server to save the basket for another table.

JUNE:
ORDER BY NUMBER.

The health-care reform law will require chains with 20 or more outlets to post calorie counts on menus. Until then, do some digging to find out how many calories are in your favorite restaurant meals. (A copy of *Eat This, Not That! 2013* can help.) A study in the *American Journal of Public Health* found that people regularly underestimate calories in foods by nearly half.

MEXICAN CHAIN

BEST:
CHIPOTLE

Think of Chipotle as Subway for Mexican food. The chain's customizable approach puts you in charge of your meal, helping you avoid a surreptitious load of fat. What's more, Chipotle is a major supporter of conscientiously raised meat and dairy, including hormone-free pork.

Top pick: Steak Burrito Bowl with black beans, cheese, and green salsa: For a robust, healthy dish with plenty of belly-filling protein and fiber, pick the Burrito Bowl instead of the regular burrito. You'll save nearly 300 calories just by skipping the tortilla.

MEAL TOTAL: 425 calories, 16 grams fat, 980 milligrams sodium

WORST:
ON THE BORDER

Grilled meat, beans, and salsa make for a healthy Mexican meal. That's why it's such a shame that On the Border tends to favor breaded fish, fried tortillas, and creamy sauces instead. Order the cheese and onion Tres Enchilada dinner, for instance, and you'll rack up about 1,600 calories. The dessert menu is just as bad. Pick one at random, and odds are you'll net an additional 1,000 calories or more. Just say no mas.

Survival strategy: Remember this formula: two soft tacos with a side of beans or vegetables, or both.

---

calendar flips and be leaner in a year.

JULY:
SLOW DOWN AND THEN DECIDE.
A study published in *Psychological Science* reveals that the mere sight of a fast-food sign on the side of the road is enough to make people feel rushed, which can lead to impulsive decisions—and dangerous nutritional choices. Sidestep your impulses the next time you eat out: Plan your order before you walk through the door.

AUGUST:
DON'T EXAGGERATE THE OCCASION.
You're 45 percent less likely to make healthy choices when you identify a meal as a "special occasion," according to a 2008 study in the *International Food Research Journal*. The problem is, study participants identified "special occasions" several times a week. Unless you know what you're celebrating, stick to your healthy habits.

SEPTEMBER:
KEEP IT SIMPLE.
Beware of menu verbiage. The longer the name of an item, the more fattening it tends to be. IHOP's original French toast has 920 calories, but its Strawberry Banana French Toast has 1,060. At Applebee's, a burger has 770 calories while the Steakhouse Burger with A.1. Sauce swells to 1,190. If you can't check calories, have the simply named entrées.

OCTOBER:
AVOID PEER PRESSURE.
What your friend eats might be making you fat. A study in the *New England Journal of Medicine* found that your risk of obesity jumps 171 percent when a close friend becomes obese. Friends might influence your eating habits, the study authors suggest. Don't let them dictate your meal ("Let's share the chili cheese fries!") when you eat out.

NOVEMBER:
LISTEN TO YOUR GUT.
Try ordering a smaller meal; you might be surprised at how full you feel. In a Penn State study, people ate 30 percent more food when they were served bigger portions, yet felt no more satisfied than those who'd received smaller portions. Start by ordering less than usual (the Whopper Jr., say), and then gauge how satisfied you feel before ordering more.

DECEMBER:
WATCH THE ALCOHOL.
Your booze buzz just might be making you eat more. A study in the *Journal of Psychology and Behavior* found that drinking alcohol before a meal prompted people to consume 19 percent more calories. In the mood for a drink with dinner? Save yourself from calorie overload by holding off on your drink order until you've settled on a healthy meal.

FAMILY RESTAURANT

BEST:
RUBY TUESDAY

Sometimes the "best" restaurant is the one that inflicts the least damage, and that's the situation here. The chow coming from family restaurants—think T.G.I. Friday's, Outback, and Applebee's—is notoriously bloated. Ruby Tuesday boasts the most numerous healthy options with its Fit & Trim menu—more than a dozen entrées come in under 700 calories. (Applebee's has a healthy menu, but it offers just five options.) Venture onto the rest of the Ruby Tuesday menu, and you'll find more smart choices. The chicken and seafood entrées are fairly safe, and a half rack of Memphis Dry-Rub Ribs has 460 calories—about half what a half rack of ribs at Applebee's has.

Top pick: Barbecue Grilled Chicken with white cheddar mashed potatoes and fresh steamed broccoli: The barbecue chicken and cheesy potatoes pack plenty of indulgence, and broccoli adds a bit of greenery.

MEAL TOTAL: 621 calories, 25 grams fat, 1,012 milligrams sodium

WORST:
CHEESECAKE FACTORY

No restaurant chain exemplifies America's portion problem more than Cheesecake Factory. One of the leanest regular dinner items is a hulking cheeseburger called the Factory Burger, which delivers just about as many calories as a Double Quarter Pounder with Cheese. What's more, the average full-size sandwich contains nearly 1,400 calories, and the average pasta dish clocks in at 1,835. Worst of all, you'll find a measly four entrées spotlighted as "healthy."

Survival strategy: The Small Plates & Snacks menu items are generally the leanest fare.

CHINESE RESTAURANT

BEST:
PANDA EXPRESS

Given Panda's penchant for blanketing breaded meats with syrupy sauces, it's surprising to note how many entrées are under 300 calories. Because you can put together your own meal, it's easy to eat healthy. Pair an entrée with a side of vegetables and a chicken egg roll—a formula almost guaranteed to net a meal with fewer than 700 calories.

Top pick: Broccoli Beef with Mixed Veggies (instead of rice or noodles) and a chicken egg roll: Make Broccoli Beef your go-to entrée to keep the calorie total at 400.

MEAL TOTAL: 400 calories, 16.5 grams fat, 1,660 milligrams sodium

WORST:
P.F. CHANG'S

The entrées at this higher-end Chinese restaurant will cost you twice: once when the check arrives, and again when your body deals with the high-calorie payload. It's hard to find an entrée under 600 calories. The chain tries to pass the buck by claiming that its dishes are meant to be shared, but that's never specified on the menu. And unlike other chains, Chang's doesn't help you find the healthy items on the menu. You'd assume a dish called Lemongrass Prawns with Garlic Noodles would be relatively lean, but it delivers 970 calories. It's the luck of the draw—just call it Chinese roulette.

Survival strategy: Seafood is safest. The two salmon-based entrées are both under 700 calories. On the appetizer side, your best bets are the spring rolls and seared ahi tuna.

BURGER JOINT

BEST:
WENDY'S

The Wendy's menu is built on the same bedrock foods as every other burger joint: beef, cheese, and fat-fried potatoes. But the chain trounces the competition in two ways. First, several of its burgers, including the Double Stack and nearly the entire line of Jr. Burgers, fall below the 400-calorie threshold. Not enough beef for you? Not a big deal. The quarter-pound Single has only 470 calories, and if you add bacon but hold the mayo, you're facing a still-reasonable 550. Wendy's sides also surpass the competition's. The chili strikes a perfect balance between flavor and nutrition, and customers can replace fries with chili, a side salad, or a baked potato in a standard value meal at no extra charge, which is a courtesy that's rarely granted in the world of fast-food restaurants.

Top pick: Jr. Cheeseburger and a Chili (small): For great flavor and smart portion control, order two satisfying favorites—chili and a cheeseburger—for under 500 calories.

MEAL TOTAL: 490 calories, 18 grams fat, 1,560 milligrams sodium

WORST:
DAIRY QUEEN

DQ is the only fast-food chain that specializes in both burgers and ice cream, and both sides of the menu are driven by the same excess that gives fast food a bad name. Granted, burger-and-shake joints are bound to have calorie-dense choices, but there's no reason they need to inject each food item with egregious amounts of sodium and spike the desserts with trans fats. The indulgences at DQ include basket meals that rack up at least 49 grams of fat each, large malts with 1,300-plus calories, and the iconic Blizzard, a blended soft-serve sundae that averages over 800 calories for a medium serving. It's even served from a beverage cup, the better to scarf down alongside your burger and fries.

Survival strategy: Stick to entrées under 500 calories, like the Original Cheeseburger or any regular-size hot dog. If you want a treat, order a small ice-cream cone.

America's Best Burgers

Check out four more of the healthiest fast-food burgers.

BEST SMALL BURGER
Burger King's Whopper Jr. (no mayo): Skip the 80-calorie glob of mayo and this becomes one of the noblest fast-food burgers in the country. 260 calories, 10 grams fat, 460 milligrams sodium

BEST DOUBLE BURGER
McDonald's McDouble: McDonald's modest patties allow the chain to boost the beef-to-bun ratio without inflicting the heavy fat tariff of a typical double burger. Plus, it's only 1,390 calories, 19 grams fat, 920 milligrams sodium

BEST QUARTER POUNDER
Hardee's Little Thick Cheeseburger: The Hardee's quarter pounder with cheese stays under 500 calories. Just don't mistake it for the Little Thickburger, which has an extra 120. 450 calories, 23 grams fat, 1,180 milligrams sodium

BEST LOW-CARB BURGER
In-N-Out Protein Style Double-Double: "Protein-style" means you skip the bun in favor of lettuce. This low-carb burger succeeds where other versions fail, by avoiding oversize patties and mayo. 520 calories, 39 grams fat, 1,160 milligrams sodium

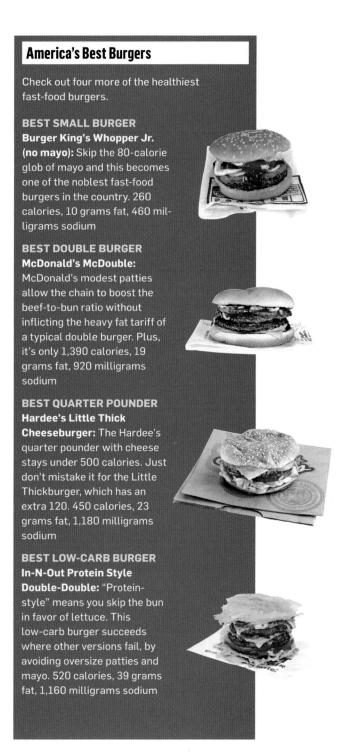

The Last 10— Lost!

Blast that last bit of fat with this meal-by-meal plan.

Lonnie Lowery, PhD, RD, leads a double life. In his 40s, he's not only a competitive bodybuilder but also a professor of exercise and nutrition science at Winona State University in Minnesota. In the classroom and in the weight room, Lowery has learned to use every waking hour to stay leaner than people half his age.

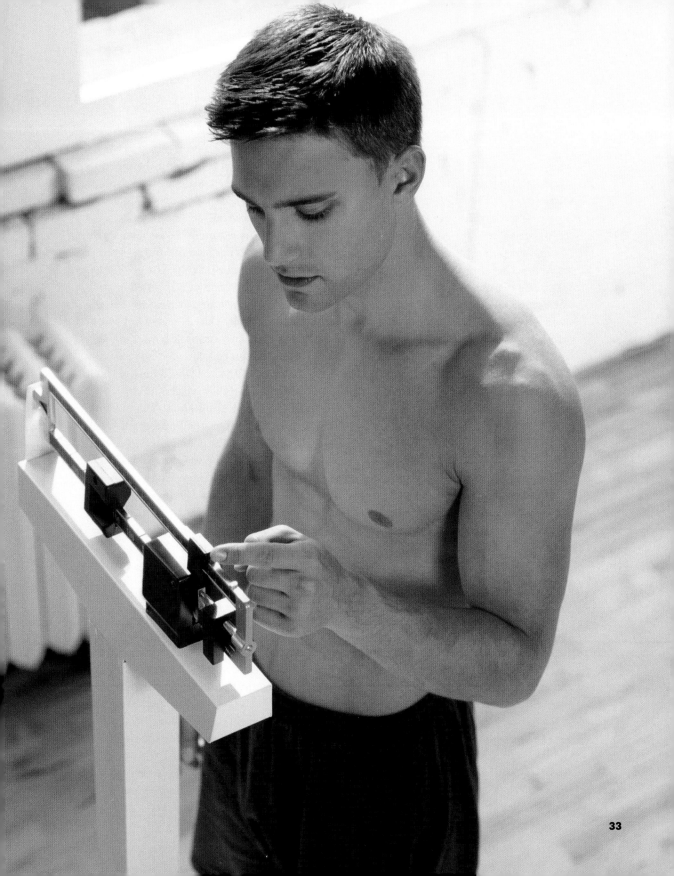

Some of Lowery's tactics actually go against the advice you might have read in *Men's Health* over the years. But as we follow his daily routine, we'll point out these tactics and explain why he's using them. As they say in the fitness biz, it's okay to break the rules as long as you know what they are and why you're breaking them.

Just keep in mind that nobody eats and exercises this way year-round. Lowery uses this regimented, disciplined approach only when he's trying to become extremely lean for one specific event. (A good approach for you too.) He doesn't exactly pig out the rest of the year, but he does eat more to allow his body to recover.

Consider this your graduate seminar in waist management.

Morning

Kick-start your metabolism, manage your blood sugar, and prepare for a heavier afternoon workload.

FIRST THING IN THE MORNING

Caffeine and cardio: Nobody wakes up ready to exercise. But morning is prime workout time, says Lowery.

"You're burning a higher percentage of fat before eating breakfast," he says, because your body's supply of available carbohydrate energy is depleted and the hormonal state makes body fat more accessible. And coffee might help squeeze even more from your fat cells.

On Lowery's plan, this workout is nothing fancy: an hour of low- to medium-intensity walking or jogging after a cup of java. If you try to do more than that, you won't have enough left for your strength workout later in the day.

This is the first big deviation from traditional *MH* advice—in this case, to eat before exercise. All things being equal, you'll probably train with more intensity if you have something in your stomach, and that leads to better long-term benefits. But in this example, Lowery isn't looking for a long-term benefit, and he's not trying to exercise intensively. The goal is to target stored body fat. In a 2006 study in *Applied Physiology, Nutrition, and Metabolism*, people who exercised following an overnight fast used more fat for energy, even though they burned no more total calories than they would have if they'd eaten before their workout.

One more point about this morning workout: It's not the main event for Lowery. That happens later in the day, when he hits the weight room. If you don't have the time to exercise twice in a day, you should choose the highly challenging weight workout over this low-intensity supplement. Just think of it this way: This exercise session is designed to enhance fat loss, but only in addition to your regular workout.

BREAKFAST

Protein and slow-burning carbs: "I keep breakfast pretty low in fat and stick with slow-acting carbs," Lowery says. Again, the low-fat breakfast is not what we usually suggest, but it makes sense in this quest for single-digit body fat. Specifically, Lowery is trying to manage the hormone insulin.

Insulin is at its lowest level in the early morning, but it comes on like a

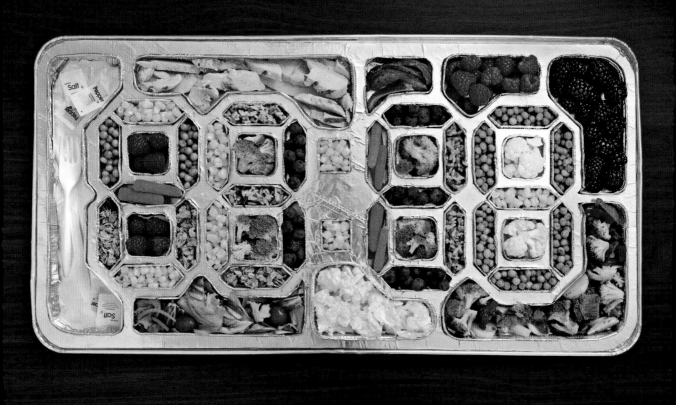

beast with the first meal of the day. If you were overeating—that is, consuming more calories than you burn—that surge of insulin could lead to greater fat storage. But in the opposite context, when you're burning more calories than you take in, fat storage is unlikely. That's why an average dieter can eat a moderate amount of insulin-inducing carbs and still lose weight.

But Lowery is playing a more complicated game than the rest of us are. He wants a rise in insulin to push protein and carbohydrates to his muscles. Carbs, when stored as glycogen within the muscles, bring water with them; that helps his muscles fill out and might also help improve their function. But if he adds

more than a few grams of fat to the mix, there's a slim chance that the fat would end up back in the fat cells that he's trying to drain by exercising in the morning on an empty stomach. Extra fat might also interfere with his body's ability to metabolize carbohydrates properly. And that's a chance he won't take.

An ideal breakfast might be two whole eggs with four egg whites, for a total of 24 grams of protein. A carb source, like whole-grain toast, oatmeal, or an apple, completes the meal.

"SECOND BREAKFAST" AND LUNCH

Protein and fiber: For a midmorning snack, Lowery likes oatmeal and berries with a scoop of vanilla protein powder.

Lunch, 2½ to 3 hours later, might be a grilled chicken breast accompanied by a high-fiber vegetable (such as broccoli) along with a cup of brown rice (for even more fiber, toss in some black beans) or two small red potatoes. Meals like this require a lot of chewing, which slows your appetite and gives your brain time to send the "stop eating" signal. The high protein content can also speed your metabolism.

Afternoon

Fuel up, work out, and recover.

PREWORKOUT MEAL

Protein and fast-burning carbs: In mid- to late afternoon, it's time to put away some fuel before you hit the weight room. Half a turkey-breast sandwich and a banana will do the trick. The turkey's protein gives your muscles some material to work with in the never-ending process of repairing and rebuilding, and the fast-burning carbohydrates provide easy energy for the coming workout.

This combination also raises your insulin levels, which opens up blood vessels and allows for a better pump in your working muscles. Not only is a pump a nice reward for your hard work, but it also squeezes nutrients into your muscles to speed recovery.

WORKOUT

Strategic destruction of muscle fibers: It's hard but not impossible to build muscle mass while you're following a strict diet and limiting calories. The key is to do

The Fat Burning Exercise Secret

Want an all-new way to blast fat? "Try tempo exercises," says Bill Hartman, PT, CSCS, co-owner of Indianapolis Fitness and Sports Training. "They'll help train your muscles to burn more fat for energy."

The idea is to perform an exercise at a slow but steady tempo from start to finish. You can use this technique with almost any exercise, including the squat, pushup, and inverted row. Simply take 2 seconds to lower the weight (or your body), and 2 seconds to lift it—all without pausing at the top or the bottom of the exercise.

HOW IT WORKS
Let's use the barbell tempo squat as an example. As you do this exercise, your leg muscles are under constant low-level tension. This tension restricts bloodflow to the working muscles, depriving them of oxygen during the exercise. Your muscles react to these lower oxygen levels by increasing the size of your slow-twitch fibers, which contain a high volume of mitochondria.

Mitochondria are tiny powerhouses in your muscle cells that produce energy from fat. So the more mitochondria you have, the more body fat you can burn. And because you're able to produce more energy, you can also exercise harder and longer before you run out of gas. The upshot: You burn more total calories.

HOW TO USE IT IN YOUR WORKOUT
Perform an exercise for 40 to 60 seconds using the tempo technique. Rest 40 to 60 seconds and repeat two more times. One note: If you're using barbells or dumbbells, you'll need to use a light weight—about 50 to 60 percent of what you could normally lift for 10 reps.

as much as you can without compromising your ability to recover in time for the next workout. Lowery suggests splitting up your exercises so you're rarely working upper-body and lower-body muscles on the same day. Instead, push the targeted muscles to exhaustion, always working from "the center of the body outward." So he starts by training his chest and back (the center), moves outward to his shoulders, and finishes up with arms.

To work your upper torso with his system, begin with basic, heavy lifts— 3 or 4 sets of 5 reps of barbell bench presses and dumbbell rows, for example. Next perform 3 sets of 10 to 12 reps of dumbbell shoulder presses and lat pulldowns. Then finish with 1 or 2 sets of 20 reps of biceps curls and triceps extensions.

POSTWORKOUT SHAKE

More fast-acting nutrients: You don't need a lot of protein and carbs following your workout; a small protein shake or smoothie should work, or even a glass or two of low-fat or nonfat milk. (Don't worry about fat, because the timing of when you eat fat doesn't matter in the way it does for protein or carbs.)

Evening

Relax, refuel, and wind down.

DINNER

Protein and fat: A couple of hours after your strength workout, it's time for your final meal of the day. Lowery typically eats more fat at this meal than at any other. That's because, as a fuel, fat appears to be preferable to carbohydrates at this time. The whole insulin-carbohydrate system isn't working as well late in the day. Plus, his daily dietary variety is increased by including healthy fats, and he's had little of them up until now.

A stir-fry with vegetables and chicken or steak hits the spot, along with a green salad, lightly dressed. The protein and fat, along with the fiber in the vegetables, help you feel full until you fall asleep—which will probably be very soon, considering how hard you've worked.

Lean for Life

Use the new science of weight maintenance to keep your new waistline right where it is.

You've probably heard that 95 percent of all diets fail. In other words, almost everyone who loses weight eventually regains it. This isn't true, but it's easy to understand why so many of us believe it.

The problem isn't really with diets. It's with a lack of guidance after your diet. Christopher Sciamanna, MD, discovered this the hard way. After losing 30 pounds, he described his new, lower weight as "shockingly challenging" to maintain.

Luckily for him—and for the rest of us—Dr. Sciamanna has the perfect job for learning how to deal with this challenge. He's physician and professor at Penn State University's Milton S. Hershey Medical Center. He and his colleagues decided to study weight-loss maintenance.

For the past two decades, this field of research has focused on a single group of people: those who choose to join the National Weight Control Registry (NWCR). To qualify, they have to lose at least 30 pounds and keep the weight off for at least a year.

And when experts study NWCR participants, their efforts reveal this bleak checklist of post-diet strategies that nobody enjoys.

- Exercise at least an hour a day, almost every day.

- Follow a low-fat, low-sugar, low-calorie diet.

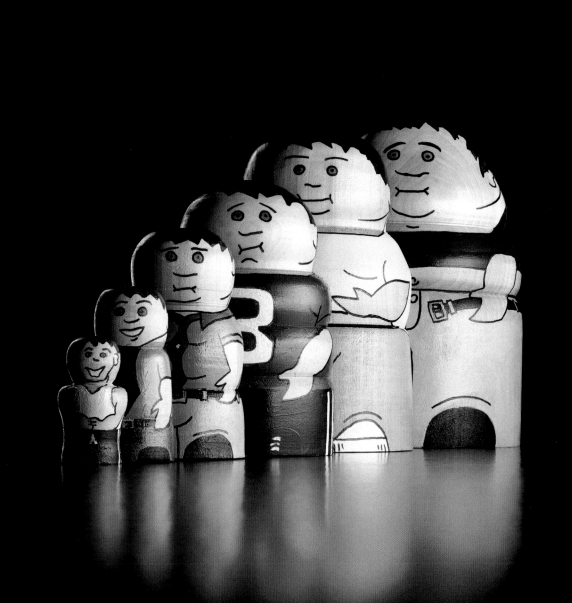

- Eat more or less the same stuff all the time.

- Minimize TV watching.

- Eat breakfast.

Ugh (mostly). You can understand why dieters continue searching for alternatives, and why dieters and nondieters alike believe permanent weight loss is virtually impossible.

But it's not. Dr. Sciamanna's team found that more than a third of people who lost at least 5 percent of their initial body weight kept it off. About a sixth of those who lost at least 10 percent were able to do the same.

These results should be encouraging. Remember, even if you fall short of your original weight-loss target, permanently downsizing by 5 to 10 percent of your birth offers substantial health benefits, and almost certainly improves your appearance as well.

To keep the weight off, you have to adjust. You'll require skills and practices that are different from the ones you used to drop the pounds in the first place.

"Maintenance requires a specific focus," Dr. Sciamanna says. "It's like an exit strategy to a war. Once you lose weight, it's not 'mission accomplished.' You need to rethink how you're going to maintain the weight loss." Here are three ways to keep lost pounds off for good.

Find Your New Normal

When you begin a weight-loss program, says Dr. Sciamanna, you're willing to make enormous, zero-to-60 changes. A drive-thru addict might quit cold turkey. A careless chowhound might start weighing his food and tracking his calorie intake religiously.

"But at a certain point you want your old life back," he says. "There's a huge fatigue that sets in. How long do you want to spend on that one problem?" You can't literally have your old life back, because that's how you gained so much weight in the first place. But you can create a "new normal" with these three practices.

Weigh yourself regularly. Sounds too simple, but Dr. Sciamanna's research confirms what we first learned from the National Weight Control Registry. People who weigh themselves most often and most consistently are best at catching and releasing new pounds before those interlopers acquire residency status.

When Can You Stop Dieting?

Make the shift from weight loss to weight maintenance when you see these signs.

You've been dieting for 6 months. Research shows that every diet stops working around the 6-month mark. In studies lasting a year or longer, most dieters typically regained a significant amount in the second 6 months.

You've lost only a pound or two in the past month. When your rate of weight loss slows to a crawl, it's a sign that the diet is no longer working or that you're unable to stick with it. Either way, it's time for a change.

You've continually cut back on your daily calories. Long-lasting calorie deficits slow your metabolism. And as your muscles become more efficient, your workouts burn fewer calories and your weight loss stalls.

You're weaker in the gym. Losing strength is a sign you're losing muscle mass, failing to recover between workouts, or both. Your muscles may not be receiving the fuel they need.

Many diets can help you maintain your weight.
Just pick one and stick with it.

Plan your meals. You can maintain your weight with a low-fat, a low-carb, or a well-balanced diet; just pick one and stick with it. That takes planning. The Penn State team confirmed that people who successfully maintain their weight tend to eat the same things most of the time, but they vary what goes with these foods. A grilled-chicken salad will taste different if you use mixed greens with mustard vinaigrette instead of spinach with raspberry vinaigrette. Add chopped vegetables to the former and sliced fruit to the latter for even more variety. You're still having "a salad" for dinner. A standard meal that you can modify allows you to be consistent without being boring.

Make a list before you shop. The "plan your meals" bit works only if you also write down everything you need before you shop. Again, it's common sense, but it's uncommonly used.

Focus on Process, Not Outcome

When you're losing weight, you think of an outcome and then find a process that takes you there. For weight maintenance, it helps to start with the process. Try these sustainable habits.

Eat the same number of meals a day. It doesn't matter if you have three, four, or six. You just can't skip a meal or a planned snack. It disrupts your hunger cues and puts you at risk of eating stuff you'd typically avoid, or of overeating when you finally do eat.

Include fruits, vegetables, and/or lean protein in every meal. A large body of research, including Dr. Sciamanna's, shows the importance of eating protein and fresh, fiber-rich foods among those who successfully manage their weight.

Follow a consistent exercise routine. You don't have to crush it every time, but you do have to show up. Alwyn Cosgrove, CSCS, owner of Results Fitness in Newhall, California, suggests setting a monthly goal for workouts. Tell yourself you'll go to they gym 20 times, and you'll force yourself to do four or five workouts a week.

Think Like a Winner

The latest research from the Penn State team shows a major attitude adjustment among people who win at permanent weight loss. Here's how to join their ranks.

Reward yourself. Weight loss is about deprivation. Weight maintenance works best when you occasionally give in to temptation.

Remind yourself why you need to stay vigilant. You might be thinner on the outside, but inside you still have billions of depleted fat cells longing to return to their days of greasy glory. It helps to keep mementos of your inflated past. A photo on the fridge should work.

Remember your accomplishment. When you need a confidence boost, go to the mall to observe the well-fed fauna. Isn't it nice to know you're no longer a member of that herd?

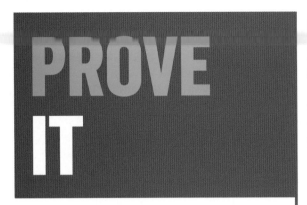

PROVE IT

WAKE UP AND SMELL THE PROOF

People with a history of skipping breakfast have larger waists—by nearly 2 inches—than those who eat in the a.m., according to research in the *American Journal of Clinical Nutrition*. Pass on breakfast and you may pig out later, the study warned. Over time, this can cause your body to store more fat. Shoot for 20 to 30 grams of protein at breakfast.

Hit your protein goal with eggs (6 grams each); bacon, sausage, or cheese (2 to 7 grams per slice or link); milk (8 grams per cup); yogurt (8 to 12 grams per 8 ounces); peanut butter (4 grams per tablespoon); or cereal (oatmeal, 6 grams per cup; Kashi GoLean, 13 grams per cup).

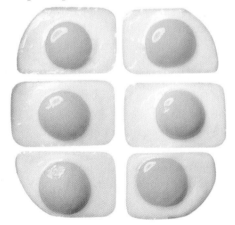

OVERCOME YOUR GENES

Don't blame DNA for your gut. A British study found that even if you've inherited a genetic susceptibility to obesity, regular exercise can reduce this risk by 40 percent. In fact, people who have obesity-prone genes might benefit from increased physical activity more than people whose genes guard against it, according to researchers.

GO ON A CASH DIET

The next time you go food shopping, hit the ATM first. In a simulated shopping session, people using credit or debit cards spent 70 percent more on junk food than cash customers did, but spent about the same amount on healthy foods, a study in the *Journal of Consumer Research* found.

Scientists observed the same pattern among real-life shoppers too. The researchers think that you feel less "wallet pain" when you use abstract forms of payment (such as credit and debit cards), and this might weaken your ability to control impulse purchases, according to the study.

SLOW DOWN TO LOSE BIG

Slow = skinny

Scarfers, beware. Greek researchers report that eating slowly can boost levels of two hormones that make you feel fuller. They compared blood samples from diners who took 30 minutes to eat with those from people who took 5 minutes. Pacing yourself might make your small intestine produce more of these hormones for a longer period of time, the study authors say.

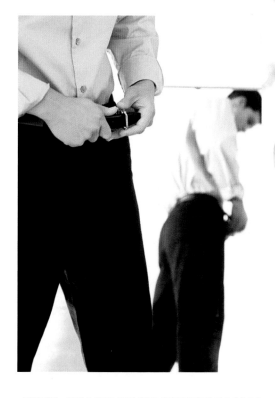

GET MORE MILK

Calcium, which might prevent some dietary fat from being absorbed, is a weight-loss weapon. In an *American Journal of Clinical Nutrition* study, dieters with the highest calcium intake from dairy foods lost 60 percent more weight than those with the lowest. Aim for 1,000 milligrams a day. The foods below are good sources. Avoid supplements; a U.K. study showed that they raise your heart-attack risk.

Food	Amount	Calcium (mg)
Canned baked beans	1 cup	86
Canned sardines	3 ounces	325
Collard greens	1 cup cooked	357
Canned salmon	3 ounces	181
Spinach	1 cup cooked	245
Oranges	1 large	74
Almonds	1 ounce	75
Peas	1 cup cooked	94
Black-eyed peas	1 cup cooked	211

JUMP-START YOUR METABOLISM

A little exercise can go a long way. Just 15 minutes of weight training can help flatten your belly, say researchers from Southern Illinois University at Edwardsville. They found that performing a single set of a 10-exercise circuit boosted metabolism as much as doing 3 sets of the same routine.

"The longer you train, the more calories you burn," says study author Erik Kirk, PhD. "The first set of an exercise turns on the hormones that control your metabolism, and additional sets don't seem to increase that process."

YOU ASKED

Q: Are any of those home body-fat scales really accurate?

A: They're not even in the body-fat ballpark.

"Even the best home machines can be 5 points off in terms of your body-fat percentage," says Pete McCall, CSCS, a personal trainer and exercise physiologist at the American Council on Exercise.

The problem is that most monitors work by sending an electric current through your body and calculating how much resistance it encounters. Flab impedes the current because it contains little water, while muscle, which has high water content, lets the current zip through. But because these monitors are essentially measuring water, your overall hydration level can significantly skew the result, says McCall.

His advice: Have your fat measured using a 5-point skin caliper test. Just make sure that the person doing the pinching has done at least 30 of these tests—that's the minimum amount of practice necessary to master the technique. Or you can take human error out of the equation by sitting in a Bod Pod for about 2 minutes. This pressurized chamber calculates your body fat by correlating your weight with how much air you displace. Find one locally at bodpod.com ($30 to $45 per test).

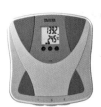

THE SCALE SMACKDOWN

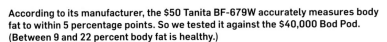

TANITA BF-679W VS. BOD POD

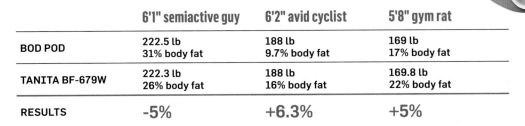

According to its manufacturer, the $50 Tanita BF-679W accurately measures body fat to within 5 percentage points. So we tested it against the $40,000 Bod Pod. (Between 9 and 22 percent body fat is healthy.)

	6'1" semiactive guy	6'2" avid cyclist	5'8" gym rat
BOD POD	222.5 lb 31% body fat	188 lb 9.7% body fat	169 lb 17% body fat
TANITA BF-679W	222.3 lb 26% body fat	188 lb 16% body fat	169.8 lb 22% body fat
RESULTS	-5%	+6.3%	+5%

The bottom line: "Muscle is about 75 percent water," says exercise physiologist Pete McCall, CSCS, "and a person who is lean and exercises often could be dehydrated. A scale like the Tanita might misinterpret that dehydration as having more fat."

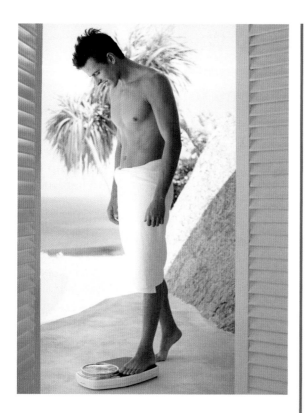

Q: What's the single most important thing I can do to avoid gaining weight?

A: We fired this chestnut at our weight-loss advisor, David Katz, MD, MPH, director of Yale's Prevention Research Center. Surprisingly, his response had nothing to do with calories or exercise.

"You need a prenuptial agreement with your food. A prenup says, 'I love you, but we need to have some rules in place ahead of time so we're not left to make decisions when we are less composed.' Do the same for food." Identify your particular diet vulnerability by reviewing which foods you've overeaten and why, and make a list of key foods and situations. (You're familiar with the common saboteurs: soda, beer, white bread and other empty carbs, and desserts.) Then tailor your prenup to prevent a recurrence of those specific hazards.

The more specific the decision, the more it boxes you in and the more reliable it becomes, says Dr. Katz. For instance, if you binge on bread, commit to eating low-calorie, nutrient-rich stuff—like raw vegetables—instead. If you know you eat more when you drink beer, commit to drinking no more than two and then swigging seltzer. Then, to give your strategy teeth, weigh yourself once a week. You'll have a more intimate knowledge of your own body, and there will be no scale shock in 3 months.

Q: Is fasting really a good way to lose weight?

A: The research on fasting and weight loss is a little thin. But in one study in the *American Journal of Clinical Nutrition*, obese adults who fasted every other day for 8 weeks shed about 3 percent of their body fat. The mechanism: When you swear off food, you're depriving your body of its usual fuel source, so you burn more fat instead, says Mike T. Nelson, CSCS, PhD(c), of the University of Minnesota. He recommends fasting only 1 day a week; any more can make it harder to recover from training.

Start out by delaying your breakfast 1 day a week. If you normally eat at 7 a.m., hold off until 10 a.m. (Stay on your usual caffeine schedule to avoid headaches.) Then stretch the interval between meals until you can last 24 hours. Have a craving? Drink some water or green tea, says Nelson. Finally, to avoid a binge at the end of your fast, resume eating with a high-protein, high-fiber meal. Nelson's suggestion: grilled salmon with 2 cups of broccoli, and a cup of blueberries for dessert.

YOU ASKED

Q: What's the best indicator of healthy weight?

A: You can't beat a $2 tape measure. "Determining your waist-to-hip ratio can help indicate your level of visceral fat, the dangerous belly fat linked to heart disease, diabetes, and cancer," says George Blackburn, MD, PhD, associate director of Harvard Medical School's Division of Nutrition.

The problem with body mass index (BMI) is that it can't tell the difference between a well-muscled 5-foot-10, 180-pound man and a guy with a gut who's the same height and weight. So to measure your waist, wrap the tape around your body at the midpoint between your lowest rib and your hip bone. Then check your hip circumference by measuring at the widest part of your hips—usually around your butt. Divide waist by hip for your ratio. Aim for 0.9 or lower. While you're at it, calculate your waist-to-height ratio, which may be an even more meaningful number. A 2010 study in the *Journal of Clinical Endocrinology and Metabolism* showed that waist-to-height ratio is better than BMI, waist circumference, or waist-to-hip ratio for predicting your risk of a heart attack, a stroke, or death from heart disease. Aim for a waist-to-height ratio of 0.5.

Q: What are some healthy chip options for game day snacking?

A: You'll never conquer your chip addiction unless you understand why you're hooked. The salt jolts your taste buds, and the crunch amplifies the flavor, making you desire more chips, says Valerie Berkowitz, MS, RD, director of nutrition at the Center for Balanced Health in Manhattan.

Our picks meet these craving criteria by delivering flavor and crunch, and also hit the health parameters chosen by Berkowitz and Alan Aragon, MS, a *Men's Health* nutrition advisor: One ounce should come in at 150 calories or less, pack at least 2 grams of fiber, and contain 150 milligrams of sodium or less.

"The more fiber a snack has, the less calorie-dense and more nutrient-dense it tends to be," Aragon says.

Q: Do any of those weight-loss supplements really work?

A: You might drop a few pounds by taking one, but you might also drop dead. Supplements are not regulated by the FDA, so their active ingredients can stray from what's printed on the labels. In fact, since 2008, the government has had to recall 72 weight-loss supplements because they contained prescription drugs such as sibutra-

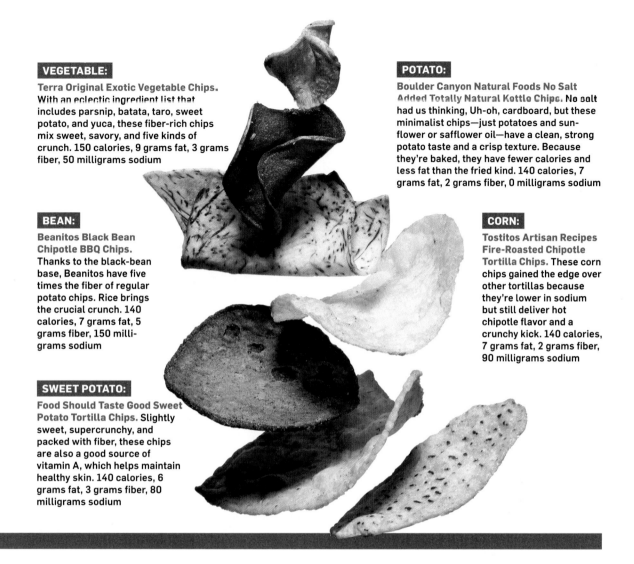

VEGETABLE:

Terra Original Exotic Vegetable Chips. With an eclectic ingredient list that includes parsnip, batata, taro, sweet potato, and yuca, these fiber-rich chips mix sweet, savory, and five kinds of crunch. 150 calories, 9 grams fat, 3 grams fiber, 50 milligrams sodium

POTATO:

Boulder Canyon Natural Foods No Salt Added Totally Natural Kettle Chips. No salt had us thinking, Uh-oh, cardboard, but these minimalist chips—just potatoes and sun-flower or safflower oil—have a clean, strong potato taste and a crisp texture. Because they're baked, they have fewer calories and less fat than the fried kind. 140 calories, 7 grams fat, 2 grams fiber, 0 milligrams sodium

BEAN:

Beanitos Black Bean Chipotle BBQ Chips. Thanks to the black-bean base, Beanitos have five times the fiber of regular potato chips. Rice brings the crucial crunch. 140 calories, 7 grams fat, 5 grams fiber, 150 milli-grams sodium

CORN:

Tostitos Artisan Recipes Fire-Roasted Chipotle Tortilla Chips. These corn chips gained the edge over other tortillas because they're lower in sodium but still deliver hot chipotle flavor and a crunchy kick. 140 calories, 7 grams fat, 2 grams fiber, 90 milligrams sodium

SWEET POTATO:

Food Should Taste Good Sweet Potato Tortilla Chips. Slightly sweet, supercrunchy, and packed with fiber, these chips are also a good source of vitamin A, which helps maintain healthy skin. 140 calories, 6 grams fat, 3 grams fiber, 80 milligrams sodium

mine, an appetite suppressant. At high levels, like the dose found in some of those recalled weight-loss pills, sibutramine can raise your risk of heart attack and has even been linked to a few deaths.

Even when the labels are accurate, these supplements can produce serious side effects that outweigh any benefits. For instance, many have stimulants, such as caffeine and bitter orange, that are effective at revving your metabolism temporarily. But there's no strong evidence that this translates to weight loss, and it can cause spikes in blood pressure and heart rate, says Judith Stern, ScD, a professor of nutrition at the University of California at Davis. "The vast majority of people do not lose weight by taking a supplement."

If you want to shed pounds, stick to the only safe, proven method: Monitor the calories you eat and the calories you burn, and make sure your daily balance is in the red.

YOU ASKED

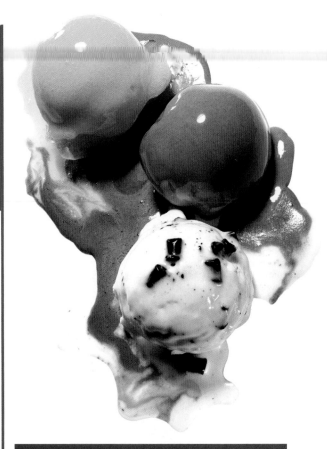

Q: How can I satisfy my cravings for ice cream without packing on pounds?

A: So you want to have your ice-cream cake and eat it too? The obvious step is portion control. Limit yourself to a serving of about 200 calories, says Heather Bauer, RD, founder of Nu-Train nutrition counseling center.

How many scoops is that? It depends, but to achieve a satisfying quantity-to-calories ratio, you'll need to go low on the butterfat and sugar. Alas, these two ingredients give ice cream its rich flavor and velvety thickness, says Edgar Chambers IV, PhD, a professor of sensory analysis at Kansas State University. "To mimic that combination at lower calorie counts, manufacturers cut the cream, add thickeners, and use artificial sweeteners," he says. The result: wretched. But we found exceptions that hit the frozen-treat trifecta of great flavor, low calories, and even a smidgen of nutrition. Note: All nutritional data is based on a ½-cup serving.

GOAT'S MILK ICE CREAM:

Laloo's Deep Chocolate—5 stars. Smooth, flavorful, and low in calories, this ice cream is made with goat milk and rich, 77 percent cacao Scharffen Berger chocolate. Goat milk's fat content is similar to cow milk's, but it has smaller fat molecules—so there's no need to add cream. **160 calories, 5 grams protein, 6 grams fat, 17 grams sugars**

Muscle Ice Cream!

Alan Aragon, MS, *MH*'s nutrition advisor, whips up this chocolate-almond treat to eat after workouts. The almond butter provides thickness and accents the chocolate flavor.

MAKES 1 SERVING

- 1 TABLESPOON UNSALTED ALMOND BUTTER
- 1 SCOOP CHOCOLATE PROTEIN POWDER
- ¼ CUP 2% MILK
- ¼ CUP WATER

In a bowl, mix the almond butter, protein powder, milk, and water. Freeze for 3 hours.

Per serving: 222 calories, 26 grams protein, 8 g carbohydrates, 11 g fat, 1.5 g saturated fat, 1 g fiber, 103 mg sodium

½ FAT ICE CREAM:

Breyers Smooth & Dreamy Mint Chocolate Chip—4 stars. To slash calories while maintaining flavor, Breyers folds in more air during the final mixing and limits the number of ingredients, most of which are natural. 130 calories, 3 grams protein, 5 grams fat, 18 grams sugars

ICE CREAM:

Häagen Dazs Five Vanilla Bean—4 stars. The additive-free Häagen Dazs Five line has less cream and more milk than regular HD, saving you 70 calories and 7 grams of fat in an ice cream that's still rich and smooth. 220 calories, 5 grams protein, 11 grams fat, 22 grams sugars

GELATO:

Ciao Bella Strawberry—4 stars. Gelato has 4 to 8 percent butterfat, versus at least 10 percent for ice cream, so it typically has fewer calories. Streaks of strawberry add texture and flavor. 190 calories, 2 grams protein, 9 grams fat, 18 grams sugars

FROZEN YOGURT:

Ben & Jerry's Cherry Garcia—3 stars. By combining a splash of cream with low-calorie yogurt, Ben & Jerry's delivers a fro-yo that tastes like real Cherry Garcia, but with 40 fewer calories and 10 fewer grams of fat. 200 calories, 8 grams protein, 3 grams fat, 27 grams sugars

SORBET:

Julie's Organic Mango Passion—3 stars. Zero-fat, zero-dairy sorbets can taste like cheap flavored ice, which is why Julie's stands out: It's a full-bodied blend that receives a luscious lift from a generous infusion of mango. 100 calories, 0 grams protein, 0 grams fat, 24 grams sugars

FROZEN KEFIR:

Lifeway Pomegranate–3 stars. Fans of frozen yogurt will appreciate this new kefir creation: It's refreshing, tart, and higher in calcium than ice cream, plus it serves up 10 different probiotics. 90 calories, 4 grams protein, 1 gram fat, 16 grams sugars

Q: I do intervals and lift weights. Would it be smart to use a heart-rate monitor?

A: More like brilliant.
"Most men don't know their bodies very well. They think they're going all out, but they're not," says David Jack, general manager at Competitive Athlete Training Zone. "A heart-rate monitor tells you exactly how hard you're going."

That's critical whether you're hammering out intervals or doing strength training. For instance, short intervals are best done at 90 percent of your maximum heart rate and heavy lifts at 60 percent of your max, says Jack. Use these tips to find the right monitor and squeeze more out of your sessions.

Setup: Expect to spend 5 to 20 minutes customizing your device. Also, if you plan to keep an online diary, visit the manufacturer's Web site to find out how to upload your workout data.

Running: Check to see if your monitor has an intervals setting. There are two ways to measure speed and distance: an accelerometer that attaches to your shoe, and a GPS (which usually costs more).

Fitness: To find your max heart rate, Jack recommends this test, although you should consult with your doctor first if you have heart problems: After warming up, sprint up a hill (or a treadmill set on an incline of 8). Keep checking your monitor and note when your heart rate stops rising: That's your max. Now catch your breath.

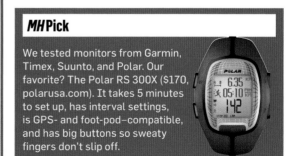

MHPick

We tested monitors from Garmin, Timex, Suunto, and Polar. Our favorite? The Polar RS 300X ($170, polarusa.com). It takes 5 minutes to set up, has interval settings, is GPS- and foot-pod–compatible, and has big buttons so sweaty fingers don't slip off.

YOU ASKED

Q: Can I trust the calorie data provided by chain restaurants?

A: No more than you can trust that they'll remember to hold the pickles or put the dressing on the side. In other words, it's hit or miss.

When USDA researchers tested food samples from 42 chains, they found that some restaurants played by the rules while others broke them. In general, the calorie data at fast-food joints tended to be more accurate, while data from sit-down restaurants varied—sometimes by a lot. About one in five samples had at least 100 more calories than stated, and one in 10 had more than 275 extra calories.

"Fast-food workers usually just field food shipments and then reheat and serve them, while restaurant employees have to assemble dishes," says study author Susan Roberts, PhD, director of the Energy Metabolism Laboratory at Tufts University.

"By adding more dressing or sauce, a chef can skew the calorie count."

Here's a safe bet: Use the nutrition numbers at a chain restaurant as a guide, not gospel, and be especially careful with salads and soups. Their calorie counts were underreported most often, the USDA study found.

THE FIVE WORST DISHES

Beware: The following dishes deviated most from the stated calorie data. Stated calories are based on the restaurants' listed nutritional information, which the researchers converted to gross energy for their lab tests. Averages used where available.

RESTAURANT: DISH	RESTAURANT CLAIM	LAB TEST ACTUAL DATA
ON THE BORDER: Chips and Salsa	451 calories	1,462 calories
OUTBACK STEAKHOUSE: Classic Blue Cheese Wedge Salad (side)	376 calories	1,035 calories
HUNGRY HOWIE'S PIZZA: Pizza Special Sub	1,186 calories	1,728 calories
DON PABLO'S: Chicken Chile Rellenos (2)	517 calories	1,018 calories
BOB EVANS: Cranberry Pecan Chicken Salad (with dressing)	841 calories	1,274 calories

Q: What's a great workout I can do in half an hour to fry fat and help my heart?

A: That two-for-one special calls for a hybrid workout that redlines your ticker and stokes your metabolism. The high-intensity interval circuit on this page, designed by Rachel Cosgrove, CSCS, owner of Results Fitness in Newhall, California, does that by mixing bursts of rowing with explosive body-weight moves.

"Rowing demands more strength than most cardio training does. Plus, it's great for a guy who sits at a desk because it targets his back muscles. Squat thrusts and split jumps work your entire body."

Each interval is 30 seconds on, 30 off: That's short enough to max your intensity, yet it also gives you time to recover. Studies show that high-intensity intervals strengthen your heart's muscles, increase your blood's ability to carry oxygen, and make your arteries more flexible. They can also increase the size and number of your mitochondria, the powerhouses that burn fat and provide energy to your cells. In fact, a recent study in the *Journal of Applied Physiology* found that people who did intervals for just 2 weeks fried 36 percent more fat in subsequent workouts than those who did traditional exercises.

ROW

ROW AS HARD AS YOU CAN FOR 30 SECONDS, AND THEN REST FOR 30 SECONDS.

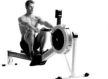 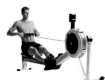

Choose a resistance setting that allows you to row at 85 percent of your maximum heart rate for 30 seconds. Grab the handle using an overhand grip, arms straight. Bend your knees and slide the seat as close to your heels as possible. Push off explosively while pulling the handle to your chest.

SQUAT THRUST

SQUAT THRUST FOR 30 SECONDS, AND THEN REST FOR 30 SECONDS.

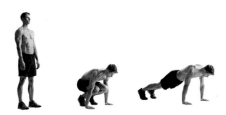

Stand with your feet shoulder-width apart. Push your hips back and drop into a deep squat. Then place your hands on the floor and kick your legs back so you're in a pushup position. Do a pushup, spring back into the squat, and then stand up.

ROW

AGAIN, ROW AS HARD AS YOU CAN FOR 30 SECONDS, AND THEN REST FOR 30 SECONDS.

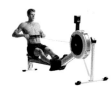

ROWING TIPS:

1. Maintain good posture; don't let your back and shoulders round. "Pull your shoulder blades back and down as you row," says Cosgrove.
2. Keep your core engaged by tensing your abs, and push through your heels.

SPLIT JUMP

SPLIT JUMP FOR 30 SECONDS, AND THEN REST FOR 30 SECONDS.

 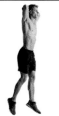 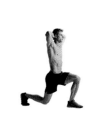

Step forward with your left foot and lower your body into a lunge. Then jump and switch leg positions in midair. Land in a lunge, with your right leg in front of your left. Repeat, alternating back and forth.

REST FOR 2 MINUTES, AND THEN REPEAT THE SEQUENCE FOUR MORE TIMES.

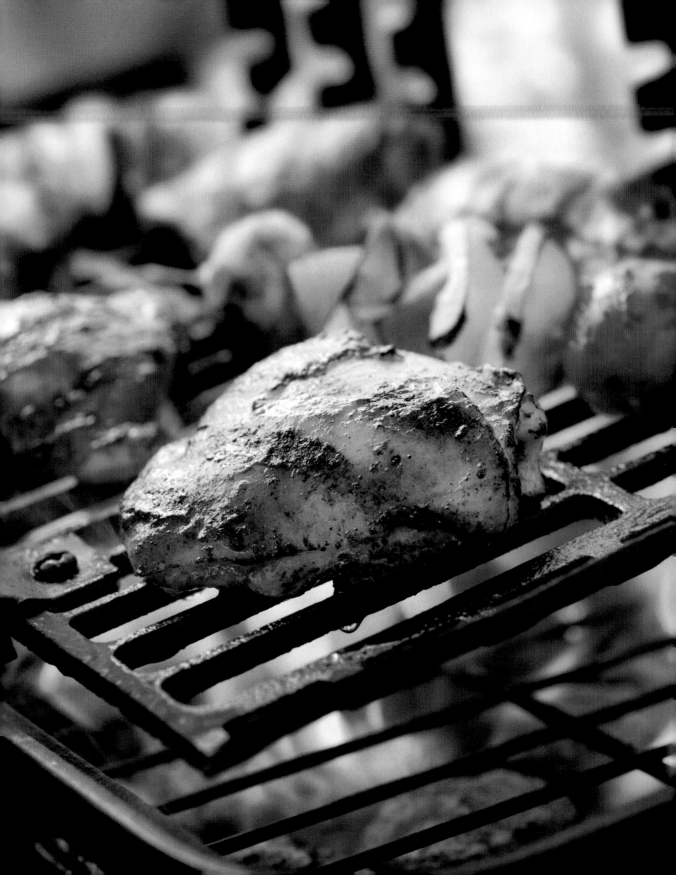

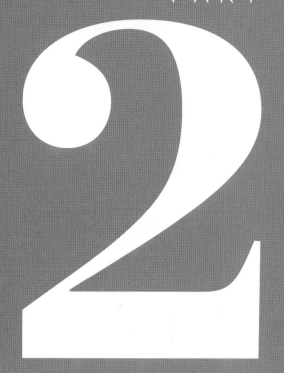

Eat Flat-Belly Foods

The Food You Need to Eat Now

Every diet needs plenty of variety. But that doesn't mean every choice is a good choice. Armed with our top picks, you'll be empowered to make the healthiest choices.

The *MH* Top Picks

Here are our top picks for readily available fresh foods, based on criteria from Alan Aragon, MS, *Men's Health* nutrition advisor.

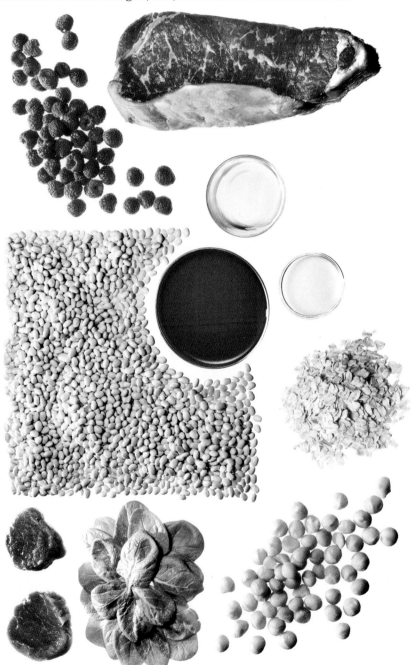

BEEF AND GAME
GRASS-FED BEEF STRIP STEAK
Best combo of vitamin B_{12} and iron, low in calories

HEALTHY FATS
OLIVE OIL
Best combo of high monounsaturated fatty acids and a good ratio of omega-3 to omega-6 fatty acids

DAIRY
1% MILK
Best combo of high protein and calcium with low calories

WINE
RED WINE
Best combo of antioxidant activity and heart-protective effects

WHOLE GRAINS
OATS
Best combo of fiber, folate, and magnesium

NUTS
MACADAMIA NUTS
Best combo of monounsaturated fatty acids and zinc

SEAFOOD
MACKEREL
Best combo of omega-3 fatty acids, vitamin D, and zinc

GREEN VEGETABLES
SPINACH
Best combo of vitamin A, potassium, and folate

POULTRY AND PORK
PORK TENDERLOIN
Best combo of zinc and iron, low in calories

FRUIT
RASPBERRIES
Best combo of fiber and antioxidants, low in calories

STARCHY VEGETABLES AND LEGUMES
NAVY BEANS
Best combo of magnesium, potassium, and vitamin C

The *MH* Nutrition Spectrum

Here's what you need to eat, how often, and why you'll be a better man for it.

Fad diets come and go. But eating right doesn't have to be complicated. "The best diet known to man—a diet that can help you lose weight, build muscle, and live longer—is simple," Aragon says. "Eat mostly whole and minimally processed foods, and start cooking at home more often."

But just how much of these foods should you eat? Hit the goals shown here, and you'll accelerate your path to optimal health.

WHAT THEY DO
Improve blood cholesterol levels, lower blood pressure, and fight cancer.

NUTS

1 TO 2 SERVINGS PER DAY

WHAT THEY DO
Aid muscle functioning, build muscle, and improve blood pressure

EGGS

WHAT THEY DO
Improve blood cholesterol levels, lower blood pressure, and fight cancer

HEALTHY FATS

WHAT THEY DO
Helps your heart, fights cancer, boosts brain function, prevents eye damage and age-related macular degeneration, aids muscle functioning, and build muscle

SEAFOOD

WHAT THEY DO
Promote satiety, aid muscle functioning, and build muscle

POULTRY AND PORK

WHAT THEY DO
Promote healthy blood cells, promote satiety, aid muscle functioning, and build muscle

BEEF AND GAME MEAT

1 TO 2 SERVINGS PER DAY

1 serving = ¼ cup nuts or seeds, or 2 tablespoons nut butter

1 serving = 1 egg

1 serving = 2 tablespoons oil, ½ small avocado, 2 grams fish oil, or 1 pat butter

1 serving = 3 ounces

1 serving = 3 ounces

HEALTHY FATS

QUICK IDEAS
- Use grapeseed oil for high-heat cooking (such as stir-frying) or as your go-to oil for grilling.
- Halve an avocado, fill it with canned crabmeat, and scoop to eat.
- Mix softened butter with minced fresh herbs and garlic; use it to top grilled steak.

SEAFOOD

QUICK IDEAS
- Grill salmon until done and flake it into pasta, along with extra-virgin olive oil, freshly ground pepper, and fresh herbs.
- Buy canned sardines and eat with hearty bread or with mustard and Triscuits.
- Keep shrimp shells on, brush with olive oil, and grill until pink. Peel and eat.

POULTRY AND PORK

QUICK IDEAS
- During the last few minutes of grilling, cover skinless chicken breasts with the sauce from a can of chipotle peppers in adobo.
- Grill pork chops until done and serve with grilled apples and peaches.
- Skip the turkey lunch-meat. Roast a turkey breast, and eat in sandwiches, wraps, and salads.

COFFEE

0 TO 3 SERVINGS PER DAY

WHAT IT DOES
Might reduce risk of Parkinson's, dementia, and Alzheimer's; improves short-term memory

1 serving = 8 ounces

GREEN TEA

0 TO 3 SERVINGS PER DAY

WHAT IT DOES
Might fight cancer, promotes satiety, and prevents tooth decay and gum disease

1 serving = 8 ounces

WINE, BEER, SPIRITS

0 TO 2 SERVINGS PER DAY

WHAT THEY DO
Might prevent diabetes, lower blood pressure, and fight cavities

1 serving = 5 ounces wine, 12 ounces beer, 1.5 ounces hard liquor

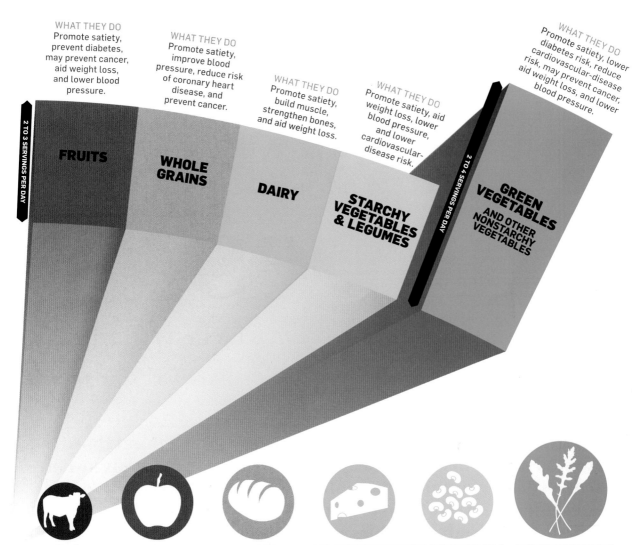

WHAT THEY DO Promote satiety, prevent diabetes, may prevent cancer, aid weight loss, and lower blood pressure.

WHAT THEY DO Promote satiety, improve blood pressure, reduce risk of coronary heart disease, and prevent cancer.

WHAT THEY DO Promote satiety, build muscle, strengthen bones, and aid weight loss.

WHAT THEY DO Promote satiety, aid weight loss, lower blood pressure, and lower cardiovascular-disease risk.

WHAT THEY DO Promote satiety, lower diabetes risk, reduce cardiovascular-disease risk, may prevent cancer, aid weight loss, and lower blood pressure.

2 TO 3 SERVINGS PER DAY

FRUITS

WHOLE GRAINS

DAIRY

STARCHY VEGETABLES & LEGUMES

2 TO 4 SERVINGS PER DAY

GREEN VEGETABLES AND OTHER NONSTARCHY VEGETABLES

---

2 TO 3 SERVINGS PER DAY

2 TO 4 SERVINGS PER DAY

---

1 serving = 3 ounces

QUICK IDEAS

- The best seasonings for beef are rosemary, cumin, and smoked paprika. Season and grill.
- Marinate lamb kebabs in a mixture of plain yogurt, lemon juice, a little ground cinnamon, chopped fresh parsley, and a few cloves of minced garlic.
- Try adding ground venison to chili for a robust flavor upgrade.

1 serving = 1 baseball-size fruit, 2 egg-size fruits, 1 cup fresh fruit, or 1/4 cup dried fruit

QUICK IDEAS

- Chop an apple and add it to 1/2 cup uncooked rolled oats, along with slivered almonds and milk. Cook as usual.
- Slice strawberries and add them to a spinach salad, along with some balsamic vinegar and crumbled goat cheese.
- For breakfast, top whole-wheat bread with peanut butter, raisins, cinnamon, and banana slices.

1 serving = 1 cup cold cereal, 1/2 cup hot cereal, 2 bread slices, or 1/2 cup rice

QUICK IDEAS

- For an Asian rice bowl, layer grilled salmon, scallions, and sautéed shiitakes over brown rice. Drizzle with soy sauce and sriracha hot sauce.
- Season unflavored popcorn with pepper and Parmesan.
- Toss cooked quinoa with roasted peppers, cubed mozzarella cheese, and chopped basil.

1 serving = 1 cup milk, 1 cup yogurt, or 1 ounce cheese

QUICK IDEAS

- Chocolate milk fuels muscle growth: Add it to your protein shake to make it taste better, and drink up!
- Eat blue cheese with walnuts and dried apricots as an easy cheese plate.
- For an awesome taco topping, flavor sour cream with fresh lime juice and sriracha.

1 serving = 1 cup cooked legumes or 1 baseball-size portion of potatoes or yams

QUICK IDEAS

- For salsa, mix black beans with cilantro, chopped scallions, minced jalapeño peppers and garlic, and lime juice. Season with salt and pepper.
- Toss cooked green peas with a drizzle of extra-virgin olive oil, and season with sea salt.
- Bake whole sweet potatoes until tender; drizzle with maple syrup.

1 serving = 1 cup raw or 1/2 cup cooked

QUICK IDEAS

- Try arugula in salads and on sandwiches to add bite.
- Steam bok choy until tender and then toss with hoisin sauce and sesame oil. Garnish with sesame seeds.
- For instant coleslaw, combine thinly sliced cabbage with red onions, carrots, rice-wine vinegar, crushed red-pepper flakes, and a little sugar.

Subzero Heroes

Raid the freezer section to whip up tasty meals.

Approach the frozen-food aisle with caution. Behind those frosted doors lurk sodium-tsunami pizzas, dangerously sweet frozen desserts, and boxed entrées sauced with chemical cocktails. But you can also find your shortcut to stellar meals: frozen fruits and vegetables.

Think of frozen produce as your secret weapon, held in suspended animation until you need it. Pre-prepped frozen produce can be the foundation of a range of superfast dishes, from smoothies and soups to stews and sides.

Here's an unexpected bonus: In winter, frozen produce can be more nutritious than the anemic fresh fruits and vegetables on display in other areas of the supermarket. That's because the frozen stuff was harvested at peak ripeness, when it was dense with nutrients, says Barry Swanson, PhD, a food science professor at Washington State University and spokesman for the Institute of Food Technologists. "The subsequent flash-freezing during the first 24 hours of harvest locks the fruit or vegetable into a nutrient- and antioxidant-rich state." So go ahead. Crack open a cold one.

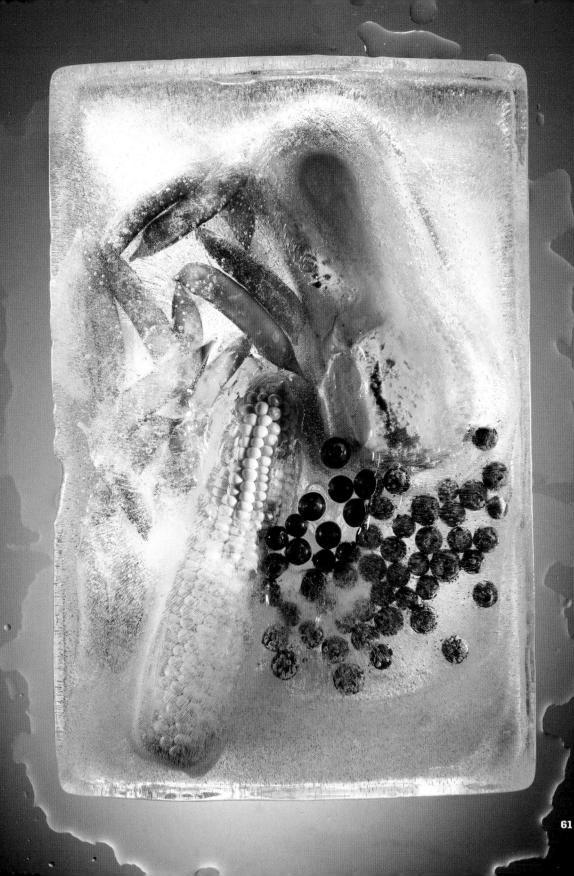

Corn

Compared with lowly canned kernels, frozen corn is king when it comes to taste, texture, and nutritional power.

Health bonus: Although it's thought of as a nutritional dud, corn is chockablock with yellow-orange carotenoids called xanthophylls, which have been shown to protect against cataracts and age-related macular degeneration.

Corn Tomato Succotash

MAKES 4 SERVINGS

- 1 tablespoon oil
- 1 onion, chopped
- 2 cups frozen lima beans
- 2 cups frozen corn kernels
- 2 cloves garlic, minced
- 1 cup diced tomatoes
- 1 jalapeño pepper, seeded and chopped
  Salt
  Ground black pepper

In a large skillet, heat the oil on medium heat and cook the onion until it's soft, about 4 minutes. Stir in the beans, corn, and garlic. Cook until the beans are tender, about 12 minutes.

Add the tomatoes and pepper. Cook, stirring occasionally, for 3 minutes. Season with salt and pepper to taste.

PER SERVING: 223 calories, 9 g protein, 40 g carbohydrates, 4 g fat, 0.5 g saturated fat, 7 g fiber, 196 mg sodium

Corn Pudding Cups

MAKES 6 SERVINGS

- 2 cups frozen corn kernels, thawed
- 2 eggs
- ½ cup plain dried bread crumbs
- ½ cup low-fat sour cream
- 1 small jalapeño pepper, seeded and chopped
- ¼ teaspoon salt

Preheat the oven to 350°F. Pulse 1 cup of the corn in a food processor until it breaks down. Remove the blade and stir in the remaining 1 cup of corn, the eggs, bread crumbs, sour cream, pepper, and salt.

Spoon the mixture into 6 greased muffin cups. Bake until they start to turn golden, about 25 minutes.

PER SERVING: 137 calories, 6 g protein, 18 g carbohydrates, 5 g fat, 2 g saturated fat, 1 g fiber, 202 mg sodium

Creamy Corn-Potato Chowder

MAKES 4 SERVINGS

- 1 tablespoon oil
- 1 onion, chopped
- 1 red bell pepper, chopped
- 2 cloves garlic, minced
- 2 cups frozen corn kernels
- 1 pound Yukon Gold potatoes, chopped
- 1½ cups low-sodium vegetable broth
- 2 bay leaves
- 1 tablespoon chopped fresh rosemary
- 1 teaspoon red-pepper flakes
- 1 cup 1% milk
  Salt
  Ground black pepper

Your Freezer Rules

From store to stove, here's how to make the most of your frozen produce.

Test the bag. Make sure you can feel the individual fruits and vegetables.

"A bag that feels like a block of ice has most likely been thawed and refrozen, degrading the flavor and nutrients," says Barry Swanson, PhD.

Go fancy. If you can, choose bags or boxes of frozen produce with the USDA "U.S. Fancy" shield, not those with the lower-grade "U.S. No. 1."

Stay pure. Steer clear of frozen fruits and vegetables with added sweeteners, salt, or sauces. The only ingredient should be the fruit or vegetable itself.

Toss some. Those peas you've had since Super Bowl XLII should be compost. Frozen fruits last about 6 months, and frozen vegetables about 1 year, before their flavor, texture, and nutrients begin to degrade, says Swanson.

Thaw not. If you're making smoothies, soup, chili, or stir-fry, there's no need to defrost your produce.

In a large saucepan, heat the oil over medium heat. Cook the onion, bell pepper, and garlic for 4 minutes. Toss in the corn, potatoes, broth, bay leaves, rosemary, red-pepper flakes, and milk, and add salt and pepper to taste. Bring to a boil and then reduce the heat and simmer, covered, until the potatoes are tender, about 15 minutes.

Remove the bay leaves. Ladle half the soup into a blender, puree it, and return it to the pot.

PER SERVING: 237 calories, 7 g protein, 44 g carbohydrates, 5 g fat, 1 g saturated fat, 4 g fiber, 129 mg sodium

Green Peas

Even in season, truly delicious fresh peas are elusive. Their sweetness turns starchy almost immediately after they're picked. Frozen peas retain their flavor for months.

Health bonus: Each cup of peas contains a laudable 6 grams of fiber. A diet high in fiber (35 grams a day or more) has been linked with a reduced risk of heart disease.

Buttermilk Pea Soup

MAKES 4 SERVINGS

- 1 tablespoon oil
- 1 leek or onion, thinly sliced
- 2 cloves garlic, minced
- 4 cups reduced-sodium chicken broth
- 3 cups frozen peas
- 1 teaspoon ground cumin
- 2 teaspoons dried thyme
- 1/4 cup fresh mint leaves
  Salt
  Ground black pepper
- 3/4 cup buttermilk

In a large saucepan, heat the oil on medium heat. Add the leek or onion and the garlic and cook for 4 minutes. Stir in the broth, peas, cumin, thyme, and mint, and add salt and pepper to taste. Simmer for 15 minutes, and then puree in a blender until smooth.

Return to the pan, stir in the buttermilk, and simmer 5 minutes longer.

PER SERVING: 193 calories, 13 g protein, 24 g carbohydrates, 6 g fat, 1 g saturated fat, 6 g fiber, 228 mg sodium

Pea Fritters

MAKES 4 SERVINGS

- 1 cup frozen peas
- 1/4 cup whole wheat flour
- 2 tablespoons chopped scallions
- 2 tablespoons butter
  Salt
  Sour cream, for garnish

Cook the peas according to the package directions, drain, and mash them with a fork. Stir in the flour, scallions, and salt to taste. Form into 4 patties.

In a skillet, heat the butter on medium heat. Add the patties and cook until lightly golden, 1 1/2 minutes on each side. Serve as an appetizer with sour cream.

PER SERVING: 103 calories, 3 g protein, 10 g carbohydrates, 6 g fat, 3 g saturated fat, 3 g fiber, 117 mg sodium

Chicken Pea Curry

MAKES 4 SERVINGS

- 1 tablespoon oil
- 1 onion, chopped
- 1 pound chicken breasts, cubed
- 1 sweet potato, chopped
- 1 carrot, sliced
- 2 cloves garlic, minced
- 1 tablespoon minced ginger
- 1 tablespoon curry powder
- 1/2 teaspoon red-pepper flakes
- 1/4 teaspoon salt
- 1/4 teaspoon ground black pepper
- 1 cup frozen peas
- 1 15-ounce can coconut milk
- 1/2 cup water
- 1 teaspoon fresh lime juice
  Cilantro, for garnish

In a large saucepan, heat the oil on medium heat. Add the onion and chicken, and cook until the chicken is no longer pink, about 5 minutes.

Stir in the sweet potato, carrot, garlic, and ginger and cook for 3 minutes. Stir in the curry powder, red-pepper flakes, and salt and pepper and cook for 1 minute. Then stir in the peas, coconut milk, and water. Bring to a boil, then lower the heat and simmer for 15 minutes. Stir in the lime juice and garnish with the cilantro.

PER SERVING: 449 calories, 29 g protein, 20 g carbohydrates, 29 g fat, 21 g saturated fat, 5 g fiber, 359 mg sodium

Winter Squash

Even if fresh winter squash is available, choose frozen instead. There's no need to peel, cut, seed, or puree. It's ready to go straight from the box.

Health bonus: The orange glow of winter squash is a sign of its beta-carotene, which your body converts to immunity-boosting vitamin A.

Squash-Apple Soup

MAKES 4 SERVINGS

- **1** tablespoon oil
- **2** shallots, chopped
- **1** tablespoon minced ginger
- **2** 10-ounce packages frozen squash puree
- **3** cups reduced-sodium vegetable broth
- **1** apple, chopped
- **1** tablespoon dried sage
  Salt
  Ground black pepper
  Sour cream for garnish

In a large saucepan, heat the oil on medium heat. Add the shallots and ginger, and cook for 3 minutes. Add the squash puree, broth, apple, sage, and salt and pepper to taste.

Bring to a boil, then simmer, covered, for 15 minutes. In batches, process the soup in a blender until smooth. Serve with a swirl of sour cream.

PER SERVING: 171 calories, 4 g protein, 37 g carbohydrates, 4 g fat, 1 g saturated fat, 4 g fiber, 145 mg sodium

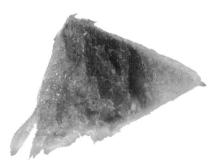

Penne with Winter Squash and Ricotta

MAKES 4 SERVINGS

- **8** ounces whole-grain penne pasta
- **2** shallots, chopped
- **2** cloves garlic, minced
- **1** tablespoon oil
- **10** ounces frozen squash puree, thawed
- **½** cup light ricotta cheese
- **½** cup grated Parmesan cheese plus additional for topping
- **½** cup water
  Juice of ½ lemon
- **¼** teaspoon ground nutmeg
  Salt
  Ground black pepper
  Chopped parsley for garnish

Cook the pasta according to package directions.

Meanwhile, sauté the shallots and garlic with the oil in a skillet on medium heat for 3 minutes. Stir in the squash puree, ricotta, Parmesan, water, lemon juice, nutmeg, and salt and pepper to taste. Simmer for 5 minutes. Drain the pasta and toss it with the sauce. Serve topped with the parsley and more Parmesan.

PER SERVING: 408 calories, 18 g protein, 63 g carbohydrates, 11 g fat, 4 g saturated fat, 6 g fiber, 242 mg sodium

Pan-Seared Pork Chops with Maple-Squash Polenta

MAKES 2 SERVINGS

- **4** cups water
- **1** cup coarse cornmeal
- **2** bone-in pork chops
  Salt
  Ground black pepper
- **1** tablespoon oil
- **1** cup frozen squash puree, thawed
- **¼** cup grated Parmesan cheese
- **2** teaspoons pure maple syrup

In a medium saucepan, bring the water to a simmer, and then whisk in the cornmeal until it begins to thicken, about 1 minute. Reduce the heat to medium-low and cook until thick, whisking frequently, about 15 minutes. Meanwhile, season the pork chops with salt and pepper. Heat the oil in a skillet on medium heat and sear the chops until cooked through, about 5 minutes on each side. When the polenta is done, stir in the squash puree, Parmesan, and maple syrup. Add salt and pepper to taste.

PER SERVING: 626 calories, 47 g protein, 70 g carbohydrates, 18 g fat, 4 g saturated fat, 12 g fiber, 291 mg sodium

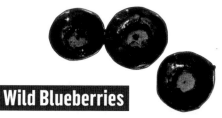

Wild Blueberries

During the summer, intensely flavorful wild blueberries sell for sky-high prices at local farmers' markets. Frozen ones, though, are priced right—and available year-round.

Health bonus: Cornell researchers who ranked the antioxidant power of 25 fruits found that wild blueberries had the highest overall levels, and a study in the *Journal of Agricultural and Food Chemistry* found that wild blueberries pack about 50 percent more antioxidant power than regular cultivated blueberries.

Wild-Blueberry Cornmeal Pancakes

MAKES 2 SERVINGS

- $1/3$ cup yellow cornmeal
- $2/3$ cup whole-wheat flour
- $1/2$ cup frozen wild blueberries plus additional thawed berries for garnish
- $1/2$ cup milk
- 1 ripe banana, mashed
- 1 egg
- 1 teaspoon ground cinnamon
- 1 teaspoon baking powder
- 1 tablespoon butter
  Pure maple syrup for topping

In a large bowl, combine the cornmeal, flour, blueberries, milk, banana, egg, cinnamon, and baking powder (stir in more milk if the batter is too thick to pour).

Heat the butter in a large skillet on medium heat. Drop the batter in, $1/3$ cup at a time. Cook until the pancakes are golden brown, about 3 minutes per side. Serve topped with pure maple syrup and thawed blueberries.

PER SERVING: **408 calories, 13 g protein, 69 g carbohydrates, 12 g fat, 6 g saturated fat, 10 g fiber, 633 mg sodium**

Seared Chicken with Blueberry Salsa

MAKES 4 SERVINGS

- 1 cup frozen wild blueberries, thawed
- 1 small red onion, chopped
- 1 red bell pepper, chopped
- 1 jalapeño pepper, seeded and chopped
- $1/2$ cup torn basil leaves
  Juice of 1 lime
- 1 teaspoon honey
- $1/4$ teaspoon salt
- 4 6-ounce skinless chicken breasts

In a bowl, combine the blueberries, onion, bell pepper, jalapeño pepper, basil, lime juice, honey, and salt.

Serve over seared chicken or fish.

PER SERVING: **238 calories, 37 g protein, 11 g carbohydrates, 5 g fat, 1 g saturated fat, 3 g fiber, 346 mg sodium**

High-Protein Blueberry-Yogurt Shake

MAKES 2 SERVINGS

- 1 cup frozen wild blueberries
- $1/2$ cup plain Greek yogurt
- 1 scoop plain or vanilla whey protein powder
- 1 banana
- $1/2$ cup pomegranate juice
- $1/4$ cup walnut pieces
- $1/2$ teaspoon vanilla extract

In a blender, combine the blueberries, yogurt, protein powder, banana, pomegranate juice, walnut pieces, and vanilla.

Whirl until smooth.

PER SERVING: **312 calories, 17 g protein, 39 g carbohydrates, 11 g fat, 1 g saturated fat, 6 g fiber, 31 mg sodium**

The Best Food You'll Ever Eat

Five of the world's best chefs make your favorite meals better than you've ever tasted. Join writer Paul Kita as he meets the chefs and discovers their secret techniques.

Ribs. Grilled cheese. Bacon and eggs. Barbecue chicken. Burgers. These are the meals men love. You've been devouring these foods all your life. Maybe you even think you've mastered cooking them.

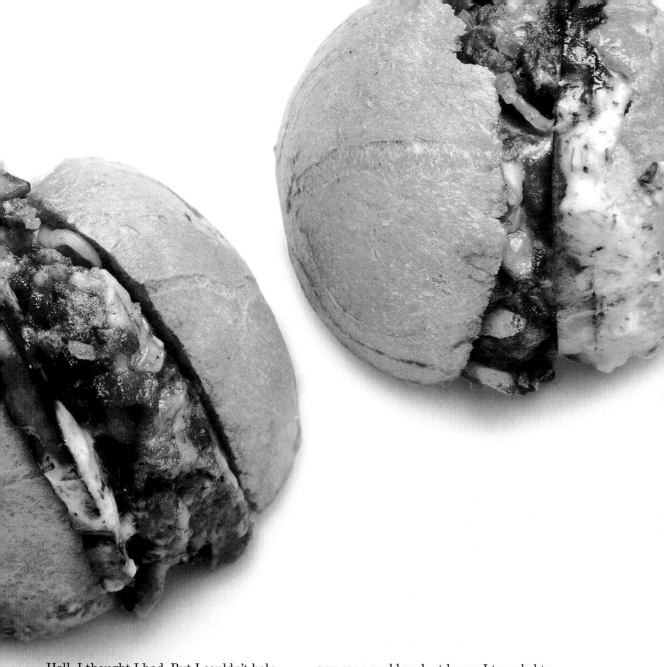

Hell, I thought I had. But I couldn't help wondering if my favorite chefs—guys known more for working with fine caviar and microgreens than for flipping burgers—could make these standards even better. So *Men's Health* challenged five of the nation's preeminent chefs to transform iconic guy foods into mind-blowing meals any man could cook at home. I traveled to their kitchens to chronicle their secrets. What those chefs came up with may forever change your approach to your go-to meals. Sharpen your knife and prep your palate: With these new techniques and incredible recipes, you'll be ready to give your favorite foods a four-star upgrade.

The Burger

At Grant Achatz's temple to avant-garde cooking, Alinea, he's garnered an almost obscene pile of accolades by creating food that challenges the senses. During my last visit there, I tasted mozzarella foam, created by crystallizing the cheese with liquid nitrogen.

Two years later, I'm back in Chicago, challenging Achatz to use his creative, analytical approach to engineer the ultimate burger. He accepts the challenge, invites me to his home, and dives in.

"Classic burgers usually have the same group of ingredients, and they're all there for a reason," Achatz says. So he reconfigures the elements, taking a bit of extra inspiration, he points out, from the flavors of French charcuterie. Instead of topping the beef patty with bacon and cheese, he folds the ingredients directly into the raw beef to infuse it with smoky richness. Then he creates a traditional French gribiche sauce, which is the perfect burger condiment, he says, because it incorporates traditional burger enhancements such as mayo, mustard, onion, and pickle. A final inspired touch: He uses a topping of tangy sautéed apple instead of ketchup, adding an extra layer of nuance.

As Achatz leans against his kitchen counter, I devour the whole thing in seconds, speechless. Achatz smiles. The guy's done it again.

Don't work too hard. Avoid overworking the beef and making it tough: Chilling the meat briefly helps it blend with the dry burger ingredients.

Cap Your Apples

No need to buy a corer. Slice the apples crosswise and then use the cap from a liquor bottle to punch out the hard, seeded center.

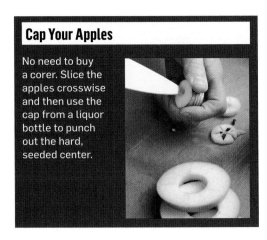

> ## "This burger has all the traditional components, but **it's unlike any burger you've ever eaten**."
>
> —Grant Achatz, executive chef, Alinea, Chicago

Charcuterie Burger

MAKES 4 SERVINGS

Sauce Gribiche

- **3** tablespoons finely chopped hard-boiled egg whites
- **3** tablespoons mayonnaise
- **1½** tablespoons Dijon mustard
- **1** tablespoon finely chopped cornichon pickles
- **1** tablespoon finely chopped nonpareil capers
- **1** tablespoon finely chopped white onion
- **1** teaspoon finely chopped parsley
- **1** teaspoon finely chopped tarragon

  Pinch of kosher salt

The Burgers

- **2½** teaspoons canola oil
- **8** slices hickory-smoked bacon, sliced crosswise into ¼"-thick lengths
- **½** cup finely diced shallots
- **1** tablespoon caraway seeds, ground in a spice grinder
- **1** pound ground beef (80% lean)
- **2** medium Granny Smith apples, cored and sliced ½"thick
- **½** teaspoon unsalted butter
- **½** cup grated Gruyère cheese
- **1½** teaspoons (plus a pinch) kosher salt

  Ground black pepper
- **1** sprig thyme
- **3** garlic cloves, crushed with the flat side of a chef's knife
- **4** sourdough hamburger buns, split and toasted

Combine the gribiche ingredients in a medium bowl and refrigerate. In a large pan, heat ½ teaspoon of oil on medium. Add the bacon and sauté until partially cooked, about 3 minutes. Add the shallots and caraway seeds and cook until the shallots are translucent, about 3 minutes more. Using your fingers, gently break apart the beef into another bowl. Place the bowl of beef, the bacon mixture, and a fork in the freezer for 10 minutes.

Meanwhile, heat 1 teaspoon of oil in a skillet over very high heat until it begins to smoke. Immediately add the apple slices and cook until well browned on one

> ### Fat = Flavor
>
> For burgers, skip lean ground meat like sirloin. Pick ground meat with at least 20 percent fat (also labeled 80 percent lean), such as chuck. If a burger isn't juicy, you might as well serve a hockey puck.

side, about 4 minutes. Flip them and cook until browned on the other side, another 2 minutes or so. Add the butter and cook until the apples are very soft, about 2 minutes more. Remove them from the pan.

Preheat the oven to 375°F. Remove the beef, bacon, and fork from the freezer. Add the bacon mixture to the beef along with the Gruyère, 1½ teaspoons of kosher salt, and a few grinds of black pepper. Using the cold fork, gently mix the ingredients together. Form the meat into four ¾"-thick patties.

Heat 1 teaspoon of oil in a large ovenproof sauté pan on high until the oil begins to smoke. Add the burger patties, thyme, and garlic. Cook, without moving the meat, until the bottoms of the burgers caramelize and develop a crust, about 2½ minutes. Using a thin metal spatula, flip the patties and cook for 1 minute more. Transfer the pan to the oven and cook for 2 to 3 minutes to finish the burger. Remove the burgers from the pan and set on paper towels to drain the excess fat.

Place the burger patties on the bottom half of each bun. Spread a generous helping of sauce gribiche on each burger. Add a few pieces of roasted apple and then the bun tops, and serve.

PER SERVING: 829 calories, 35 g protein, 44 g carbohydrates, 57 g fat, 19 g saturated fat, 4 g fiber, 1901 mg sodium

TEST YOUR BURGER

To check how well you've packed your patty, place it on your fingertips so a few inches of patty hang off the edge. If it starts to break apart, you need to compress it more. If it droops slightly without breaking, it's good to go.

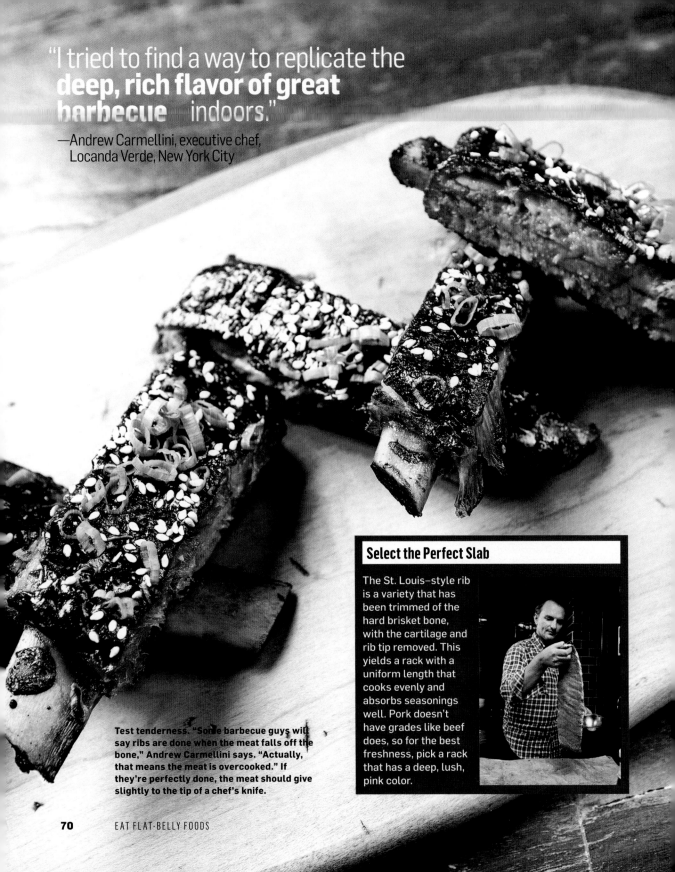

> # "I tried to find a way to replicate the **deep, rich flavor of great barbecue** indoors."
> —Andrew Carmellini, executive chef,
> Locanda Verde, New York City

Test tenderness. "Some barbecue guys will say ribs are done when the meat falls off the bone," Andrew Carmellini says. "Actually, that means the meat is overcooked." If they're perfectly done, the meat should give slightly to the tip of a chef's knife.

Select the Perfect Slab

The St. Louis–style rib is a variety that has been trimmed of the hard brisket bone, with the cartilage and rib tip removed. This yields a rack with a uniform length that cooks evenly and absorbs seasonings well. Pork doesn't have grades like beef does, so for the best freshness, pick a rack that has a deep, lush, pink color.

The Ribs

Andrew Carmellini has already mastered refined French cuisine; now he draws crowds to his Tribeca restaurant, Locanda Verde, with rustic, modern Italian cooking. But make no mistake: The man also knows ribs.

He traveled the South to research recipes for his latest cookbook, *American Flavor*, and his SoHo restaurant, the Dutch. Along the way, Carmellini sampled succulent smoked pork from a pantheon of pitmasters. But when I challenge him to create the ultimate rack, he turns to his local Chinese takeout joint for inspiration.

"Great spareribs are just as tender and flavorful as old-fashioned barbecue," he says, "and the best part is you don't need a smoker to cook them."

To prove his point, he cooks up a batch for me in the compact kitchen of a two-story suite at the Greenwich Hotel, next door to Locanda Verde. He showers the ribs with a rub dominated by the anise notes of Chinese five-spice powder, and then bakes them until they're pull-apart tender.

The savory pork scent wafts through the suite as Carmellini glazes the rack with a tangy, slightly sweet sauce. The result is remarkable—rich, smoky, addictive. Ribs you'll want to make all year long.

Wrap It Up

The foil packet creates a high-moisture environment, which helps the meat self-baste and prevents it from drying out during cooking.

New-School Asian Ribs

MAKES 4 APPETIZER SERVINGS

Ribs

- **2** tablespoons Chinese five-spice powder (available in the spice aisle or at penzeys.com)
- **1** teaspoon chipotle pepper powder (available in the spice aisle or at penzeys.com)
- **½** teaspoon garlic powder
- **½** teaspoon salt
- **⅛** teaspoon cayenne pepper
- **1** full rack St. Louis ribs

Sauce

- **⅓** cup hoisin sauce
- **⅓** cup ketchup
- **⅓** cup rice-wine vinegar
- **2** tablespoons black-bean sauce

To finish

- **3** scallions, thinly sliced
- **1** tablespoon sesame seeds

In a small bowl, mix the dry ingredients together to make a rub. Cut a piece of foil a little longer than the rib rack; place the foil on a baking sheet and lay the ribs on top. Sprinkle both sides of the meat with the rub, massaging it in. Refrigerate the ribs, uncovered, for 2 hours so the rub infuses the meat.

Preheat the oven to 250°F. Fold the foil around the ribs so all the meat is covered, but leave a small vent on top. Place the baking sheet in the oven and bake for 3 hours. Then reduce the heat to 225°F and bake until the meat is very tender, about 2 hours more. Meanwhile, in a bowl, whisk the sauce ingredients with 2 tablespoons of water.

When the ribs are done, unwrap them and place the rack directly on the baking sheet. Pour any cooking juices into the bowl with the rib sauce and stir them in. Brush both sides of the ribs generously with the sauce.

Raise the oven temperature to 400°F. Return the ribs to the oven and bake them until the sauce caramelizes slightly, 5 to 10 minutes. Brush the ribs with more sauce, sprinkle with scallions and sesame seeds, and serve with the remaining sauce for dipping.

PER SERVING: 812 calories, 42 g protein, 20 g carbohydrates, 63 g fat, 19 g saturated fat, 1 g fiber, 831 mg sodium

Grilled Cheese

It's a few hours before lunch service at Per Se, the New York restaurant that Thomas Keller, executive chef, helms along with its equally acclaimed California counterpart, the French Laundry. The immaculate kitchen is humming with activity as the brigade prepares confits, gelées, and mousses.

I'm standing in the middle of it all, talking to one of the most acclaimed chefs in the country about grilled cheese. Is it sacrilege, I wonder, to ask Thomas Keller to turn his attention to this humble, almost retro sandwich?

"Why not?" he asks. "Everyone loves grilled cheese." Of course, defaulting to Kraft Singles and spongy white bread—that would be sacrilege. Keller starts with buttery brioche and selects two cheeses for nuance.

Then he chars mild and spicy peppers and tucks them into the sandwich for a stealth hit of sweetness and heat. A few minutes on the griddle, and grown-up grilled cheese is born.

Spicy Pepper, Monterey Jack, and Cheddar Grilled Cheese

MAKES 2 SANDWICHES

- **1** or 2 jalapeño peppers
- **1** red bell pepper
  Butter, softened at room temperature
- **4** slices brioche, whole wheat, or sourdough bread (¾" thick)
- **4** slices Monterey Jack
- **4** slices Cheddar

Fill a bowl with ice water. Place the jalapeño and bell peppers on a metal baking sheet, and fire up a small butane torch (we like the Weller Table Top butane torch; $24 at sears.com) until the flame burns blue. Carefully blister the skins of the peppers with the blowtorch, turning them with a fork as you work.

Pull on a pair of plastic gloves and plunge the peppers into the ice water for a few seconds. Remove them and rub off their skins. Then halve them lengthwise, remove the seeds, and chop the peppers.

Heat a cast-iron skillet on medium. For each sandwich, liberally butter both sides of two bread slices. Place two slices of Monterey Jack on one piece of bread, with a heaping tablespoon of the pepper mixture in the middle. Place two slices of Cheddar on the other piece of bread, and put the bread slices together.

Place the sandwiches in a skillet over medium heat, and cook until the bread is golden brown and the cheeses melt together, 3 to 5 minutes a side. Cut them in half diagonally and serve with beer.

PER SANDWICH: 679 calories, 34 g protein, 35 g carbohydrates, 46 g fat, 28 g saturated fat, 5 g fiber, 1028 mg sodium

THE PERFECT SLICE:
Don't squash the bread slices: Freeze the loaf first, and use a bread knife to cut it.

Build it right. Leaving a border of cheese around the peppers prevents them from spilling out as you eat the sandwich.

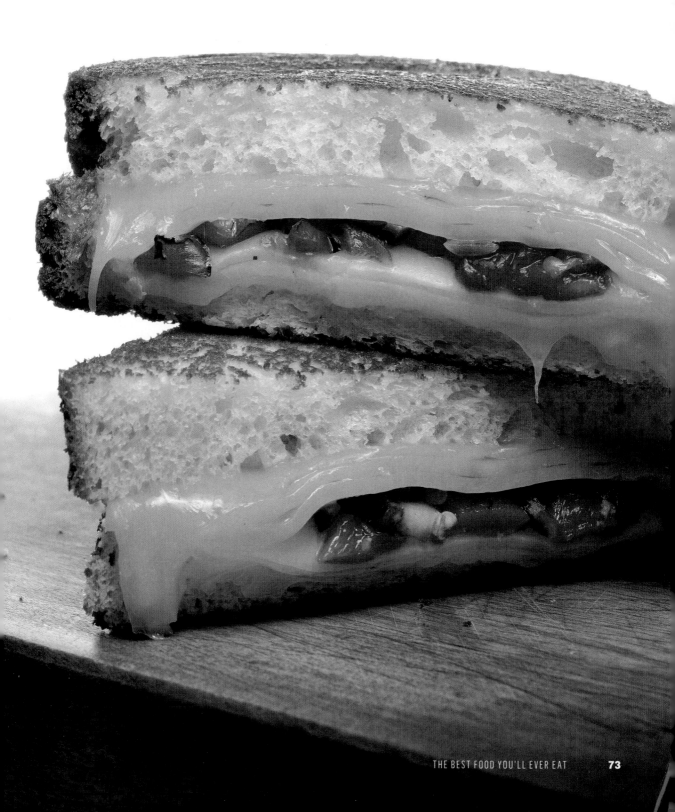

Barbecue Chicken

Some men don sunglasses, spike their hair, and call themselves rock-star chefs. David Chang, frontman of the Korean-inspired Momofuku restaurants, lets his food put on the performance. Chang's menus are filled with gutsy, innovative dishes like roasted corn with miso butter, foie gras terrine with pickled blueberries, and seared scallops with kimchi and black rice. But when he brings me into his kitchen to reinvent "barbecue chicken," he turns to his childhood for inspiration.

"When I think of barbecue chicken, I think of the Korean barbecue chicken I grew up eating," Chang says. "We used to sit in the park and grill, and the smell of that spicy meat was so intense."

So he decides to re-create those flavors, stirring together a quick marinade based on gochujang, a sweet, pungent Korean chili-bean paste. A hit of apple juice goes in too: "It adds some sweetness to a traditionally very spicy dish," he explains. The sour malic acid in the juice helps open up the flavors in the chicken, while the sugars in the marinade help the meat turn a rich brown when it hits the grill. There's a reason the marinade is a Korean barbecue classic, Chang says: "It's delicious, it's quick, and it's really easy."

Skip the Skin

Removing the skin from your chicken does more than just cut calories. It also helps it to cook more quickly, and it allows the sugars in the honey and the apple juice to caramelize more easily.

Spicy Korean Barbecue Chicken

MAKES 4 SERVINGS

- **8** skinless, boneless chicken thighs
- **2** tablespoons gochujang (available at Asian markets) or sriracha hot sauce
- **2** tablespoons grapeseed oil, plus more for cooking
- **½** cup apple juice
- **1** tablespoon honey
- **1** tablespoon Korean miso or Japanese shiro (white) miso (available at Asian markets)
- **1** teaspoon minced ginger
- **2** garlic cloves, roughly chopped
- **1** teaspoon kosher salt, plus more to taste
- **1** cup water
- **1** medium yellow onion, thinly sliced
- **½** cup chopped scallions
  Grapeseed oil for grilling

Place the chicken in a large resealable plastic bag. In a medium bowl, mix together the gochujang or sriracha, the oil, apple juice, honey, miso, ginger, garlic, and salt. Add the water and mix thoroughly. Mix in the onion and scallions. Pour half the marinade mixture into the plastic bag with the chicken, seal, and refrigerate for at least 2 hours or up to a day. Refrigerate the remaining marinade in a small covered saucepan.

When you're ready to eat, remove the chicken from the fridge. Place the saucepan with the reserved marinade on medium heat and simmer until the mixture is thickened and saucelike, about 20 minutes.

Brush a grill or grill pan with grapeseed oil and set the heat to medium high. When the grill is ready, cook the thighs until the undersides have charred grill marks and release easily from the grill, about 5 minutes.

Flip the thighs and cook until a meat thermometer inserted in the middle reads 165°F, about 5 minutes more. Let them rest for 2 to 3 minutes, and serve with white rice and grilled vegetables like scallions, mushrooms, or bok choy.

PER SERVING: 297 calories, 29 g protein, 14 g carbohydrates, 14 g fat, 2 g saturated fat, 2 g fiber, 780 mg sodium

CHAR YOUR CHICKEN
To create cross-hatched grill marks on your chicken, use tongs to give the meat a quarter turn halfway through cooking each side.

"**So many flavors are going on at once in this recipe**, and each of them spicy, sweet, salty, bitter, earthy—helps create a complex but balanced dish."

—David Chang, executive chef, the Momofuku restaurants, New York City

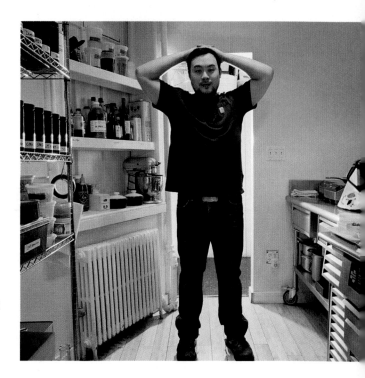

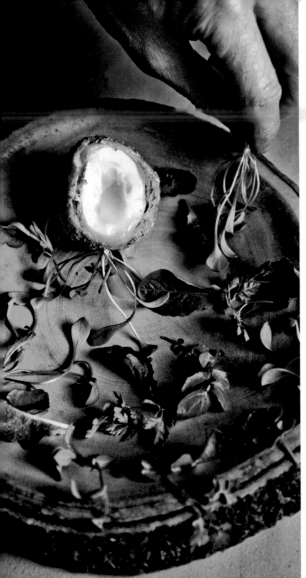

Bacon and Eggs

As I tour the acres of farmland and pasture that surround Blue Hill at Stone Barns, it's easy to see why Dan Barber knows bacon and eggs. The eggs he uses at the restaurant come from portable chicken houses at the Stone Barns Center for Food and Agriculture. Back in the restaurant's kitchen, Barber mentions that his bacon is cured and smoked in-house. So it's no surprise that when he sets out to make a bacon-and-egg breakfast, he isn't content with simply frying them up in a skillet.

"It's about creating a play off the classic combination of ham, eggs, and cheese," he says. So he soft-boils those superlative eggs, wraps them in thin rashers of beautiful bacon, and coats the whole deal in cheese and bread crumbs. A quick minute in hot oil and the eggs emerge crispy on the outside but molten within.

"I call these eggs 'green' because that's how you should buy your eggs—pasture-raised and organic," Barber says. He cuts into the center of an egg, and bright-orange yolk spills out over a plateful of mixed greens. "You'll see and taste the difference."

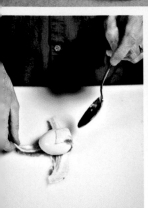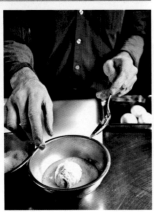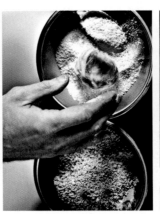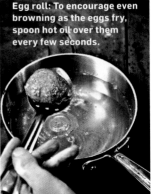

Egg roll: To encourage even browning as the eggs fry, spoon hot oil over them every few seconds.

"It's egg meets pig, and both are at their best."

—Dan Barber, executive chef, Blue Hill at Stone Barns, Pocantico Hills, New York

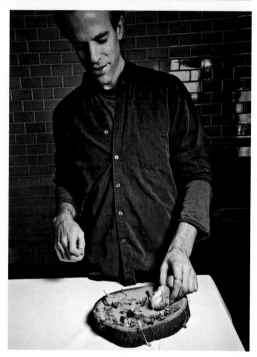

"Green" Eggs and Ham

MAKES 2 SERVINGS

Grapeseed oil for frying
- **4** whole eggs plus 1 beaten egg
- **2** tablespoons panko bread crumbs
- **2** tablespoons ground toasted almonds
- **2** tablespoons finely grated Parmesan
- **¼** cup flour
- **4** slices thin-cut bacon, halved crosswise to make 8 pieces (see "Flatten Your Pork")
  Salt
  Ground black pepper
- **2** cups Mesclun greens for serving

Fill a small pot with enough oil to submerge an egg (about 3 cups), and set it over medium heat (use a cooking thermometer; the oil should eventually hover at 370°F). Meanwhile, bring a medium pot of water to a boil and prepare a large bowl of ice water. Using a slotted spoon, carefully lower the four eggs into the water and cook them for 6 minutes. Remove them with the slotted spoon and place them into the ice bath. When they're cool, carefully peel and set them aside.

Arrange your breading station: In a small bowl, combine the bread crumbs, almonds, and Parmesan. Place the flour in another small bowl and beat the remaining egg in a third bowl.

Lay a slice of bacon on a cutting board. Place an egg at one end of the slice and roll it, wrapping the bacon around the egg as you go. Place a second slice of

bacon on the board and roll the same egg down it; the second slice should wrap any uncovered area. Do the same with the remaining three eggs.

Dip each egg first into the flour, then into the beaten egg, and finally into the bread crumb mixture, shaking off the excess. Using the slotted spoon, lower two of the eggs into the hot oil and fry until golden brown, about 1 minute. Place them on paper towels to drain, and season them well with salt and pepper. Repeat with the remaining two eggs. Serve hot on a bed of mesclun.

PER SERVING: 783 calories, 31 g protein, 20 g carbohydrates, 65 g fat, 18 g saturated fat, 2 g fiber, 976 mg sodium

FLATTEN YOUR PORK
For the bacon to cook in the time it takes the egg to fry, you'll need superthin slices. Ask the butcher to cut them for you, or flatten pre-sliced bacon at home. Place the slices between two sheets of plastic wrap and flatten them with a wine bottle.

TOAST YOUR OWN
Golden-brown ground almonds add a deep, rich note to the eggs. To make them, toast a handful of skinned whole almonds in a dry skillet over medium-low heat, stirring occasionally, until lightly browned, 5 to 10 minutes. Toss them into a clean coffee grinder and pulverize.

Umami Power

Miso adds a ton of umami, the savory, meaty "fifth taste" that's integral to great food. For this dish, stick with a less salty white or Korean variety of miso rather than using a darker, saltier type.

The Science of Steak

Want to craft the best
meat-and-potatoes meal
you've ever tasted?
Time to enroll in
Food Science 101

Cooking a great steak at home isn't rocket science. It's more like advanced chemistry, with a focus in biology. Master the principles of meat and heat, and you can construct a dinner worthy of serving to a Nobel laureate—or any lucky Friday-night guest.

That's where Nathan Myhrvold, PhD, the former chief technology officer at Microsoft, comes in. After leaving the tech world, Myhrvold pursued his passion for food, training as a chef and then building the Intellectual Ventures lab in Bellevue, Washington. There, he and his team apply high-tech ingenuity to solving age-old cooking challenges.

"Understanding how and why cooking works helps us do a better job. And it's fascinating," Myhrvold says.

In *Modernist Cuisine: The Art and Science of Cooking*—the six-volume, 2,400-page work he co-wrote with chefs Chris Young and Maxime Bilet—he shares his most essential discoveries. Follow his principles and you'll create the best slab of beef you've had outside a steakhouse.

Age Your Rib Eye—at Home

The aging process is what separates top-dollar steakhouses from sit-down chains.

"As beef ages, the longer protein chains within the muscles break down," Young says. "As aging creates more of these protein fragments, the meat becomes more tender and flavorful."

Most high-end chophouses age their beef for at least 30 days, but you can tenderize your beef simply by being lazy. Just leave your steaks in their packaging in the refrigerator for 5 days before cooking, says Young. They'll change color but won't go bad. No time? That's okay. Myhrvold's innovative cooking method will still ensure tenderness.

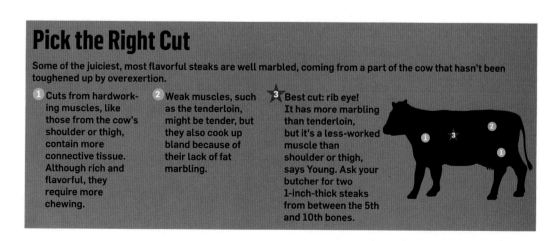

Pick the Right Cut

Some of the juiciest, most flavorful steaks are well marbled, coming from a part of the cow that hasn't been toughened up by overexertion.

1. Cuts from hardworking muscles, like those from the cow's shoulder or thigh, contain more connective tissue. Although rich and flavorful, they require more chewing.

2. Weak muscles, such as the tenderloin, might be tender, but they also cook up bland because of their lack of fat marbling.

3. Best cut: rib eye! It has more marbling than tenderloin, but it's a less-worked muscle than shoulder or thigh, says Young. Ask your butcher for two 1-inch-thick steaks from between the 5th and 10th bones.

Cook Your Steak

One secret to a remarkably tender steak is to cook it at a very low temperature. Doing this activates enzymes that soften the meat. (Don't worry, it won't turn out raw.) To achieve the effect, Myhrvold and Young developed a low-tech version of a French technique called sous vide. So don't slap your steaks in a pan. Be a mad scientist: Throw them in plastic bags, cook them gently in water, and then sear them quickly to brown. Here's how.

1. Fill a large pot three-quarters full of water and attach a digital thermometer to its inside edge. Adjust your stove's heat to low or medium low to raise the water temperature to between 118° and 122°F.

2. Do not preseason the meat. Place each steak inside its own large resealable bag. (Use a BPA-free brand, such as Ziploc.) Squeeze out as much air as possible from each bag, and then seal. Place the bagged steaks in the water and cook them for 30 minutes. Then raise the water temperature to between 136° and 140°F and cook them for another 15 minutes.

Steakhouse Sides

While the steaks are cooking in their bags, prep these classic side dishes to round out the plate.

GREEN BEANS

BUY THE BEST. Search for young specimens (which should be as narrow as #2 pencils). As green beans grow, they add more fibrous cellulose to their structure, and that makes them tougher. Figure on half a pound of green beans for every two people.

BOIL THE BEANS. Salt your water with a pinch of kosher salt for flavoring. Table salt and sea salt often contain magnesium and calcium, which can break down chlorophyll, diminishing the beans' bright-green color. Cook the beans at a rolling boil until they're tender, about 5 minutes.

TAKE THE PLUNGE. Pectin, a gel that helps plant cells maintain their structure, dissolves when exposed to high heat and water. To keep cooked green beans crisp-tender, bathe them in ice water for 10 seconds right after they're cooked. The cold water will firm up the dissolved pectin and add more bite to your beans. Drain thoroughly, then top them with a pat of butter and season with salt.

BAKED POTATOES

CHOOSE YOUR TUBER. Russet potatoes (also known as Idaho potatoes) contain cells that separate easily when cooked, yielding a light and fluffy interior. Steer clear of Yukon Gold or red potatoes, both of which are too waxy for the result you want.

SPEAR THE SPUDS. Cut the cooking time by as much as half by stabbing a clean aluminum-based nail (60d will do) lengthwise through the center of each potato. Make sure at least an inch of nail is sticking out of the potato. The nail will conduct heat, boosting the spud's internal temp, says Young.

BAKE 'EM. Preheat the oven to 400°F. Lightly coat two potatoes with oil, which slows the escape of moisture and helps gently fry the skins. Place the spuds on a baking sheet and bake them until the skins are crisped and you can pierce them easily with a fork, about 45 minutes. Wearing an oven mitt, carefully remove the nails. Make a shallow cut lengthwise in each potato and fluff the inside with a fork, gradually adding about a tablespoon of cubed cold butter. Season with salt and pepper.

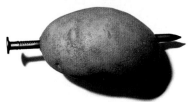

3. Remove the bags from the water and transfer the steaks to paper towels to blot excess moisture. (The meat will look grayish pink until it's seared.) Use a small butane torch to brown the exteriors, or brush the steaks with vegetable oil and sear them in a hot skillet for 20 seconds on each side.

Finish the Steak

Let the steaks rest for 15 minutes—Myhrvold and Young have proved that allowing meat to rest before serving it dramatically improves its juiciness, but not for the reason you might have heard. "Resting doesn't redistribute juices that have been squeezed from the center of the meat," Young says. "Instead, letting the protein-rich juices cool slightly helps them thicken."

Then slice thinly across the grain. Want a sauce for your steaks? Whisk the juices from the bags over low heat with a pat of butter and a hit of sherry vinegar, and season with salt and pepper.

Salt your meat after slicing, and use kosher salt, not table salt. Kosher salt's larger crystals carry more flavor and extra crunch when you bite into the steak. And always use freshly ground black pepper. Pre-ground is bland; peppercorns lose pungency quickly when pulverized.

Follow the Flame

Once you've cooked your steak, crank a small butane torch (we like the Weller Table Top butane torch; $24 at sears.com) to sear the meat on a metal baking sheet until it's browned. Be sure to light the torch away from the food.

If You Don't Have Time . . .

. . . to sous vide and sear, you can still use science to create a better steak. Heat a large pan on medium high and add a bit of oil. Add the steaks and cook, flipping every 30 seconds, until they form nice crusts and their interiors register 134°F, about 15 minutes total for inch-thick steaks.

"This method works as a rotisserie would, with each side quickly taking turns on the direct heat and then resting, allowing excess heat at the surface to diffuse evenly to the core of the steak," says Chris Young, a chef and coauthor of *In Modernist Cuisine: The Art and Science of Cooking*. The result: tender beef cooked to a perfect medium rare.

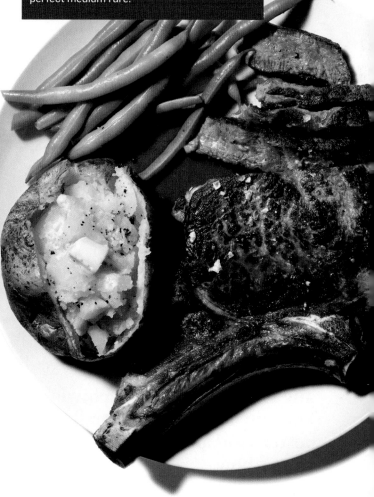

Short-Order Cook

These super quick meals come together in a flash, no cooking experience necessary.

Why brave the traffic, the weather, and the crowds? You can make tastier, healthier, better food at home. Seriously! Here's how.

Huevos Rancheros

MAKES 4 SERVINGS

These "ranch-style" eggs make a rib-sticking breakfast, but they're just as delicious for dinner

- **1** can (16 ounces) whole peeled tomatoes, with juice
- **½** small onion, chopped
- **1** clove garlic, minced
- **1** canned chipotle pepper in adobo sauce, minced (about 1 tablespoon)
  Juice of 1 lime
- **¼** cup fresh cilantro sprigs
  Salt
  Freshly ground black pepper
- **1** can (15 ounces) low-sodium black beans, drained
  Pinch of cumin
- **8** large eggs
- **8** soft corn tortillas

In a bowl, combine the tomatoes, onion, garlic, chipotle pepper, half the lime juice, and cilantro. In a food processor, pulse until well blended but still slightly chunky. Season with salt and pepper to taste.

In a mixing bowl, combine the beans with the cumin and the remaining lime juice. Add salt and pepper to taste. Use the back of a fork to lightly mash the beans, adding a splash of warm water if the mixture looks dry.

Coat a nonstick skillet with cooking spray and heat the pan on medium. Crack in the eggs and cook them until the whites have set but the yolks are still runny.

In another skillet heated on medium, toast the tortillas about a minute on each side.

Spread the beans on the tortillas and top with eggs and salsa. Serve immediately.

PER SERVING: 377 calories, 22 g protein, 29 g carbohydrates, 12 g fat, 3 g saturated fat, 9 g fiber, 489 mg sodium

Beans don't have to be refried to be tasty. Here the flavor comes from lime juice and cumin. Because canned tomatoes are precooked, your body may absorb more of their lycopene, an antioxidant. The protein from the eggs (along with the fiber from the beans) will keep you satisfied for hours.

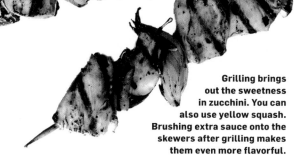

Grilling brings out the sweetness in zucchini. You can also use yellow squash. Brushing extra sauce onto the skewers after grilling makes them even more flavorful.

Sweet and Sour Chicken Skewers

MAKES 4 SERVINGS

Drop the takeout menu and make this Chinese classic on the grill.

- **1** pound boneless, skinless chicken breast, cut into bite-size chunks
- **2** medium zucchini, cut into large chunks
- **2** cups large pineapple chunks
- **2** medium red onions, cut into large chunks
- **2** red bell peppers, cut into large chunks
  Salt
  Freshly ground black pepper
- **3** tablespoons ketchup
- **1** tablespoon maple syrup
- **½** tablespoon soy sauce
- **1** tablespoon vinegar (rice wine or cider)
- **1** teaspoon sriracha hot sauce
  Fresh chopped cilantro (optional)
- **8** wooden skewers, soaked in cold water for 20 minutes

Preheat a grill or grill pan on medium high. Thread the chicken, zucchini, pineapple, onion, and pepper chunks onto the skewers and season them with salt and pepper.

In a mixing bowl, stir together the ketchup, maple syrup, soy sauce, vinegar, and sriracha. Set aside half the glaze in a separate container, and brush the rest onto the skewers.

Grill the skewers until the chunks are lightly charred and the chicken is cooked through, about 4 minutes on each side. Then use a clean brush to coat the skewers with the extra sauce. Top with cilantro, if using.

PER SERVING: 254 calories, 27 g protein, 29 g carbohydrates, 4 g fat, 1 g saturated fat, 4 g fiber, 497 mg sodium

Guinness-Braised Short Ribs

MAKES 4 SERVINGS

Beer and beef make a masterful match in this easy, hearty, slow-cooker stew. This is delicious over soft polenta or mashed potatoes.

- **2** pounds boneless beef short ribs
  Salt
  Freshly ground black pepper
- **1** tablespoon canola oil
- **2** cans or bottles Guinness Draught
- **2** cups beef broth
- **3** large carrots, peeled and cut into large chunks
- **2** onions, quartered
- **2** celery stalks, cut into large chunks
- **8** garlic cloves
- **2** bay leaves
  Gremolata, optional (See box at right)

Season the short ribs with salt and pepper.

In a large sauté pan, heat the oil over high heat. When the oil is hot, add the ribs and cook them, turning occasionally, until they're browned all over, about 10 minutes total. Transfer the ribs to a slow cooker.

While the pan is still hot, deglaze it by pouring in the beer and scraping up any brown bits. Then pour the beer and bits over the ribs in the slow cooker.

Add the broth, carrots, onions, celery, garlic, and bay leaves to the slow cooker and turn it on high. Cook the ribs until they're nearly falling apart, about 4 hours. Sprinkle with the gremolata if using.

Per serving: 547 calories, 47 g protein, 18 g carbohydrates, 27 g fat, 10 g saturated fat, 3 g fiber, 789 mg sodium

Fast Flavor

The name gremolata might sound fancy, but it's simply a quick mix of three ingredients. Use it to add a final hit of flavor to a stew.

GREMOLATA
MAKES 4 SERVINGS

- **¹/₂** cup chopped parsley
- **2** cloves garlic, minced
  Grated zest of 2 oranges or lemons

In a small bowl, combine the parsley, garlic, and zest.

PER SERVING: 6 calories, 0 g protein, 1 g carbohydrates, 0 g fat, 0 g saturated fat, 1 g fiber, 5 mg sodium

For a quick polenta, whisk ³/₄ cup cornmeal into 4 cups simmering water. Stir until thick (about 15 minutes) and add salt to taste. Other root vegetables, such as sweet potatoes, parsnips, or celery root, work as well as carrots.

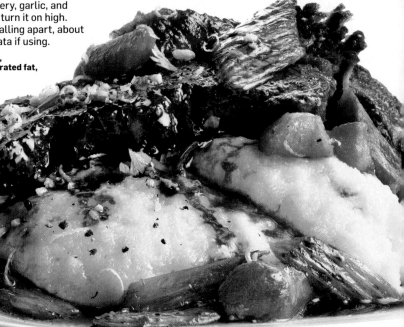

Porchetta-Style Pork Loin with White Beans

MAKES 6 SERVINGS

This Italian-inspired recipe lends deep, rich flavor to a lean cut of pork.

3 cloves garlic, minced
Grated zest of 2 oranges
1 tablespoon fennel seeds
1½ tablespoons chopped fresh rosemary
1 tablespoon olive oil
1 pork loin (about 2 pounds), preferably with a thin layer of fat still attached
Salt
Freshly cracked pepper
2 16-ounce cans cannellini beans (also called white beans), drained
2 tablespoons lemon juice

Preheat the oven to 450°F.

On a cutting board, combine the garlic, orange zest, fennel seeds, and 1 tablespoon of the rosemary. Chop the mixture until it forms a paste. Scoop it up into a small bowl and add the oil.

Season the pork with salt and pepper and rub it all over with the paste. (If you like, you can let it marinate up to 4 hours in the fridge before cooking.) Then place the pork in a roasting pan and bake until a thermometer inserted into the middle reads 160°F, 25 to 30 minutes.

Take the pork out and let it rest for 10 minutes.

In a saucepan, heat the beans, lemon juice, and remaining ½ tablespoon of rosemary until warmed through. Season with salt and pepper. Slice the pork and serve with the beans.

PER SERVING: 281 calories, 35 g protein, 15 g carbohydrates, 8 g fat, 2 g saturated fat, 4 g fiber, 252 mg sodium

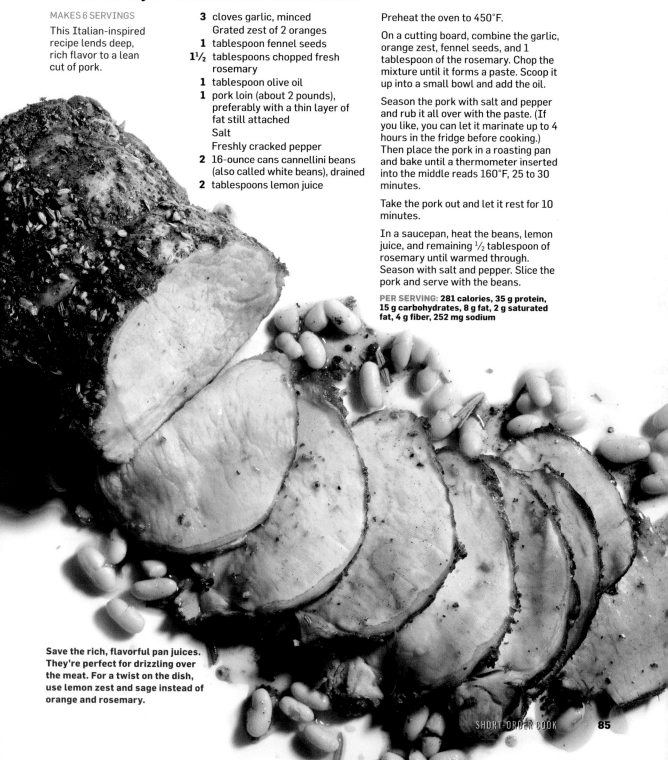

Save the rich, flavorful pan juices. They're perfect for drizzling over the meat. For a twist on the dish, use lemon zest and sage instead of orange and rosemary.

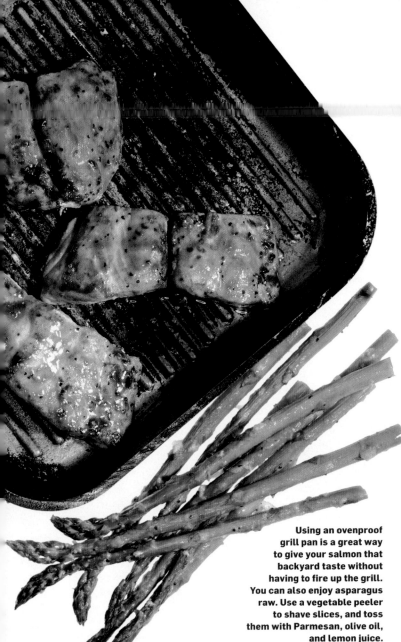

Honey-Mustard Salmon with Roasted Asparagus

MAKES 4 SERVINGS

This hearty dose of omega-3s scores big with the pickiest eaters.

- **1** tablespoon unsalted butter
- **1** tablespoon brown sugar
- **2** tablespoons Dijon mustard
- **1** tablespoon honey
- **1** tablespoon low-sodium soy sauce
- **1** pound asparagus, trimmed
- **2** tablespoons olive oil
- **¼** cup freshly grated Parmesan
  Salt
  Freshly ground black pepper
- **4** salmon fillets (6 ounces each)

Preheat the oven to 400°F.

In a bowl, combine the butter and brown sugar and microwave until they have melted together, about 30 seconds. Stir in the mustard, honey, and soy sauce.

In a bowl, toss the asparagus with 1 tablespoon of the oil, the Parmesan, and some salt and pepper. Place the stalks in a baking dish and roast until they're al dente, 10 to 12 minutes.

Meanwhile, in an ovenproof skillet, heat the remaining tablespoon of oil over high heat. Season the fillets with salt and pepper and add them to the pan, flesh side down. Cook them until browned on one side, 3 to 4 minutes. Then flip them, brush on half the honey mustard, and place the pan in the oven. Bake until the salmon is firm and flakes easily (but before white solids begin to form on the surface), about 5 minutes. Remove the fillets from the oven and brush them with more honey mustard. Serve the salmon with the asparagus.

PER SERVING: 522 calories, 39 grams protein, 34 g fat, 9 g saturated fat, 2 g fiber, 567 mg sodium

Using an ovenproof grill pan is a great way to give your salmon that backyard taste without having to fire up the grill. You can also enjoy asparagus raw. Use a vegetable peeler to shave slices, and toss them with Parmesan, olive oil, and lemon juice.

Secrets of the Stalk

PICK IT
Buy asparagus that's bright green and firm, with unopen tips, says Tal Ronnen, author of *The Conscious Cook*.

STORE IT
Wrap the ends in a damp paper towel and store in the fridge in a sealed zip-top bag. Eat within 3 days.

PREP IT
Bend each stalk like a twig. The woody portion should snap off at just the right place.

Shrimp and Spinach Salad with Bacon Dressing

MAKES 4 SERVINGS

This robust salad packs three protein sources—and hits the table in 20 minutes.

6 strips bacon, cut into ½" pieces
1 red onion, sliced
1 cup sliced mushrooms
8 ounces shrimp, peeled and deveined
  Salt
  Freshly ground black pepper
2 tablespoons pine nuts
3 tablespoons red-wine vinegar
1 tablespoon Dijon mustard
  Olive oil (optional)
6 ounces baby spinach
2 hard-boiled eggs, sliced

Heat a large skillet on medium. Cook the bacon pieces until they're crispy, 5 to 7 minutes. With a slotted spoon, transfer them onto a paper towel.

To the hot skillet, add the onion and mushrooms and cook them until the onion begins to brown, about 3 minutes.

Season the shrimp with salt and pepper and add them to the pan, along with the pine nuts. When the shrimp are pink and firm (2 to 4 minutes), stir in the vinegar and mustard and season again with salt and pepper. If the pan looks dry, add a splash of olive oil.

Divide the spinach and eggs among four plates and top with the hot shrimp mixture, some of the dressing from the pan, and the bacon.

PER SERVING: 314 calories, 20 g protein, 10 g carbohydrates, 22 g fat, 6 g saturated fat, 3 g fiber, 621 mg sodium

Investigate Your Seafood

Before you buy, check with the Blue Ocean Institute's free FishPhone service to find out if your choice is healthy and sustainable. Text 30644 with the word FISH plus your pick (shrimp or trout, say). It replies with what to eat or avoid. See bad news? Ask the restaurant or store to carry better options.

The bacon's fat helps your body absorb the antioxidant lutein from the spinach. To quickly thaw frozen shrimp, place them in a colander and rinse them.

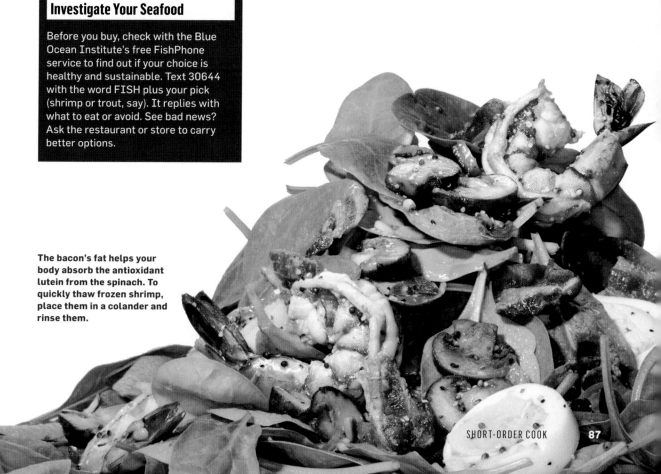

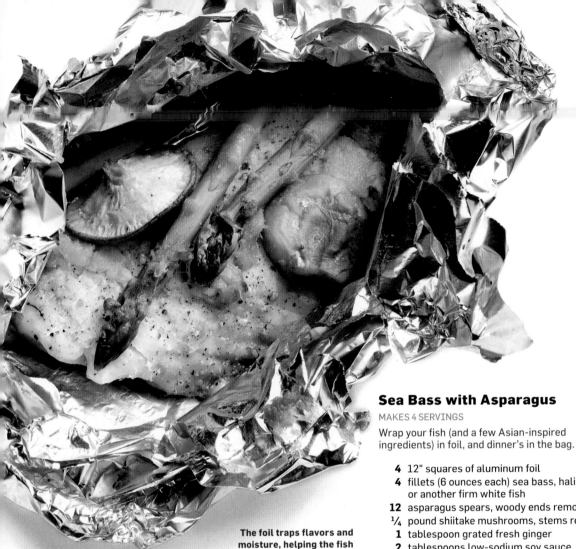

Sea Bass with Asparagus

MAKES 4 SERVINGS

Wrap your fish (and a few Asian-inspired ingredients) in foil, and dinner's in the bag.

- **4** 12" squares of aluminum foil
- **4** fillets (6 ounces each) sea bass, halibut, or another firm white fish
- **12** asparagus spears, woody ends removed
- **¼** pound shiitake mushrooms, stems removed
- **1** tablespoon grated fresh ginger
- **2** tablespoons low-sodium soy sauce
- **2** tablespoons mirin (sweetened rice wine) or sake
  Salt
  Ground black pepper

Preheat the oven to 400°F.

Lay the foil pieces on a counter and place a fillet in the middle of each one. Scatter the asparagus, mushrooms, and ginger on top of the fish.

Drizzle each fillet with soy sauce and mirin and season with a small pinch of salt and black pepper.

Fold the foil over the ingredients and crimp the edges to seal. Place the packets on a large baking sheet and bake 20 to 25 minutes, depending on the thickness of the fillets.

PER SERVING: 252 calories, 42 g protein, 7 g carbohydrates, 5 g fat, 1 g saturated fat, 2 g fiber, 417 mg sodium

The foil traps flavors and moisture, helping the fish cook perfectly.

Shiitakes work well with Asian flavors. Oyster mushrooms are a great substitute.

If the center of the fish flakes easily with a fork, it's ready to eat.

Linguine with Bacon & Clams

MAKES 4 SERVINGS

Everything's better with bacon, including this easy, flavor-packed seafood pasta.

- **4** strips bacon, thinly sliced widthwise
- **1** red onion, diced
- **2** garlic cloves, thinly sliced
  Generous pinch of red-pepper flakes
- **32** littleneck clams, scrubbed clean
- **1** cup dry white wine
- **12** ounces whole-wheat linguine
- **¼** cup chopped parsley

Heat a large sauté pan on medium and add the bacon pieces. Cook them until the fat is released and they're well browned, about 5 minutes. Using a slotted spoon, transfer the bacon to a plate. Pour out all but a thin film of the fat.

Return the pan to medium heat and add the onion, garlic, and red-pepper flakes. Cook, stirring occasionally, until the onion is translucent, about 3 minutes. Add the clams and wine and continue to cook until most of the wine has evaporated and all the clams have opened, about 10 minutes. (If the clams aren't opening, cover the pan until they do.)

While the clams cook, bring a large pot of water to a boil. Add the linguine and cook until al dente,

according to the package instructions. Drain the noodles (but keep ¼ cup pasta water) and pour them into the pan with the opened clams. Add the browned bacon and the parsley and cook, tossing, for 30 seconds. Add a bit of the pasta water if the noodles look dry.

Divide the clams and pasta among four warm bowls and serve immediately.

PER SERVING: 515 calories, 25 g protein, 70 g carbohydrates, 12 g fat, 4 g saturated fat, 11 g fiber, 239 mg sodium

Score Some Clams

Josh Even, chef de cuisine at Manhattan's John Dory Oyster Bar, shares his rules for clams: Buy from a fishmonger; supermarket clams may not be in good condition. Store them in the fridge for a day, max; clams need to be alive when cooked. If a raw clam doesn't close when tapped, it's dead. Toss it.

Can't find clams? This recipe also works well with medium shelled shrimp.

Bacon adds a hit of savory smokiness. Avoid chemicals: Use a variety without added nitrites.

Whole-wheat pasta overcooks easily. You'll want to taste and test frequently.

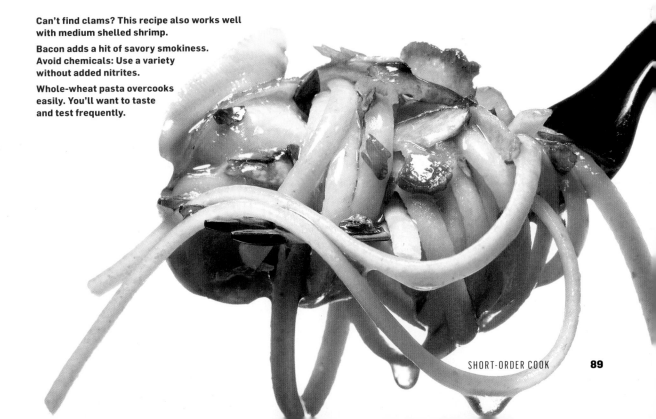

Buffalo Chicken Sandwich

MAKES 4 SERVINGS

Pack in the protein but skip the mess of frying with this lean, easy-to-eat take on hot wings.

¼ cup crumbled blue cheese

½ cup Greek yogurt

Juice of ½ a lemon

Salt

Ground black pepper

4 boneless, skinless chicken breasts (4 to 6 ounces each)

½ tablespoons chili powder

1 red onion, sliced

2 tablespoons butter, melted in the microwave for 20 seconds

2 tablespoons hot sauce (Frank's Red Hot is our pick)

4 romaine lettuce leaves

4 sesame buns, toasted

Quickly grilling the onions intensifies their flavor while softening their bite.

A crusty bun is perfect for this hefty sandwich. Pick whole wheat for extra fiber.

Greek yogurt gives the sauce creaminess without adding a lot of excess calories.

Preheat a nonstick grill or grill pan. As it's heating, combine the blue cheese, yogurt, and lemon juice, plus a pinch of salt and pepper. Stir and set aside.

Season the chicken breasts with salt, pepper, and chili powder. Add the breasts to the hot grill and cook for 5 to 6 minutes on one side before flipping them.

Add the onion to the grill's perimeter. (If you're using a grill pan, you'll need to wait to remove the chicken before grilling the onions.) Cook the chicken until firm and springy to the touch, 4 to 5 minutes more. Remove it to a plate, along with the grilled onions.

Combine the butter and hot sauce and brush the mixture all over the chicken. Place a leaf of romaine on the base of each bun. Top with a chicken breast and spoon on some blue-cheese sauce. Add grilled onions and the top half of the bun.

PER SERVING: 580 calories, 50 g protein, 49 g carbohydrates, 21 g fat, 8 g saturated fat, 3 g fiber, 1,169 mg sodium

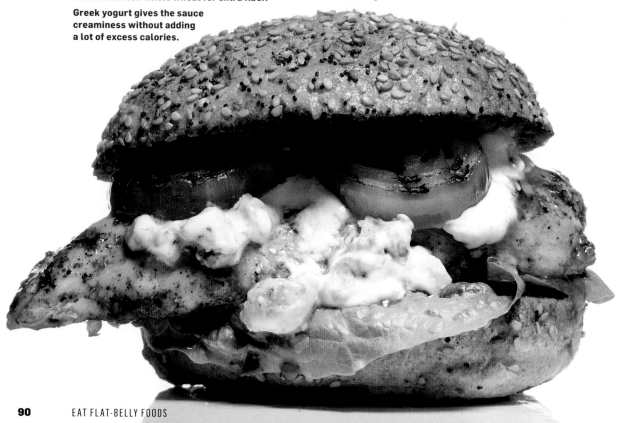

Bloody-Mary Skirt Steak

MAKES 4 SERVINGS

For sure fire juicy steak, treat your beef to a cocktail-inspired marinade.

- **2** cups tomato juice (V8 Spicy Hot works best)
- **2** tablespoons prepared horseradish
- **4** garlic cloves, minced
- **10** shakes (or more) Tabasco sauce
- **½** tablespoon Worcestershire sauce
  Juice of 1 lemon
- **1** skirt steak or flank steak (1 pound)

Add the tomato juice, horseradish, garlic, Tabasco, Worcestershire, and lemon juice to a baking dish; whisk. Add the steak, cover the dish with plastic wrap, and let the meat marinate in the refrigerator for at least 2 hours but no more than 12.

Fire up the grill. Take the steak out of the marinade and use a paper towel to pat most of the liquid off its surface. (Discard the remaining marinade.) When the grill is very hot, put on the steak and let it cook until medium rare, 3 to 4 minutes on each side.

Let the meat sit at least 5 minutes before slicing it across the grain.

PER SERVING: 267 calories, 33 g protein, 8 g carbohydrates, 11 g fat, 4 g saturated fat, 1 g fiber, 470 mg sodium

Skip the sauce. The only thing this steak needs after grilling is a hit of cracked black pepper.

While the steak rests after grilling, char some scallions for a quick side dish.

Put an Egg on It

Take the Bloody-Mary theme to the next level and transform this steak into a killer brunch dish. Just top each serving with a perfectly fried egg. Heat a 12-inch nonstick skillet over medium heat, coat the bottom with olive oil, and crack in 4 eggs. Cook until the edges start to curl and the whites are set, 2 to 3 minutes.

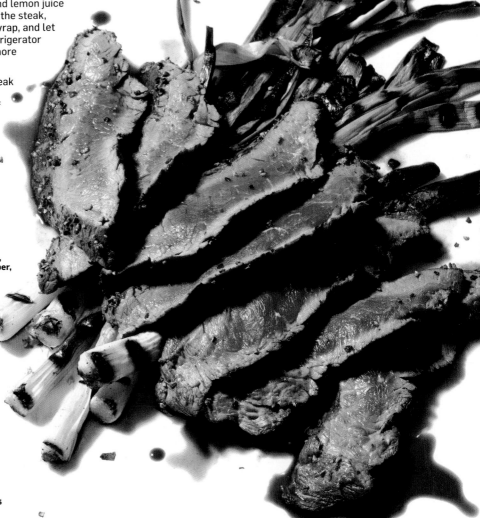

Eat This, Not That

Life is all about choices. Here, we make your choices at favorite restaurants infinitely easier. Yes, it really is this easy.

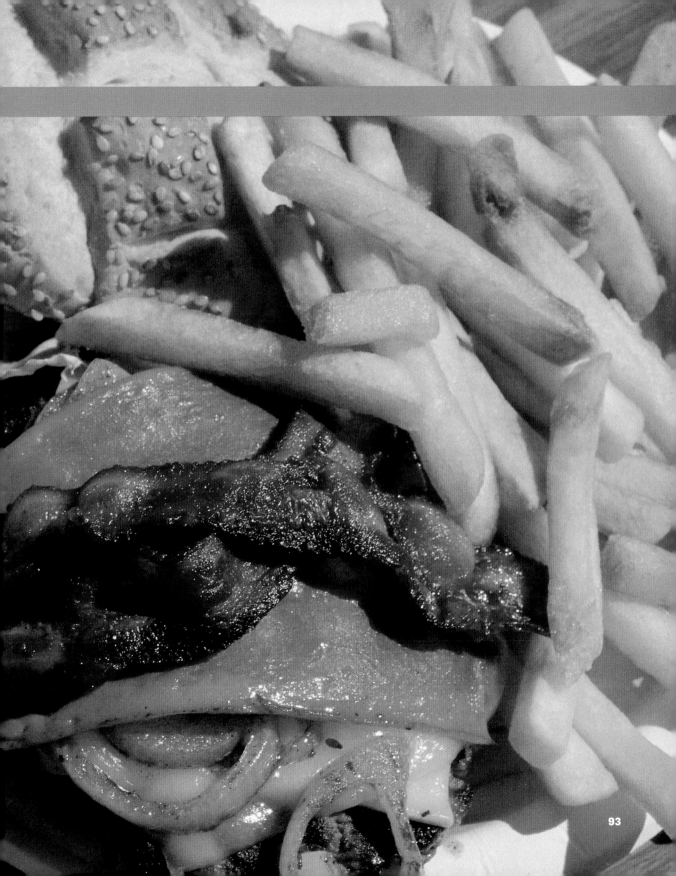

Walk into a fast-food joint or table-service eatery and the menu options can be dizzying. Here, we cut through the confusion to make ordering less onerous.

At Panera Bread: "You Pick Two" Menu

EAT THIS	NOT THAT
Half Asiago Roast Beef Sandwich + Broccoli Cheddar Soup (cup)	Half Chipotle Chicken Sandwich + New England Clam Chowder (cup)
540 calories	800 calories
32 grams protein	31 grams protein
48 grams carbohydrates	55 grams carbohydrates
24 grams fat	50 grams fat
6 grams fiber	4 grams fiber
1,660 milligrams sodium	1,870 milligrams sodium

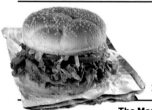 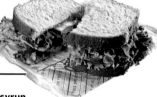

Watch your soup picks—the broccoli Cheddar soup is made with milk, while the clam chowder is made with cream (and packs 117 more calories of fat).

At Arby's

EAT THIS	NOT THAT
Super Roast Beef	Market Fresh Roast Beef & Swiss Sandwich
420 calories	770 calories
23 grams protein	38 grams protein
45 grams carbohydrates	78 grams carbohydrates
17 grams fat	35 grams fat
3 grams fiber	5 grams fiber
1,080 milligrams sodium	1,680 milligrams sodium

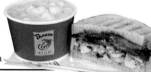

The Market Fresh sandwich has 380 calories in bread alone. Blame the bread's 14 grams of sugar, most of which come from high-fructose corn syrup.

At The Cheesecake Factory

EAT THIS	NOT THAT
The Factory Burger	Grilled Turkey Burger
730 calories	1,200 calories
52 grams carbohydrates	63 grams carbohydrates
15 grams saturated fat	27 grams saturated fat
1,016 milligrams sodium	1,544 milligrams sodium

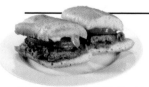 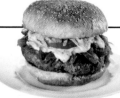

Ground turkey might sound healthier, but it has the same potential for excess as any burger meat. This beef version is the leanest full-size sandwich on the menu.
Note: The Cheesecake Factory doesn't supply protein, total fat, or fiber counts.
Go to thecheesecakefactory.com to ask the company for more dietary data.

At Red Lobster

EAT THIS | NOT THAT

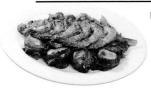

Peach-Bourbon BBQ Shrimp and Scallops
540 calories
36 grams carbohydrates
27 grams fat
1,440 milligrams sodium

Steak, Lobster, and Shrimp Oscar
1,170 calories
20 grams carbohydrates
77 grams fat
2,770 milligrams sodium

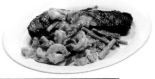

The Oscar's problem isn't just the 14-ounce steak—it's also the butter sauce. The Peach-Bourbon BBQ, served over onion rings, is indulgent, but its barbecue sauce helps save you hundreds of calories.

At Jamba Juice

EAT THIS | NOT THAT

Fresh Banana Oatmeal
280 calories
9 grams protein
57 grams carbohydrates
6 grams fiber
19 grams sugars
4 grams fat
20 milligrams sodium

Chunky Strawberry Topper (small, 12 ounces)
520 calories
14 grams protein
82 grams carbohydrates
9 grams fiber
50 grams sugars
17 grams fat
150 milligrams sodium

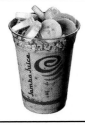

Choosing Jamba's oatmeal earns you cholesterol-lowering beta-glucan (a soluble fiber) and eliminates 31 grams of sugar.

At Applebee's

EAT THIS | NOT THAT

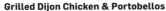

Grilled Dijon Chicken & Portobellos
450 calories
54 grams protein
30 grams carbohydrates
6 grams fiber
15 grams fat
1,790 milligrams sodium

Fiesta Lime Chicken (with rice and pico de gallo)
1,250 calories
60 grams protein
97 grams carbohydrates
9 grams fiber
70 grams fat
4,380 milligrams sodium

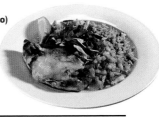

Be cautious: Applebee's can be heavy-handed with cheese and sauce, pushing the average chicken entree to about 1,100 calories.

A Matter of Taste

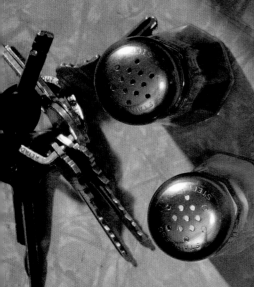

Writer Jason Feifer lost his sense of smell in childhood. Since then, food has been flavorless. So he went on a quest—one that can teach you a whole new way to enjoy what you eat.

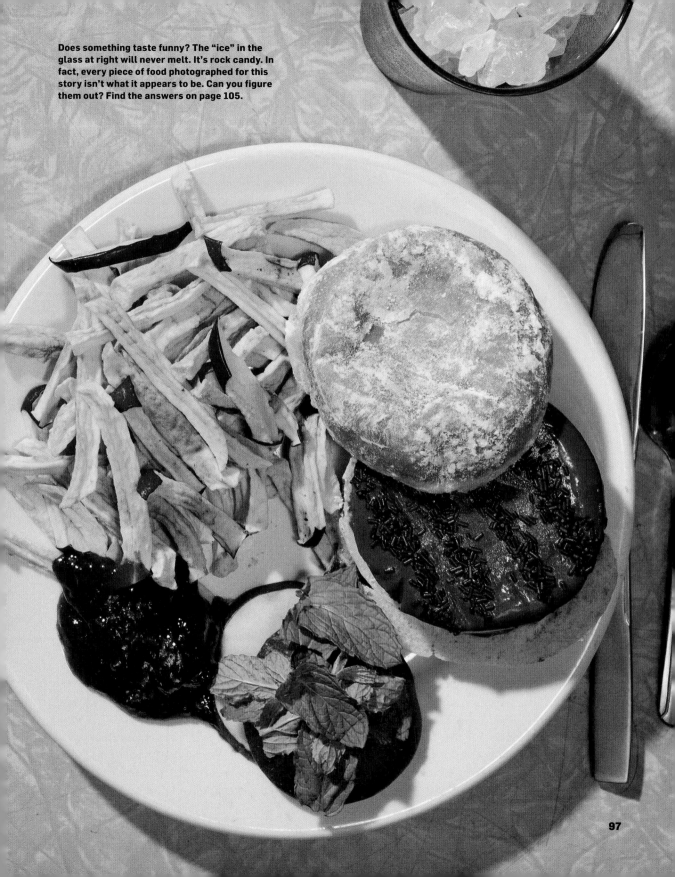

Does something taste funny? The "ice" in the glass at right will never melt. It's rock candy. In fact, every piece of food photographed for this story isn't what it appears to be. Can you figure them out? Find the answers on page 105.

I'm about four spoonfuls into a bowl of ice cream when I realize everyone is watching me.

My friend Joe had fetched us dessert from the shop down the street, and I had asked, as I always did, for mint chocolate chip. I love mint chocolate chip. It's frozen joy: creamy and sweet, with hard flecks playing over my tongue. But he'd returned instead with plain chocolate chip.

They were out of the mint, he said.

Oh well, I said.

So now I am eating my chocolate chip, and it is apparently a comical performance. My friends are rapt, choking on smiles. And so I slow my chewing and consider what's inside my mouth: creamy and sweet, with flecks of hardness.

And then I say, "This isn't vanilla, is it?"

Now, finally, they can laugh. Joe, that sly bastard. He'd bought me mint chocolate chip—the white variety.

To me, vanilla is chocolate is peanut butter is custard is the jelly from a jelly doughnut. These things are sweet and nothing more, a spine of drumbeats with no harmony to surround it. I eat. I feel hunger, and I satisfy it. But I have never truly tasted a meal.

Technically speaking, I have severe hyposmia—a sense of smell so diminished that it's basically nonfunctional. But to really understand my relationship with food, you have to reconsider a sensation you think you know well: taste. Yes, you taste food. So do I. That's because taste is not the full experience you think it is. It is rudimentary, a paper-pushing job performed by a lumbering, simplistic

tongue. When food enters your mouth, your tongue decides if it is sweet, salty, sour, bitter, or some combination. (Scientists largely agree on a fifth taste, umami, or savoriness. Less acknowledged is a sixth taste, kokumi, which is a sort of heartiness.) Then your tongue sends its report to your brain. Job done.

At the same time, odor molecules from the food in your mouth—the same sort of microscopic chemical compounds that would enter your nostrils—go up the back of your throat and are read by a tiny strand of nerve cells called olfactory neurons. These nerves are responsible for your sense of smell, but when those signals are combined with the tastes from your tongue, they create what we think of as flavor.

Think of it this way: When you chomp down on a Hershey's bar, your tongue says "sweet." That's taste. Your olfactory neurons say "chocolate." That's flavor. And that's why, when you're sick and your nose is clogged, you think your food doesn't taste as good. I remember elementary school teachers using the clogged nose as an explanation for how our sense of smell works. All my classmates said, "Oooh." But a thought popped into my little mind that I was too embarrassed, or too confused, to say out loud: But wait, for me there's no difference.

My problem is more common than you might think. Studies estimate that as many as 16 percent of us have some degree of smell loss—but it's hard to say

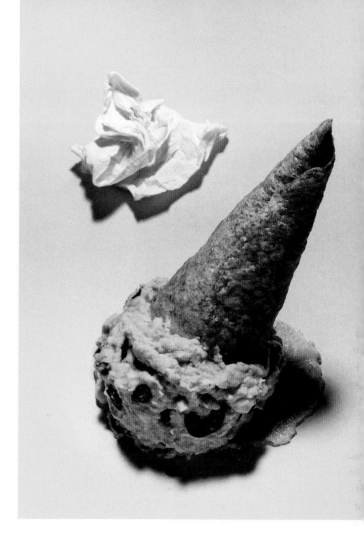

for certain, because smell can be diminished by an alarmingly broad range of conditions, from nasal polyps to brain tumors. Worse still, many people never realize that the loss occurred.

"There is a subset of the population for whom fast food is their primary diet, and they don't notice a big change," says Beverly Cowart, PhD, a researcher at the Monell Chemical Senses Center in Philadelphia. That's because fast food is largely just salty or sweet—sensations of the tongue, not of the nose.

What caused my loss? Hard to say. I have no memory of smell, which is lucky: Sometimes people who lose the sense in midlife are traumatized, but I've come to consider it an amusing oddity. I used to stuff M&M's into my grilled cheese sandwiches just because I could. But to be safe, I had myself checked out a few years ago. I went to a clinic specializing in smell and taste disorders, where doctors tested for every possible cause. One even stuck a finger up my butt, for reasons I'm still unclear on. (At least he didn't ask me to smell it.) The conclusion was a shrug: Something had broken my fragile olfactory system, but the culprit was long gone.

My parents think the damage happened when a babysitter accidentally dumped me out of a stroller. I spent an hour in traction. There's no way to really know, but there's one thing that's certain, considering my 30 years of smell-free living: My chances of recovery are very low.

Consequently, my life isn't as connected to food as yours is. Studies show that memories triggered by smells are more emotional than those triggered by any other sense, but I don't have emotional memory rushes—about anything. Food has never transported me, unless you count the time bad fish transported me to the bathroom. I've also never had a craving. No surprise: When researchers look at brain scans of people mid-crave, the same brain structures associated with recalling a memory are lit up.

And yet I look forward to eating. I have favorite foods. People ask why I spend any time contemplating a

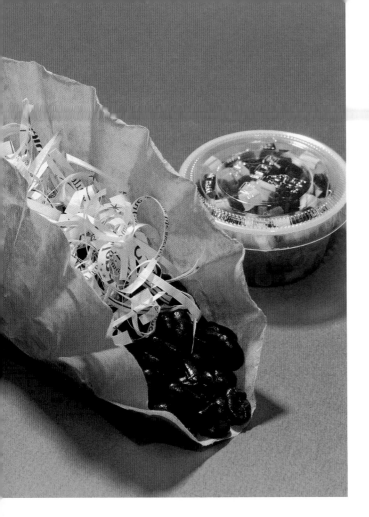

Flavor Can Fool You

I am sitting at Aldea, a modern Portuguese restaurant in Manhattan, staring at a row of inch-high bottles of essential oils. Each is the distilled pure flavor of a specific food, a liquid form of the very thing that's beyond my grasp, and just a drop from any bottle transforms 3 cups of water into a brimming taste sensation. The chef here, George Mendes, uses olive, saffron, and coriander oils, for example, to make broth come alive.

But Mendes discovered another fun use for them: messing with customers' heads. If he covers up a bottle's label with his hand and waves it under someone's nose, the person is flummoxed.

"You'd be surprised at the number of people who will say, 'Yeah, I know that's—oh my god, I know it, I know it, I know it.' And they'll say that for 15 minutes," he says.

Here's the problem: "We like to think of each of our five senses as independent—what you're hearing in your headphones is totally independent of what you're seeing in the subway—but in fact everything interacts really, really amazingly in the brain," says Daniel Wesson, PhD, a neuroscientist at the Nathan Kline Institute in Orangeburg, New York.

When you eat an olive, your eyes see the olive, your tongue picks up the salt, your mouth processes the meaty texture, and your olfactory neurons pick up those odor molecules. All of that combines in a little, fractional spot of your brain called the olfactory cortex, which is partly responsible for combining sensory information to tell you what you're eating.

restaurant menu, and I used to say it was because, well, I can't just tell a waiter to "bring me the food." But my reasons are more complex than that. The pleasure of food isn't just about flavor. In fact, what you savor often has little to do with what you think of as taste.

You—yes, you, with your nose that knows—might have been fooled by that mint ice cream, too, if the circumstances were right. But here's the big difference between us: You have a guaranteed ability to improve your senses and enjoy your food more. To do that, though, you need to pay closer attention to what you're eating.

Even the sounds you hear as you eat may alter the way you perceive your food, although Wesson and his team are only beginning to understand how.

We know this much, though: When Mendes waves a little bottle of olive essence under your nose, your brain doesn't have enough information to go on. You might love olives. You might pop them whole. It doesn't matter. Without the additional sight, flavor, and texture cues, your sense of smell is rarely enough.

And because of that, you're easily fooled.

Have you ever smelled isovaleric acid and butyric acid? Probably, yes. Used often in food, these two make a pungent combo. Once, Brown University smell researcher Rachel Herz, PhD, combined them in an unmarked jar.

"Before I handed it to people, I said, 'This is Parmesan cheese.' They opened it up and said, 'Mmm, yeah.' They said it's very pleasant and familiar, and they would eat it," says Herz, the author of *The Scent of Desire*. "A week later I gave them the exact same smell, and as I'm handing them the jar I tell them it's vomit—and they scrunch up their faces; they say it smells horrible."

This works the other way, too, and you should be mindful of it: The more real information you give your brain about the food you're eating—in other words, the more inquisitive you are with your waiter, or the more hands-on you are in your own kitchen—the more flavor you'll actually experience.

At the University of Dresden in Germany, professor and smell and taste researcher Thomas Hummel, MD, makes this point to his students with soda. "You're familiar with Coke—it has lime and this very strong cinnamon odor, ya?" he tells me, then stops. "Oh, I'm sorry, I'm talking to the wrong person."

This happens every time I talk food: Someone apologizes. Really, they need not. When you smell a fart, I don't apologize

Trick Your Taste

Flavor is relative, as these tongue twisters will show you.

EXPERIMENT #1: When cooking a dish that has mushrooms, season it with a little lemon juice. Your guests won't taste the lemon; they'll say simply that the dish tastes especially "mushroomy," says George Mendes, chef at Aldea in Manhattan. The acidity of the lemon heightens the mushrooms' taste.

EXPERIMENT #2: Have a friend plug his nose, close his eyes, and then eat a jelly bean. Without being able to see the color or allow the jelly bean's odor molecules to connect with his olfactory neurons (for more on that, see main story), every jelly bean will be the same sort of sweet, says Rachel Herz, PhD, author of *The Scent of Desire*. "Now tell him to unplug his nose and then he'll know the flavor— licorice, lime, even watermelon!"

EXPERIMENT #3: Eat an artichoke, and then drink water. You know how orange juice tastes awful after you brush your teeth? The toothpaste's foaming chemical, sodium lauryl sulfate, is temporarily dulling your tongue's ability to taste sweet. So while OJ is normally a balance of sweet and sour, you're whacked with the sour. Artichokes contain a chemical, cynarin, that does the opposite—it inhibits taste receptors, making water (and other foods and drinks) seem sweet.

for being unbothered. We're even.

And in this case, actually, I'm not the wrong person at all: Most of Dr. Hummel's students don't know about the cinnamon and lime either. So he tells them. Then they drink Coke again. "As soon as they know it's there, they'll find it," he says. "It's always the same: You find only what you're searching for."

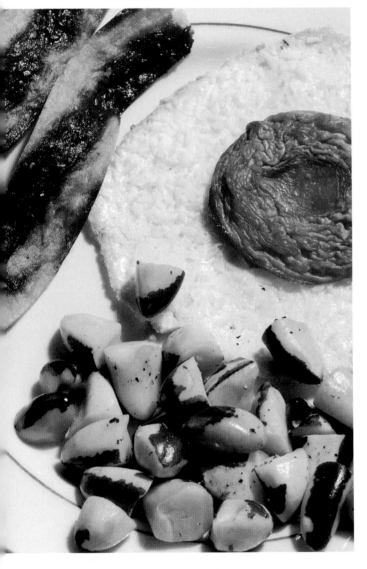

Sensation Woos You

I used to be that obnoxious beer guy, smugly ordering the one obscure brew on tap, and scolding friends for being so mass-market with their Bud Lights. But eventually, I felt foolish: I could never really taste the brews I praised.

Then I discovered whiskey, and now it's my drink. I'll only have it neat. Whiskey geeks will tell you that a little splash of water opens up the flavor or that an ice cube calms the burn, but these are affronts to the singular pleasure I can take from this liquid. I can hold that burn, weigh it, feel it. I want it to sucker punch me in the throat; I want it to tell me I'm alive. I can tell Johnnie Walker Blue from Black. Maybe they taste different—hell, I don't know—but to me it's all in the swallow.

I can do this because whiskey's burn is neither taste nor flavor, which is to say, neither tongue nor nose. It is a signal from the trigeminal nerve, a ganglion responsible for sensations inside your face. You might say Tabasco and sriracha taste different, but their heat is conveyed by this nerve, not your taste buds. Ditto for the coolness of mint.

I'm not the only one hooked on a feeling. The nerve works in concert with our other senses, says David Horrocks, a research chef at International Flavors & Fragrances, a company that major food manufacturers hire to develop products. That's why guys like him have trigeminal pleasures down to a science.

"We have this cooling technology; you add a little drop of the liquid to anything you want, and it creates a cooling effect," he says. Imagine the coolness of mint, minus the minty flavor—which is to say, exactly what I experience when I eat mint. That's what they've created. And because the coolness is free of a taste that might clash with other flavors in their foods, they can add it to anything just to create a sensation you'll remember and keep coming back for.

The same goes for heat. Horrocks and some colleagues were recently helping develop a rice product that came with a spice packet full of different peppers. The peppers weren't selected for flavor, though. They were paired up because each variety triggered the trigeminal nerve in a somewhat different way.

"White pepper hits differently on the tongue than black pepper and red pepper hit. Fresh jalapeño is a more back-of-the-throat heat," Horrocks says.

Eat them all and they begin a domino effect and provide a lesson in why you should always explore combinations of herbs and spices: Stimulate your tongue more and your taste receptors become more active. And the more active they are, the more you'll notice the other flavors in a food—or, as Horrocks puts it, "the bolder the flavor perception is going to be."

Catch that? Flavor perception.

Food Is for Feeling

When I tell someone I can't smell, I'm often asked the same first two questions. One, have my other senses become stronger to compensate? Answer: no, which has really paid off for my eye doctor. The second question is a follow-up: Because I can feel my food just fine, am I

something of a texture connoisseur?

I used to say no to that one, too. I can't lose myself in, say, "fluffy" the same way people close their eyes to savor chocolate mousse. But then I began calling researchers for this story, and they'd always ask me what my favorite foods are. So I'd say, well, pad thai, and sushi, and just about anything Indian.

"Of course!" says Marcia Levin Pelchat, PhD, a Monell researcher. "Texture is a dimension of flavor that you can appreciate, and you're naming things that have variations of texture."

Texture is a dimension of flavor. Does that sound weird? Think back to your olfactory cortex. It's factoring in your sense of touch as it converts food to flavor. Without a nice texture, flavors can fail. "In fact, one of our meat processors says that in a steak, tenderness is the number one factor, not flavor," says Horrocks, the research chef. French fries are the same: A limp fry is offensive—even though its flavor is exactly the same as a crisp one's.

But eaters aren't looking for any old texture. Many scientists believe we find a food more palatable if it has a texture that changes as we eat, says Pelchat. Chocolate melts and coats; a BLT separates, some parts crunchy, others oozing. You probably hate soggy cereal: It feels the same going in your mouth as it does after you chew it.

My condition makes textural pursuits easy. Almost every day for lunch, I head across the street from my office to a takeout buffet, where I cram a cross-cultural disaster of food into a tiny plastic container. Today, as I type this paragraph, I'm polishing off a box that contained baked ziti, blackberries, shrimp, brown rice, seaweed salad, and brussels sprouts. I shovel it into my mouth indiscriminately, a forkful of fruit and seafood, just enjoying the mix. Colleagues react with horror, but truthfully, I don't even know which of those foods clash.

You, of course, have the burden of combining foods that actually go together, arranging one to build off the next, boosting the entire sensory experience of a dish simply by cooking it to the right level of crisp or adding something that crackles. Sorry, pal. Sounds like a hassle.

Taste the Difference

If I drink apple juice and then iced tea, I never actually taste apple or tea. But I can tell they are different. If I eat apple pie and then peach pie, the same holds true. This is as much as my body will allow. They are each different in an abstract way, two shades of black.

There's a good reason for this. Different is the heartbeat of your sense of smell, its most basic function, and even my ravaged olfactory system has retained some ability to detect it.

"Our neural systems work that way: They perceive differences very well," says Donald Leopold, MD, a professor of otolaryngology at the University of Nebraska medical center.

He guesses that this is because our senses of smell and taste evolved mostly to distinguish safety from danger. They're alert to anything new. Once a food is established as safe, however, your body no longer needs to focus on it. So it doesn't. "That person who eats a whole plate of spaghetti—after the first two bites, he isn't really appreciating it. He's just shoving calories in his mouth," Dr. Leopold says.

This is why Dr. Leopold says we must begrudgingly admit that foodies are onto something—what with their servings the size of a mouthful and their 12-course meals. Each little plate is a new flavor collection, alerting your brain to come check it out. You run out of food before your brain loses interest, a trick you can reproduce at home just by making smaller portions. "It gives you a lot more bang for your sensory buck," he says.

And going mouthful by mouthful, slowly tasting, gives time for the late-breaking news that you've eaten enough to travel from belly to brain. So by savoring more, you may actually eat less—and lose weight by enjoying food.

Sniff Better, Savor More

Sometimes, unpredictably, I smell food. Months go by in darkness, and then: popcorn. Or I will walk into my apartment and know: fish for dinner. I will sniff for more, inhaling with urgency, but the smell is gone. It's like hearing people speak Japanese and knowing a single word—not in your own language per se, but simply understanding theirs. Ask the speaker to repeat it, and you can listen closely and really focus—but it's foreign again, not for your ears. Maybe it never was.

I've asked many experts why this happens to me, and everyone has a guess. The one I like the best is that in some small way I've trained myself to recognize certain smells. I don't experience them the way you do, but maybe I can put names to some faint fragments of odors. And with practice, I might be able to do it more.

Dr. Hummel, the researcher in Germany, recently guided a group of smell-loss patients through training. He gave them sticks scented with four odors—lemon, clove, rose, and eucalyptus—and asked them to smell each one for 10 seconds, every morning and night. After 12 weeks, about 30 percent of the patients were better able to identify smells.

It's not clear why that happened or how well that experience can be replicated—these are mysteries Dr. Hummel is exploring now. But at the Nathan Kline Institute, Wesson says he often sees brains respond to training.

"Your brain, even as an adult, is what we call plastic—it's very malleable, and it's always changing. So every new experience makes new synapses and strengthens cell connections, and these are considered vital for learning and memory, and even perception."

This has implications that reach beyond people who are smell challenged. Chefs learn to recognize the nuances of flavors. Sommeliers, after years of shoving their noses into glasses, can tell you about the soil a grape was grown in. Dr. Hummel's study may have involved scheduled smell training, but you don't need such rigors. You need only pause to learn about what you're eating, breaking it down to the tasty nuances. Appreciate, then repeat.

"My two words of advice are 'pay attention,'" Wesson says. "Even the sloppiest piece of pizza is a beautiful work

Does Something Taste Funny?

THE "FOOD" IN THESE PHOTOS ISN'T WHAT YOU THINK. HERE ARE THE FOOD PHOTOS, DECODED.

Page 97: Chocolate gelato "patty" with chocolate sprinkles, jelly doughnut "bun," dried apple "fries," strawberry jelly "ketchup," rock candy "ice," apple "tomato slices," mint "lettuce."

Page 99; Guacamole with black olive "ice cream," whole-grain flour tortilla "cone."

Page 100: Coffee filter "tortilla," coffee bean "black beans," cut stirrers and straws "pico de gallo," shredded Splenda pack "grated cheese."

Page 102: Coconut macaroon "egg" with dried nectarine "yolk," Brazil nut "home fries," fruit leather "bacon."

of art in terms of how your brain is decoding all the tastes and odor molecules. But if you don't attend to it, those things will never impact your brain in the same way that van Gogh's Starry Night will. You attend to that, so why not attend to smell and taste?"

With that in mind, I return to mint chocolate chip ice cream. Creamy and sweet, with flecks of hardness—yes, old friend, you're still the same. But I pause. There's something new: There's a freshness, the trigeminal effect of mint, so subtle in ice cream that I never realized it was there. Could that be why I chose it as a kid, long before I knew my nose had checked out? Most ice creams are creamy and sweet, after all, and many have bits of chocolate. But this one had a little something extra that spoke directly to me.

I only needed to take the time to notice.

PROVE IT

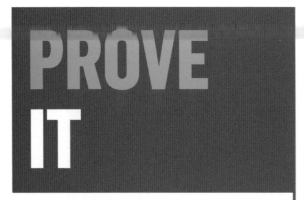

STIFFEN UP

Bananas may be the phallic fruit, but watermelons could help you have better sex. Italian researchers found that when men with erectile dysfunction took 1.5 grams of L-citrulline (an amino acid in watermelon) every day for a month, half had stronger erections.

Swallowing an L-citrulline supplement, like the 500-milligram capsules from Source Naturals ($24 for 120, vitaminshoppe.com), might boost your body's production of another amino acid that improves penile blood flow. But check with your doctor first; weak erections can be a symptom of heart disease.

BERRY YOUR BP

Have the blood-pressure blues? Try loading up on berries.

Berries are more than just summer treats: Blueberries and strawberries may help prevent high blood pressure. In a Harvard study, people who consumed the most anthocyanins—found in high amounts in these berries—had a 12 percent lower risk of developing hypertension than those who consumed the least.

GET THE ORGANIC EDGE

Strawberries are a perfect snack, if you know how to pick them.

Ignore those tasteless mass-market strawberries. According to a study in *Food Chemistry*, organic strawberries have more disease-fighting antioxidants than conventionally grown ones have. Why? Without pesticides, berries must fend for themselves naturally, which in turn boosts their antioxidant powers. And if you store berries in the fridge, their antioxidant potency increases further, a Croatian study has found. Find organic farms at pickyourown.org.

AVOID NITRATES

What do some hot dogs and spinach have in common? Nitrates. In a study in the *International Journal of Cancer*, men who consumed the most nitrates—often found in leafy vegetables—were more likely to develop thyroid cancer than men who took in the least. One theory: Excess nitrates trigger a hormone thought to promote tumors.

Play it safe by eating nitrate-free meats and organic produce, which may contain fewer of the compounds.

POP THIS PILL

Fish-oil supplements might help prevent pancreatic cancer, according to an *International Journal of Cancer* study. Participants who took at least 850 milligrams of omega-3 fatty acids a day reduced their risk of developing the cancer by 53 percent. Omega-3s may help halt the growth of cancer cells, scientists say.

AVOID SNACK ATTACK

If it's cream-filled and sold in a convenience store, skip it. The phosphorus compounds used as additives in junk food such as Twinkies might raise your risk of cardiac and kidney diseases, according to a study in the *Journal of the American Society of Nephrology*. Scan ingredient lists: The additives go by monikers such as "disodium phosphate," "monocalcium phosphate," and "sodium aluminium phosphate."

SIP A CUPFUL OF COVERAGE

Tea and coffee might protect your brain. Men who sipped as little as half a cup of coffee or tea a day were 34 percent less likely to develop brain cancer later in life than those who didn't, according to a study in the *American Journal of Clinical Nutrition*. High levels of antioxidants in these drinks may help prevent cancer cells from forming in the brain, the scientists say.

EAT UP, DRINK UP

Score another point for red wine: Ten ounces (about two glasses) of red wine after a fatty meal might shield your heart from the meal's adverse effects, say Italian scientists. Red wine reduces the postmeal rise of cholesterol oxidation products in the blood, which are linked to heart disease. Less wine might still provide the benefit.

RAISE A GLASS

Plastic is looking less fantastic every day. Even BPA-free plastics may leach estrogenic chemicals, a study in the journal *Environmental Health Perspectives* reports. It's unclear how

HARD TRUTH

66 The percentage drop in bisphenol A (BPA) in the urine of people who ate only fresh foods for three days, according to Environmental Health Perspectives

these hormone disrupters could affect you, but play it safe by using stainless-steel water bottles and glass containers, says Heather Patisaul, PhD, who studies hormones and sex differentiation at North Carolina State University.

TRY THIS TRANS FAT

A good trans fat? Maybe.

Behold the power of cheese: A naturally occurring trans fat found in dairy might be good for you. A study in the *Annals of Internal Medicine* found that a diet high in the fat, called trans-palmitoleate, is associated with up to a 60 percent reduced risk of type 2 diabetes. Researchers speculate that trans-palmitoleate might turn off the liver's production of fat and improve glucose handling by muscle cells. Try for two to three daily servings of dairy that has some fat.

This is Gouda news for cheese-heads.

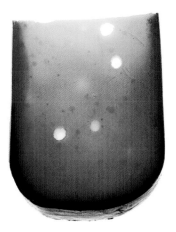

YOU ASKED

Q: What's the best day to do my grocery shopping?

A: Wednesday

Only 11 percent of shoppers hit the store on hump day, according to *Progressive Grocer*, a magazine for food retailers. You'll be able to speed through the aisles, and the produce will be less picked-over. Along with time, you can also save cash because most stores start their promotions on Wednesday, says Phil Lempert, an editor at *Supermarket News*.

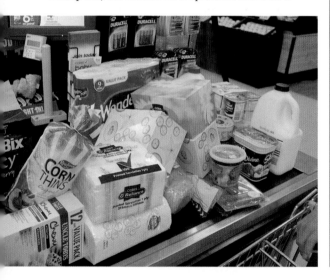

Q: I'm seeing more exotic vegetables at the grocery store. Which are the best?

A: If you think hitting the five-a-day quota is hard, chew on this: Early humans ate some 800 varieties of plant foods, says Susan Bowerman, MS, RD, of UCLA's Center for Human Nutrition. "We evolved expecting a mix of vegetables from diverse sources, not the 20 or so we average now. When you eat exotic vegetables, you introduce a wider range of health-promoting compounds to your antioxidant defense system."

That would be your defense against heart disease, diabetes, and common forms of cancer. Because the exotics broaden your options, you have a better shot at joining the elite 23 percent of adults who do eat five a day. To upgrade your vegetable rotation, include the all-stars listed here, selected because they deliver a diverse dose of phytonutrients and taste great.

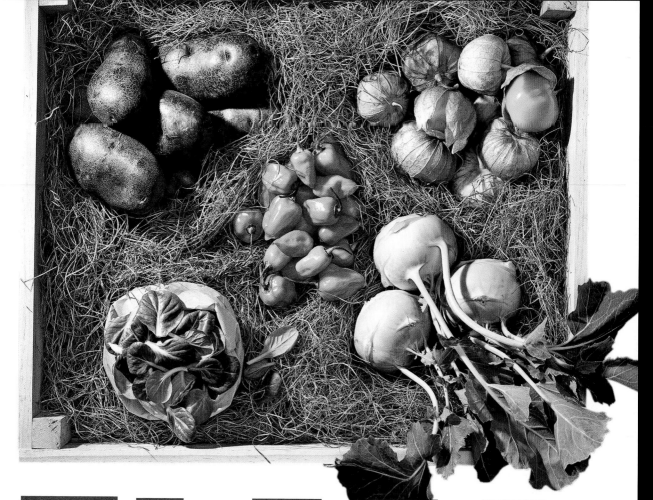

PERUVIAN PURPLE POTATO

Anthocyanins, the same brain-boosting antioxidants found in blueberries, give these superior spuds their purple color and nutritional power.

To preserve their antioxidants and bold color, steam and then dress them with olive oil and dill, says Aliza Green, author of *Field Guide to Produce*. They make a colorful bed for grilled salmon.

TATSOI

First cultivated in China, this leafy green is a crucifer—the same family as broccoli—and has a lemon-pepper taste. Crucifers contain powerful cancer-fighting phytonutri-ents, says Bowerman.

Add young leaves raw to pep up salads, or use large leaves in place of spinach in almost any cooked dish, says Green.

HABANERO

Sweeter, fruitier, and hotter than a jala-peño, the habanero is rich in vitamin C and capsaicin (the stuff that ignites your tongue), a compound that can help lower your blood pressure, according to Chinese researchers.

Mix a tablespoonful of diced habanero with diced mango, pineapple, red bell peppers, and chop-ped scallions for an antioxidant-packed salsa, says Green. Remove the white spongy membrane and seeds to keep the heat under control.

TOMATILLO

Draped in a papery husk, this caped crusader from south of the border can help fight cancer. It's high in withanolides, chemical compounds that can prevent colon-cancer cells from forming, according to research from the University of Illinois at Chicago.

Tomatillos have a tangy taste; add them raw to salsa or gazpacho, or cooked in chili.

KOHLRABI

A sweeter-tasting cousin of kale, kohlrabi has 93 percent of the recommended dietary allowance of vitamin C in 1 cup. It contains glucosinolates, potent antioxidants that fight prostate cancer, according to a German study of 11,000 men.

Kohlrabi can be eaten raw or cooked, says Green. She suggests using it in place of cabbage in summer slaws, or sautéing it with olive oil and garlic.

YOU ASKED

Q: I've heard that cooking broccoli and other vegetables reduces their nutritional value. Is this really true?

A: It isn't even entirely true for broccoli. When you've steamed this vegetable, your body is actually able to absorb more of its disease-fighting carotenoids and polyphenols, according to a report in the *Journal of Agricultural and Food Chemistry*. However, steaming broccoli does reduce its vitamin C content.

And that's the lesson: It all depends on the nutrient and the cooking method—or the lack of one, because going raw can be the most nutritious option.

Your best bet: "Balance your diet with a mix of raw and cooked vegetables," says T. Colin Campbell, PhD, a professor emeritus of nutritional biochemistry at Cornell University. When you want your vegetables hot, use the chart below to maximize your antioxidant intake.

Here's how cooking affects antioxidant levels in six vegetables.

Q: Will a can of 5-hour Energy really provide me with 5 hours of energy?

A: The source of an energy drink's "energy" is usually sugar and caffeine. "In a low-calorie brand like 5-hour Energy, it's simply a caffeine buzz," says Marion Nestle, PhD, MPH, a professor at New York University's Department of Nutrition. Specifically, 5-hour Energy claims it contains "about as much caffeine as a cup of premium coffee," which is roughly 115 milligrams. Because the average man's metabolism will gradually process half that amount in 5 hours, you'll end up with about 58 milligrams left in your system. So does that mean the company delivers on its promise? Maybe. However, the implication is that

	BROCCOLI	CARROTS	BELL PEPPERS	BRUSSELS SPROUTS	SPINACH	ASPARAGUS
BOIL	Okay	Best	Okay	Best	Okay	Best
STEAM	Best	Good	Good	Good	Best	Good
MICROWAVE*	Okay	Okay	Best	Good	Best	Best
RAW	Best	Best	Best	Good	Best	Best

* Avoid microwaving if you want to preserve the texture of your vegetables.

imbibing a can will provide 5 hours of sustained energy, not a steadily dwindling reserve.

For true lasting energy that can power you through an afternoon at the office, eat a balanced lunch that includes lean protein, vegetables, whole grains, and fruit, says Nestle. And of course, maintain a healthy sleep schedule.

Q: I know it's important to consume plenty of potassium, but I hate bananas. What else could I try?

A: Bananas are hugely overrated as a source of peelable potassium. You'd need to choke down nearly a dozen every day to hit the 4,700 milligrams recommended by the Institute of Medicine.

Why so much potassium? To help keep your BP in check, says Christine Gerbstadt, MD, RD, a spokeswoman for the American Dietetic Association. "Sodium attracts water, and potassium pushes it away. When you're low on potassium, you retain more fluid, which increases your blood volume and puts pressure on your blood vessel walls."

Use this chart to pick your potassium power players.

Q: Since the Four Loko news, I'm wondering: How many Red Bull and vodkas can I down before it's dangerous?

A: Drinking even one is a gamble: These schizophrenic cocktails contain caffeine (a stimulant) and alcohol (a depressant), a combo that plays mind games on you.

"Long before Four Loko blew up, scientists knew that combining caffeine and alcohol in carbonated form caused your body to absorb the alcohol faster while reducing your perception of your own intoxication," says David Weldy, MD, PhD, an assistant professor of family medicine at the University of Toledo's College of Medicine. What's scary about Red Bull and Four Loko is that they contain additional stimulants, such as taurine and guarana, which might amplify this process. So you're more likely to be drunk yet think you're sober. Yep, that guy.

If you like the unique buzz that a caffeinated alcoholic drink delivers, consider a rum and Coke: It has about 30 milligrams of caffeine, compared with 77 in an 8.4-ounce can of Red Bull, 95 in an Irish coffee, and 135 in Four Loko. But sip, don't slam, because your body takes an hour to metabolize the alcohol. Then switch to a beverage with no caffeine.

FOOD	POTASSIUM (MG)
Potato, baked with skin (1 large)	1,600
Spinach, boiled (1 cup)	839
Sweet potato, cooked with skin (1)	694
Yogurt, plain, skim (8 ounces)	579
Raisins, seedless (1/2 cup)	543
Brussels sprouts, cooked (1 cup)	495
Broccoli, cooked (1 cup)	457
Cantaloupe (1 cup)	427
Banana (1 medium)	422
Milk, 2% (1 cup)	342
Peaches (1 cup)	323

YOU ASKED

Q: Everything has added folic acid in it these days. Could I OD on it?

A: Not in one sitting, but if you regularly consume too much folic acid, you might be increasing your odds of developing cancer. Folic acid is a synthetic form of folate, a powerful nutrient that in small doses plays a critical role in cell division and DNA maintenance, says Jane Figueiredo, PhD, an assistant professor of preventive medicine at the University of Southern California. "However, excess folate has been associated with some cancers."

In one study in the *Journal of the National Cancer Institute*, men who took a daily 1,000-microgram folic acid supplement were 2.6 times more likely than men who took a placebo to develop prostate cancer over the next 10 years. Another study in *Cancer Prevention Research* found that people with the highest folate levels showed more potentially cancer-causing DNA changes in their colorectal tissue.

To stay healthy and safe, aim for the recommended daily amount of folate, which is 400 micrograms, says John Baron, MD, a professor of medicine at the University of North Carolina. You can probably hit that mark without taking a supplement because many foods, such as bread, cereal, and rice, have added folic acid, and lots of produce and legumes are rich in folate.

Q: Okay, I'll eat more fish. Fresh? Frozen? Wild? Farmed?

A: If you aren't trolling for tonight's dinner, choose fish labeled "frozen at sea," which means it was flash-frozen before it could begin to spoil. It will be as flavorful as fresh fish—and cost less. Same-day feast? Spring for fresh, but inspect it first: Is its flesh firm and translucent? Does it smell like the ocean? (Ask to take a whiff.) If you can't answer yes, cut bait. As for wild versus farmed, go wild: Fish that roamed the ocean usually contain more omega-3s (and higher, more beneficial ratios of omega-3s to omega-6s) than farmed fish do, says Manuel Villacorta, RD, a spokesman for the American Dietetic Association. Wild fish are also free of the antibiotics used to prevent diseases in farmed fish. These factors, and others, helped us rank widely available fish. Dive in.

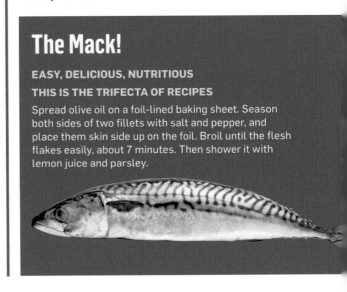

The Mack!

EASY, DELICIOUS, NUTRITIOUS
THIS IS THE TRIFECTA OF RECIPES

Spread olive oil on a foil-lined baking sheet. Season both sides of two fillets with salt and pepper, and place them skin side up on the foil. Broil until the flesh flakes easily, about 7 minutes. Then shower it with lemon juice and parsley.

Q: Could I be addicted to junk food?

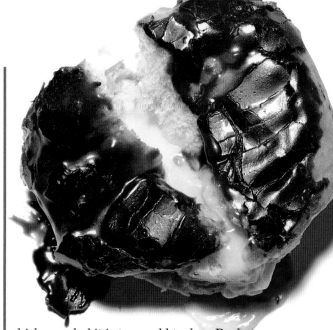

A: Until recently, scientists didn't believe people could become junk-food junkies. But a Scripps Research Institute study revealed that the same neurological and behavioral patterns seen in cocaine and heroin addicts are also present in obese rodents that are given extended access to a sweet, fatty buffet.

"High-calorie foods trigger the release of dopamine, which results in a feel-good high," says Louis Aronne, MD, a clinical professor of medicine at Weill Cornell Medical College. But eat too much junk food for too long and dopamine will overwhelm your brain, causing it to compensate by decreasing the number of pleasure receptors. This means you'll need to eat increasingly more food to achieve the same dopamine high, says Dr. Aronne. Before you know it, you'll be like a cokehead snorting a pile of powder—except you'll be inhaling a pile of powdered doughnuts instead.

Of course, for most people, the best way to kick your habit is to go cold turkey: Replace chips, ice cream, and candy with popcorn, yogurt, and fruit. When you want a filling snack, eat crunchy vegetables, such as carrots, celery, and radishes, dipped in salsa. Dr. Aronne also says it's critical to reduce consumption of sodas (even diet ones) and juices because the sweetness can trigger overeating. Wean yourself by mixing your beverages with an equal part of water or club soda.

Fish (6 ounces)	Protein (g)	Omega-3s/Omega-6s (mG)	Safe number of servings / month*	Environmental friendliness**
Alaskan salmon	46	2,420/192	4+	Best
Spanish mackerel	40	2,478/184	2	Best
Halibut (Pacific)	46	1,138/65	4+	Best
Yellowfin tuna	50	528/17	4	Good
Cod (Pacific)	40	482/14	4+	Good
Rainbow trout (U.S. farmed)	42	2,102/1,614	4+	Best
Swordfish	44	1,796/63	1	Good
Tilapia (U.S. farmed)	42	403/504	4+	Best
Catfish (U.S. farmed)	32	440/1,750	4+	Best
Salmon (farmed)	38	3,842/1,132	1	Bad

* Based on contamination with mercury and PCBs

** Source: Monterey Bay Aquarium Seafood Watch, a science-driven, peer-reviewed rating of farmed and wild seafood, based on its harm to the environment. To stay current, download the app at seafoodwatch.org

YOU ASKED

Q: New kinds of milk keep popping up in the supermarket. Are any worth trying?

A: Sure, if you want to wake up your cereal and earn a little nutrition boost to boot. We asked Andrea N. Giancoli, MPH, RD, of the American Dietetic Association, to help us select the cream of this crop. One caveat: If you view milk more as muscle fuel, then don't bother with these alternatives; their protein content is negligible. (All nutrition data is for 8 ounces.)

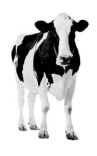

WHOLE COW'S MILK

A variety of research extols milk's benefits: Its high calcium content can lower blood pressure, and its fat can help you feel fuller longer while not clogging your arteries.

150 calories
8 grams protein
12 grams carbohydrates
8 grams fat
25 percent RDA vitamin D
30 percent calcium

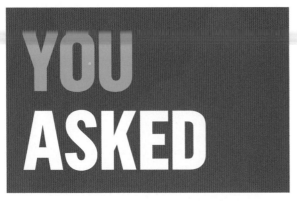

HEMP DREAM

Original

Made from (THC-free) hemp seeds, this creamy, nutty drink is a good source of the bone-strengthening minerals calcium and magnesium. Try it with cereal or in a protein shake

100 calories
4 grams protein
8 grams carbohydrates
6 grams fat
25 percent RDA vitamin D
30 percent calcium

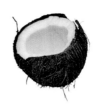

SO DELICIOUS COCONUT MILK

Unsweetened

Naturally sweet and healthy, its fat, which is composed of 65 percent lauric, capric, caproic, and capryllic acids, can boost satiety and positively affect your cholesterol. Try it straight up, with cereal, or in a protein shake.

50 calories
1 gram protein
1 gram carbohydrates
5 grams fat
30 percent vitamin D
10 percent calcium

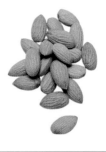

ALMOND DREAM

Unsweetened

It's low in calories and high in calcium and healthy monounsaturated fat, and it has a nutty flavor. But it has a watery, chalky consistency. Try it in a protein shake.

30 calories
1 gram protein
1 gram carbohydrates
2.5 grams fat
25 percent vitamin D
30 percent calcium

Q: Are probiotics worth it?

A: They can be, if you know what to look for. Here is a probiotics primer.

What they are: Naturally occurring microorganisms that can be good for your health. They're added to foods, especially yogurt.

What studies show: Certain probiotics can help you fight colds, diarrhea, and more. But those aren't always the ones in your food.

Source: Mary Ellen Sanders, PhD, who studies probiotic microbiology and consults in the industry

Follow this guide to make your meal count.

Step 1: Know names

See the chart below? It shows the three elements of a probiotic's name. The trouble is, most companies list only the genus and species of a strain. That's like a restaurant serving "fish" without identifying what kind it is. Not having enough information makes determining any health benefits a difficult task.

Your move: Choose products that include the full names of their probiotics. Chances are, more research is available about the benefits, which is why the food company chose to spotlight the strains it included.

Here's Lactobacillus rhamnosus HN001—the full name of a probiotic in Stonyfield Farm yogurt—dissected.

LACTOBACILLUS:	RHAMNOSUS:	HN001:
Genus	Species	Strain

Step 2: Ignore the usual suspects

Take these, for example . . .

L. BULGARICUS

S. THERMOPHILUS

Help turn milk into yogurt

Your move: Don't be impressed by foods that list only L. bulgaricus and S. thermophilus. These organisms do help you digest lactose, but they mostly just help create yogurt. To be labeled a probiotic, an organism has to have a health benefit. L. acidophilus is also common. Some companies use studied strains of it as probiotics, but others use it only for flavor.

Step 3: Vet research

Bifidobacterium lactis DN-173 010 is found only in Dannon Activia—because Dannon developed it, studied it, and patented it. (Dannon claims this strain helps regulate your digestive system.) This is common: Many strains are studied primarily by the companies that developed them. Then the companies promote the benefits.

Your move: Watch for definite claims, like "clinically proven" or "scientifically proven"—Dannon had to scrap both of these claims in a 2010 settlement and replace them with less-certain phrases, such as "clinical studies show."

Step 4: Read the label closely

Questions about probiotics shouldn't stop you from eating yogurt, a good source of protein and calcium. Hey, if the live cultures have other health benefits, that's all the better. Probiotic supplements are another story: Many may have no proven benefits. Look for products with labels that list probiotics' full names, the number of colony-forming units, and the scientifically studied benefits of each strain. Dosage and storage suggestions should also be included.

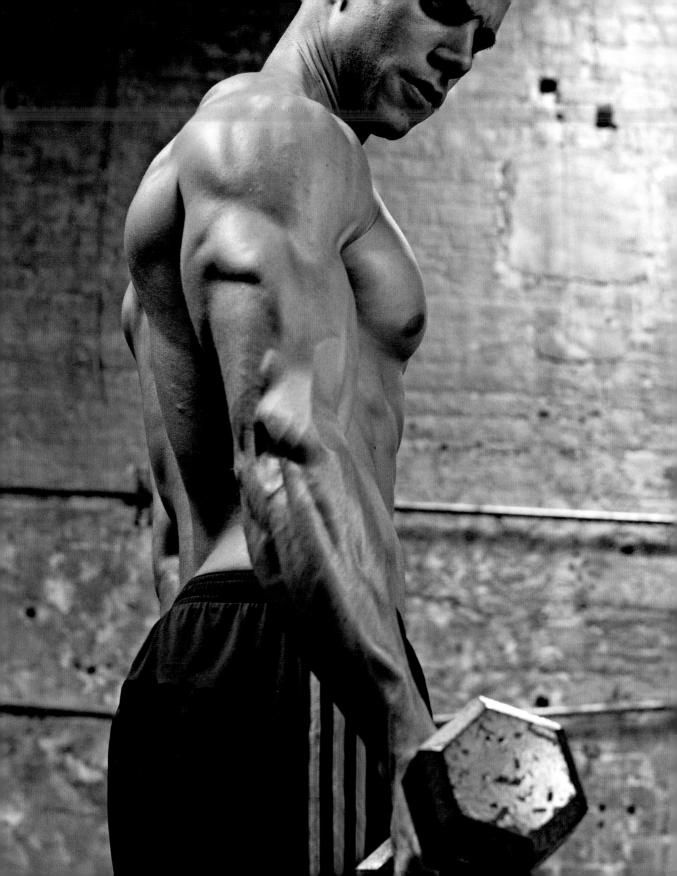

Muscle Up Fast

The Muscle Express Train

Take this simple self-test to uncover the secret to instant gains.

When it comes to building a better body, every guy is looking for an edge. And while some men might opt for a 'roid trip to an underground pharmacy, the rest of us want a safer, smarter shortcut to more muscle. We've found your advantage: fast-twitch muscle training. It's the X factor that'll help you pack on new muscle, add strength, and even burn more fat.

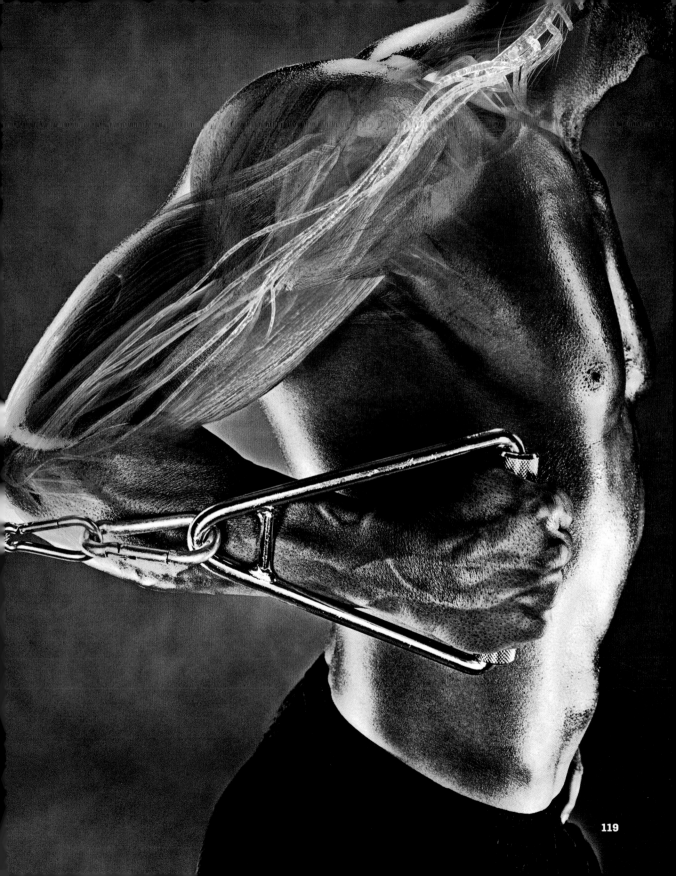

Doing bench presses is one of the best ways you can **target your fast-twitch muscle fibers**.

But before we reveal the secret, let's make one thing clear: Nothing can help you increase the quantity of your fast-twitch fibers. That was determined at birth. This leaves you with a choice: Pray that you won the genetic lottery, or find the best way to make your fast-twitch fibers bigger. Follow this two-step approach, and you'll build more muscle than you ever thought possible.

Test Your Fast-Twitch Fibers

You can activate your fast-twitch fibers two ways: by lifting heavier weights or by lifting lighter weights very quickly. Take this test to determine your fast-twitch ratio. The result will tell you how you need to lift in order to see the fastest improvement.

Step 1: Test your 1-rep max on the bench press. (See "How to Test Your 1-Rep Max," below). Then rest 5 minutes.

Step 2: Select a weight that's 45 percent of your 1-rep max. (So if your max is 225 pounds, start with one that's about 100 pounds.) Try to perform 5 reps in 5 seconds.

Step 3: If you succeed, rest 1 to 2 minutes and then repeat the test, this time using 5 to 10 percent more weight. Keep adding 5 to 10 percent until you can no longer complete 5 reps in 5 seconds.

Step 4: Calculate your fast-twitch ratio: Simply divide the heaviest weight you could lift in 5 seconds by your 1-rep max. If you lifted 135 pounds in 5 seconds and your max is 225, your ratio would be 60 percent.

5-rep test/1-rep max = **fast-twitch ratio**

How to Test Your 1-Rep Max

Using a spotter, perform a barbell bench press. Start with half of your estimated 1-rep max, or 1RM (the amount of weight you think you can press only once). Do 5 or 6 reps with perfect technique. Now add 10 percent more weight but subtract 1 rep. Rest 2 minutes. Repeat this pattern until you do 1 rep with about 90 percent of your estimated 1RM. Rest 3 to 5 minutes, and try your estimated max. If you achieve it, then that's your true 1RM. If you fail, then use the 90 percent weight; if it's too easy, add 10 percent to your estimated 1RM.

THE WORKOUT

Now that you've determined your fast-twitch ratio, select one of the workouts here to do as your upper-body routine at least twice a week, making sure you never do an upper-body routine 2 days in a row. Alternate between exercises that share the same number (1A and 1B, for example) until you complete all the exercises in the pairing. Then move on to the next exercise. Select a weight that allows you to perform at least the minimum number of reps listed. See the exercise descriptions on the opposite page.

IF YOUR FAST-TWITCH RATIO IS 60 PERCENT OR HIGHER . . .
Do this size and strength workout.

Exercise	Week 1	Week 2	Week 3	Week 4	Rest
1A Barbell bench press	3 sets of 4–6 reps	4 sets of 3–5 reps	5 sets of 2–4 reps	3 sets of 6–8 reps	2 minutes
1B Lean-away pulldown	3 sets of 8–10 reps	4 sets of 6–8 reps	5 sets of 4–6 reps	3 sets of 8–10 reps	2 minutes
2A Dumbbell incline bench press	3 sets of 8–10 reps	3 sets of 6–8 reps	3 sets of 4–6 reps	3 sets of 8–10 reps	1–2 minutes
2B Dumbbell row	3 sets of 8–10 reps	3 sets of 6–8 reps	3 sets of 4–6 reps	3 sets of 8–10 reps	1–2 minutes
3 Face pull	2 sets of 12 reps	2 sets of 12 reps	2 sets of 8 reps	2 sets of 8 reps	45–60 seconds

IF YOUR FAST-TWITCH RATIO IS LESS THAN 60 PERCENT . . .
Do this speed workout.
N = the number of sets you can perform using the dynamic bench press guidelines.

Exercise	Week 1	Week 2	Week 3	Week 4	Rest
1 Dynamic effort bench press	N × 5 reps	N × 5 reps	N × 5 reps	N × 5 reps	1 minute
2 Dynamic effort inverted row	N × 5 reps	N × 5 reps	N × 5 reps	N × 5 reps	1 minute
3A Dumbbell incline bench press	3 sets of 8–10 reps	3 sets of 6–8 reps	3 sets of 4–6 reps	3 sets of 8–10 reps	1–2 minutes
3B Dumbbell row	3 sets of 8–10 reps	3 sets of 6–8 reps	3 sets of 4–6 reps	3 sets of 8–10 reps	1–2 minutes
4A Dumbbell scaption	3 sets of 10 reps	3 sets of 8 reps	3 sets of 6 reps	3 sets of 8 reps	1 minute
4B Face pull	2 sets of 12 reps	2 sets of 12 reps	2 sets of 8 reps	2 sets of 8 reps	45 seconds

THE EXERCISES

BARBELL BENCH PRESS

Lying faceup on a bench, grab a barbell using an overhand grip that's just beyond shoulder width and hold it above your sternum with your arms straight. Lower the bar, pause, and press the bar in a straight line back to the starting position.

LEAN-AWAY PULLDOWN

Sit in a lat pulldown machine and grab the bar using a shoulder-width, underhand grip. Lean back until your body forms a 30-degree angle with the floor. Hold this position for the entire exercise. Without moving your torso, pull the bar down to your chest. Pause, and slowly return to the starting position.

DUMBBELL INCLINE BENCH PRESS

Set an adjustable bench to an incline of 15 to 30 degrees. Lie faceup on the bench and hold the dumbbells above your shoulders with your arms straight. Lower the dumbbells to your chest. Pause, and then press the weights back up to the starting position.

DUMBBELL ROW

Holding a pair of dumbbells, bend at your hips and knees and lower your torso until it's almost parallel to the floor. Let the dumbbells hang at arm's length from your shoulders, your palms facing behind you. Bend your elbows and pull the dumbbells to the sides of your torso. Pause, and slowly lower them.

FACE PULL

Attach a rope to the high pulley of a cable station and hold an end in each hand. Back a few steps away from the stack until your arms are straight in front of you. Flare your elbows, bend your arms, and pull the middle of the rope toward your eyes so your hands end up in line with your ears. Pause, and reverse the move to the starting position.

DYNAMIC EFFORT BENCH PRESS

Perform a barbell bench press. On the first set, use the heaviest weight that allows you to do 5 reps in 5 seconds. Then add 5 to 10 percent more weight and try for 5 reps in 6 seconds. Rest, and then keep adding 5 to 10 percent more weight until you can no longer complete the 5 reps in 6 seconds. Then move to the next exercise.

DYNAMIC EFFORT INVERTED ROW

Grab a barbell secured at shoulder height using an overhand, shoulder-width grip. Hang with your arms straight and your feet elevated on a bench. Pull your shoulder blades back and lift your chest to the bar. Pause, and slowly lower your body to the starting position. Do 5 reps in 5 seconds. If that's too hard, place your feet on the floor. Do as many sets as you did on the dynamic effort bench press, and move on to the next exercise.

DUMBBELL SCAPTION

Stand holding a pair of dumbbells at arm's length next to your sides, your palms facing each other and elbows slightly bent. Without changing the bend in your elbows, raise your arms at a 30-degree angle to your body (so they form a Y) until they're at shoulder level. Pause, and slowly lower the weight back to the starting position.

The *MH* Fitness Test

If you aren't seeing the results you expect from your workouts, there might be a simple reason: You're all alone. Many of us think we can do everything on our own, but sometimes you need a wingman to help you reach your potential. You see, weight training shouldn't be a one-man activity—at least not until you've perfected your form. Sure, you can hoist heavy objects until your biceps feel like they'll pop, but if you're hoisting incorrectly, you'll never look as good as you could—and you might hurt yourself in the process.

That's why we turned to Mike Robertson, MS, CSCS, and Bill Hartman, PT, CSCS, co-owners of Indianapolis Fitness and Sports Training. They provided expert tips that a buddy can use to analyze your technique on three common exercises. Open up to constructive criticism and you'll build the strength and size you want, without the pain and frustration that comes with thinking you're a gym genius. Turbocharge your fitness with these exercise fixes.

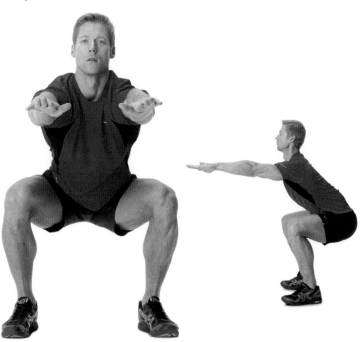

THE SQUAT

Stand with your feet slightly wider than shoulder-width apart, toes forward. Push your hips back as if you're about to sit in a chair, and lower your body. Pause, and then push back up to the starting position.

ASSESS YOUR FORM

FRONT VIEW: As you lower your body, your knees and feet should be in a straight line. If your thighs rotate inward, then your knees are moving toward each other and become vulnerable to injury. You need to strengthen your glutes and hamstrings, which will keep your legs in the correct position.
Fix it: Do the hip raise and leg curl: Lie on your back with your heels on a Swiss ball. Lift your hips so your body is straight from ankles to shoulders. Pull the ball toward your butt as you bend your knees. Reverse the move, but don't let your hips sag or touch the floor. Do 2 to 3 sets of 8 to 12 reps.
SIDE VIEW: You should be able to squat until the tops of your thighs are at least parallel to the floor (lower if you can), while keeping the natural arch in your lower back, says Hartman. If you can't, your core needs work.
Fix it: Try mountain climbers for your abs and hips. Start in a pushup position but place your hands on a Swiss ball and your toes on the floor.

Lift one knee toward your chest. Lower and repeat with the other leg. Do 2 or 3 sets of 10 to 15 reps per leg.

THE LUNCE

Stand with your feet hip-width apart and your hands on your hips. Take a long step forward and lower your body until your front knee is bent 90 degrees. Then push back to standing. Repeat with your other leg.

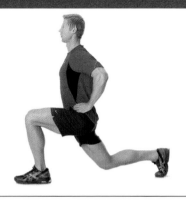

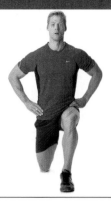

ASSESS YOUR FORM

SIDE VIEW: Your torso should be perpendicular to the floor throughout the movement. If your torso leans forward, Robertson says, you might have stiff hip flexors, which could lead to pain in your lower back or the front of your knees.
Fix it: Do the ultimate hip-flexor stretch before a lower-body

workout: Start in the lunge position with your right leg forward and left knee resting on a pad. Extend your right arm overhead, bend your torso to the left, and twist slightly to your right. Hold for 30 seconds, and repeat on the other side.
FRONT VIEW: When you're in the bottom position, your foot, knee,

and hip should be in a straight line. Hold this position for a few seconds. If your knee wobbles, you risk injury from the instability.
Fix it: The problem could be your feet, Robertson says. Take off your shoes and do 2 or 3 sets of 8 to 10 lunges per leg in socks or bare feet.

THE PUSHUP

Assume a pushup position, with your arms straight and hands below and slightly wider than your shoulders. Bend at the elbows and lower your body until your chest nearly touches the floor. Pause, and push your body back up.

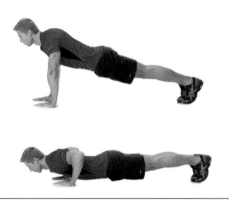

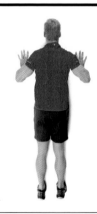

ASSESS YOUR FORM

SIDE VIEW: Does your torso sag during the exercise? Your body should be rigid, in a straight line from neck to ankles. If it isn't, you need to develop strength and endurance in your core muscles, Robertson says.
Fix it: Do planks. Start in pushup position but with your weight on your forearms. Brace your abs, and hold this position for 2 minutes.

TOP VIEW: Your shoulder blades should remain flat, Hartman says. But they shouldn't protrude above the plane of your upper-back muscles. If they stick out, it probably means your serratus anteriors are weak. These muscles are just outside your pecs alongside your rib cage, and they help control the stability and movement of your shoulder blades. A weak serratus anterior can lead to shoulder pain.

Fix it: Do incline pushups. Secure a barbell (or the bar of a Smith machine) at hip height. Grab it with your hands slightly wider than your shoulders, and do slow, controlled pushups. Push yourself up as high as you can on each rep—that ensures you're targeting your serratus. As you improve, gradually lower the bar each workout until you're doing pushups on the floor with the same form.

15 New Muscle Builders

Upgrade your workout—and transform your body—with these new fitness tips from the country's most innovative trainers.

The old reliable exercises are fine for producing old reliable results. But if you want a physique that's better than the body you have now, you need exercises that do more for you than the ones that brought you to this point. Luckily for you (and your muscles), trainers and scientists across the continent spend their days asking excellent questions, such as "Why do we do it this way?" and "What if we did it that way?" The answers they find are surprising—and useful.

Here you'll read about exercise variations and technique tweaks from some of the country's most innovative trainers. You'll refresh your workout and soon have muscle in places you didn't even know they could grow.

1 Try a New Muscle Formula

Do at least 3 sets of pulling exercises—rows, pullups, and pulldowns—for every 2 sets of chest and shoulder presses you perform, says Brian St. Pierre, CSCS, the owner of BSP Training and Nutrition in Augusta, Maine. Chances are you've been doing just the opposite, so this approach can help you build the muscles you've been neglecting. The result: Improved posture, better overall muscle balance, and faster gains.

2 Sculpt Bolder Shoulders

Strong, stable shoulders will help you lift more weight in nearly every upper-body exercise. So start each upper-body workout with the band pull-apart, suggests Shon Grosse, PT, CSCS, owner of Comprehensive Physical Therapy and Fitness in Colmar, Pennsylvania. It trains your rotator cuff and scapular stabilizers, the network of muscles that help create a strong shoulder joint. (And it counts as another pulling exercise.)

Keeping your arms straight, use both hands (palms up) to hold a stretch band out in front of your chest. Now squeeze your shoulder blades together and stretch the band out to your sides, without bending or lowering your arms, until the band touches your sternum. Reverse the move and repeat. Do 2 or 3 sets of 10 to 15 reps, resting 60 seconds between sets.

3 Beef Up Your Back

Most of the fibers in your upper-back muscles are horizontal, which is why rowing exercises work them so well. But the ones in your lats are closer to vertical. The J pull-in hits your lats from start to finish, says Lee Boyce, a Toronto-based strength coach. "And it won't take much weight for you to feel a deep contraction."

Attach a rope handle to a high pulley of a cable station. Grab an end with each hand and kneel facing the machine. Keeping your arms straight and your torso upright, pull the rope down toward your groin. (The rope's path of travel should look like a J.) Try 3 sets of 10 reps, resting 60 seconds between sets.

4 Pump Up Your Pecs

If you're unhappy with your chest development, you might have one of two problems.

You don't work your chest enough: Sometimes you just need to do more work. Boyce recommends the 1½-rep bench press, which effectively doubles the workload of your pectoral muscles. On a flat bench, lower the weight to your chest, and then press it halfway up. Lower it again, and then press it up until your arms are straight. Use 70 to 80 percent of your 1-rep max, and perform 3 or 4 sets of 8 reps.

Your shoulders are beat up: Years of dips and bench presses will do that to you, says Tony Gentilcore, CSCS, of Cressey

There's a great way to build your triceps that involves **a jackknife and a head rush**. (Read Tip 7 for details.)

Performance in Hudson, Massachusetts. To build your chest and triceps while sparing your shoulders, he recommends the close-grip board press. Duct-tape a pair of foot-long 2-by-4s together, with the 4-inch sides facing each other; secure the block under your shirt. Load a barbell onto a flat bench-press station. Lie on your back and grab the bar using an overhand grip, your thumbs 12 to 15 inches apart. Lift the bar, lower it to the block, come to a dead pause, and then push back to the starting position. You can go heavy: 3 or 4 sets of 6 to 8 reps.

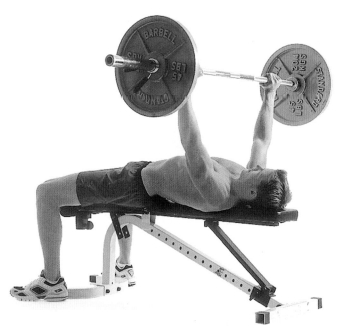

To double your workload, try the 1½-rep bench press. See Tip 4.

5 Add to Your Adductors

You wouldn't be caught dead on the inner-thigh machine. But you also don't want to ignore your adductor muscles, an area of untapped growth potential. Target them by doing pullups while holding a light weight plate between your feet, Grosse suggests. You'll force your abs and adductors to engage as you work your back, shoulders, and arms.

6 Blast Your Biceps

To hit all the muscle fibers in your biceps, you need to either lift max weight or lift at max speed—which nobody does when they work their biceps, says Chad Waterbury, MS, the author of *Huge in a Hurry*. The next time you do curls, use a weight you think you can lift just 6 or 7 times. Bang your reps out as fast as you can while maintaining good form. That means lifting the weight quickly, lowering it at a normal speed, and immediately starting the next rep. Stop the set

when one rep is clearly slower than the others. You might pull off 4 or 5 reps on your first set, and fewer on later sets. Rest for 45 seconds between sets, and shoot for 25 reps total.

7 Trick Out Your Triceps

Waterbury recommends jackknife push-ups as a triceps-building companion for the high-velocity curls (Tip 6).

Assume a pushup position but place your toes on a bench. Keep your hands on the floor, thumbs 6 to 12 inches apart, and hips up. (If you feel the blood rush to your face, you're in the correct position.) Do pushups as fast as you can without rearranging any of your favorite facial features. (That is, don't hit the floor.) Go for 35 reps total, with 7 or fewer per set.

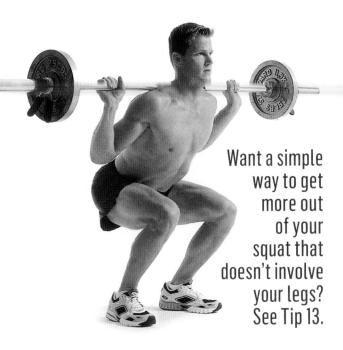

Want a simple way to get more out of your squat that doesn't involve your legs? See Tip 13.

9 Shift Your Butt into Gear

Deadlifts and squats are great for your glutes, but only if you're actually engaging those glutes. If your knees cave in toward each other, you're doing less with your butt and more with your back, says Brian Zarbatany, CSCS, co-director of the Human Performance Center in Allentown, Pennsylvania.

Here's the solution: Grab the floor with your feet, as if you're trying to twist through the outsides of your shoes. That helps you keep your knees out and your glutes working.

8 Power Up Your Legs

Supercharge any lunge variation by extending your range of motion, making your muscles work harder and grow faster. Boyce recommends these brutally effective leg builders.

Reverse lunge from step: Stand with both feet on a 6-inch-high box or step. Take a long step back with your right foot and descend until your knee almost touches the floor. Return to the starting position, and then repeat the move with your left foot.

Bulgarian split squat with front foot elevated: Place your left foot on a 6-inch step in front of you and your right foot on a bench behind you. Drop straight down until your right knee almost touches the floor. Do all your reps, switch sides, and repeat. Perform 3 sets of 12 repetitions for each leg using body weight only, or 10 reps holding dumbbells at your sides.

10 Get More from Your Core

The abdominal push press is the best ab exercise you can do in bed, although you'll probably want to try it on the floor first, says physical therapist Jonathan Fass, DPT, CSCS. Lie on your back with your knees bent and feet on the floor. Lift your right knee so your hip is bent 90 degrees, and press your left palm into your right thigh, near your knee. Now try to lift your thigh to your chest while pushing back with your hand. If you're doing the exercise properly, your core should work to produce a stalemate. Hold for 3 to 5 seconds, switch sides, and repeat until you're sick of it.

11 Mix It Up for a Hard Middle

If you have a partner, Fass recommends ab prayers, which is a core-building exercise for two that can double as foreplay. Stand facing each other in an athletic position. Put your palms together (as if praying) in front of your chest, elbows extended 6 to 10 inches from your body. Have your partner push and pull your hands in all directions, forcing you to adjust. Go for 30 seconds, and switch. You should both feel your mid-body muscles working.

No partner? Try the Swiss-ball stir-the-pot, which is a classic core exercise from spine specialist Stuart McGill, PhD. Assume a plank position with your forearms on a Swiss ball, and roll the ball around by moving your forearms and elbows in a circular pattern.

12 Build Bigger Calves

Instead of working your calves in isolation, try the bench bridge, which works them in conjunction with your hamstrings and glutes, says Nick Tumminello, a Fort Lauderdale–based personal trainer. Lie on your back with the balls of your feet on the edge of a bench and your knees slightly bent. Lift your hips. You should feel it from your calves through your glutes. Lower your hips and repeat the move for as long as you can.

13 Move More and Risk Less

Everyone wants to lift more on the classic powerlifts, and nothing beats hard work, of course. But you can also produce big improvements by incorporating even the simplest of tricks. During a barbell squat, "pull the bar down as if you're trying to rip it apart," Gentilcore says. "You'll activate your lats, which provide more spinal stability."

That means you'll move more weight with less risk of injury. And if you actually do rip the bar apart, please send us video.

14 Boost Your Bench

This one might seem "bass ackwards," but to improve your bench press, the experts would like you to start with your butt.

"Clench the bench" by contracting your glutes, and keep them contracted throughout your set, says Joe Stankowski, a personal trainer in Grand Rapids, Michigan. You'll find that this tweak solidifies your base and allows you to generate more force on the lift. Don't forget to unclench when you're done.

15 Raise Your Deadlift

Here's a gear tip: Wash your socks. Then, when you arrive at the gym, perform the deadlift with your shoes off (if your gym allows it), advises strength coach and power-lifter Eric Cressey, CSCS, co-founder of Cressey Performance. "Shoes increase the distance the bar has to travel," he says. They also lift your heels off the floor, which puts more emphasis on your quads and less on your glutes and hamstrings, where it belongs. Either barefoot or in your stocking feet is fine. If your gym frowns on this, invest in shoes with minimal heel lift. Or find a new gym.

Max weight or max speed is **the best way to build your biceps**. (See Tip 6 for the right approach.)

Lifting: The Next Level

Follow our simple tips to build the strength you need for the hardest moves in the gym.

Notre Dame football, the Situation, and crunches. **What do the three have in common? Besides making your stomach hurt, they're all overrated. Granted, the first is personal opinion, but the others? Not so much.**

Take crunches: These ab exercises can give you visible results, but focusing primarily on crunches means your muscles are missing out.

Most guys perform the same exercises—crunches, squats, bench presses, and seated shoulder presses—over and over. But when one of those guys tries a new exercise that works his body in a different way, he looks like he's never set foot in a gym.

We've identified four super-challenging exercises designed to push even the most experienced lifter to new gains. Beware: These moves might force you to use beginners' weights. But don't sweat it. You'll be adding plates in no time—and you'll be more muscular.

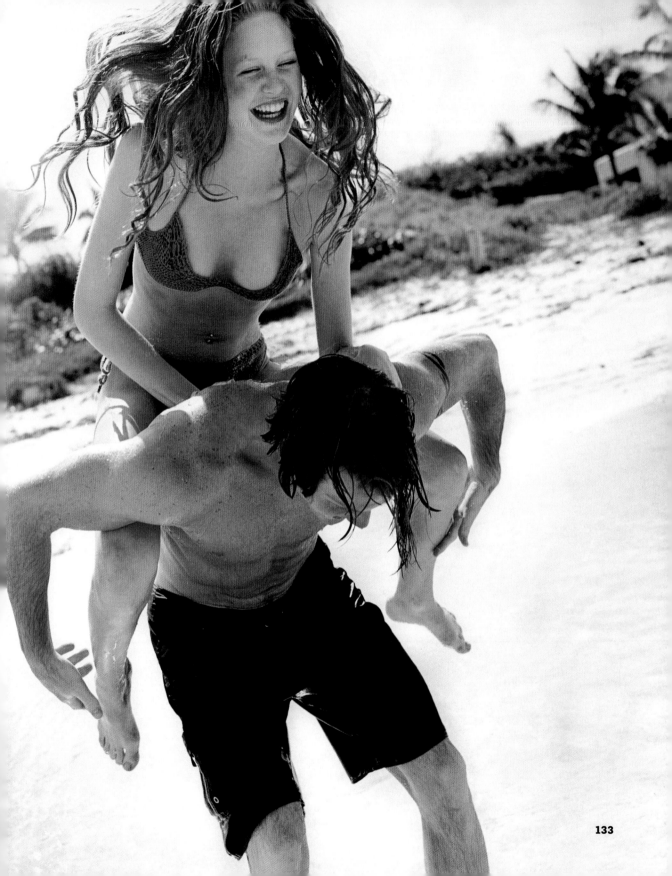

YOUR 00-TO EXERCISE: THE SQUAT

The Upgrade:
OVERHEAD SQUAT

This full-body exercise requires core strength, hip mobility, and shoulder stability. If you're weak in any of these areas, your overhead squat will look more like a slight dip of the knees. Consider yourself warned.

Hold a barbell over your head using an overhand grip that's about twice shoulder width. Your arms should be straight and your feet shoulder-width apart. Push your hips back and, while maintaining the natural arch in your lower back, squat as deeply as you can. Pause, and stand back up. Make sure the bar doesn't move forward and that your arms remain perpendicular to the floor for the entire lift. If your upper thighs aren't at least parallel to the floor, or if your heels rise, then you're either not strong enough or not flexible enough to do the exercise correctly.

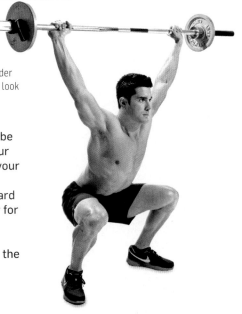

TOO Hard? Try the
FRONT SQUAT

WHY IT WORKS: This variation helps your body adjust to the stability and strength demands of removing the barbell from your back, and it builds the shoulder flexibility you need to raise the bar above your head.

ADVANCE TO THE OVERHEAD SQUAT WHEN: You can perform 3 sets of 6 to 8 reps of the front squat using at least 75 percent of your body weight.

Grab a barbell using an overhand grip, with your hands just past shoulder width. Raise your upper arms until they're parallel to the floor. Let the bar roll back so it's resting on the front of your shoulders. Push your hips back and perform a squat. Pause, and stand back up.

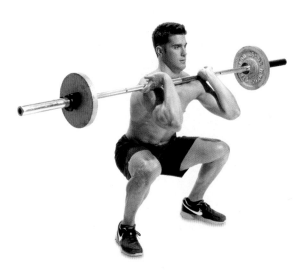

YOUR GO-TO EXERCISE: SEATED SHOULDER PRESS

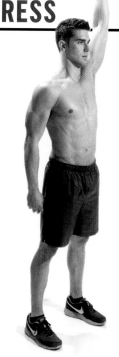

The upgrade:
STANDING SINGLE-ARM DUMBBELL SHOULDER PRESS

You're probably used to pressing weights while lying on your back (think bench press) but lack comparable strength lifting weights above your head. And if you do add overhead work, you're usually sitting, which doesn't engage your core. This move challenges every upper-body muscle, including your shoulders, traps, lats, and triceps, and even your abs. If you haven't properly trained those areas, you might find it nearly impossible to press even a light dumbbell over your head.

Stand holding one dumbbell just outside your shoulder with your arm bent and your palm facing your shoulder. Place your feet shoulder-width apart and bend your knees slightly. Press the weight overhead until your arm is straight, and then lower it back to the starting position.

TOO Hard? Try the
ANGLED-BAR SHOULDER PRESS

WHY IT WORKS: The angled version places less stress on your shoulder and rotator cuff. And by holding a weight on only one side at a time, you strengthen your core.

ADVANCE TO THE STANDING SINGLE-ARM DUMBBELL SHOULDER PRESS WHEN: You can perform the angled-bar shoulder press for 3 sets of 6 to 8 reps with 40 percent of your body weight on the bar.

Wedge one end of a bar into a weight plate on the floor. Place a plate on the other end, and hold that end in front of your shoulder so your elbow is bent 90 degrees. Press the bar up and away until your arm is straight. Pause, and return to the starting position.

YOUR GO-TO EXERCISE. LAT PULLDOWN

The Upgrade:
PULLUP

We know what you're thinking: Pullups? Those aren't tough. That's true ... when you perform them by pulling your chin up to the bar and lowering your body about 4 inches. But guess what? Those aren't real pullups. Real pullups start and end with your arms fully extended, and in between, your chest touches the bar. The truth is, when you use an overhand grip, you create two disadvantages: Your body isn't as mechanically efficient at lifting your weight, and your biceps help less—which means your back muscles are left to do the brunt of the work.

Grab a pullup bar using an overhand grip. Hang at arm's length, and then pull your chest to the bar. At the top, pause for 1 second, and then slowly lower your body back to the starting position.

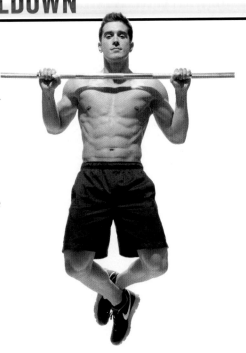

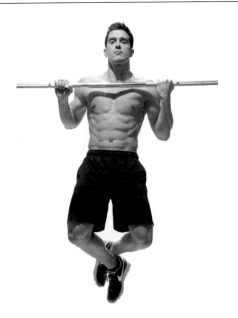

TOO Hard? Try the
MIXED-GRIP PULLUP

WHY IT WORKS: Forget lat pulldowns—this variation will improve your pullup ability by allowing the more efficient underhand grip to provide extra assistance.

ADVANCE TO THE PULLUP WHEN: You can perform the mixed-grip pullup for 4 sets (2 sets with each hand position) of 8 reps.

Perform a pullup, but use an underhand grip with one hand and an overhand grip with the other.

YOUR GO-TO EXERCISE: CRUNCHES

The Upgrade:
SWISS-BALL STIR-THE-POT

World-renowned spine specialist Stuart McGill, PhD, called this the best core exercise for a reason: It's hard. Make that really hard. That's because it combines two elements that leave your abs screaming: instability and dynamic movement. And you won't build six-pack excellence with endless crunches and leg lifts.

Assume a pushup position, but place your elbows and forearms on a Swiss ball. Move your elbows in a circle, making sure your core doesn't rotate.

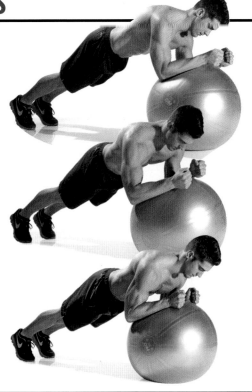

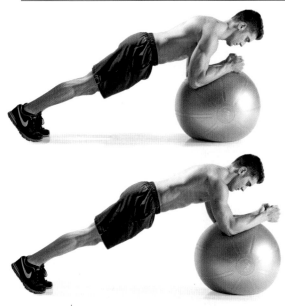

TOO Hard? Try the
SWISS-BALL BODY SAW

WHY IT WORKS: It combines instability with dynamic movement, but the motion is easier on your core muscles.

ADVANCE TO THE SWISS-BALL STIR-THE-POT WHEN: You can perform 2 sets of the Swiss-ball body saw for 60 seconds with perfect body alignment.

Assume a pushup position, but place your elbows and forearms on a Swiss ball. Then move your forearms forward and backward just a few inches in a sawing motion.

Muscle Season

Sculpt your body with this ab-shedding workout developed for Russian athletes.

Does your body look more like a blank slate than sculpted marble? This workout, based on a system developed for track-and-field athletes by Russian sports scientists, uses a combination of heavy lifting and intense "metabolic accelerators" to fatigue your muscle fibers and turn your body into a work of fine art—in just 4 weeks.

Here's how to do it: Alternate between workouts A and B 3 days a week. When two exercises have the same number (3A and 3B, for example), do 1 set of the A exercise and rest for the prescribed time; then do 1 set of the B exercise, and rest again. Repeat until you've completed all sets of each exercise. Then move on to the next pair. End each workout with the accelerator, and then wring out your shirt and go home.

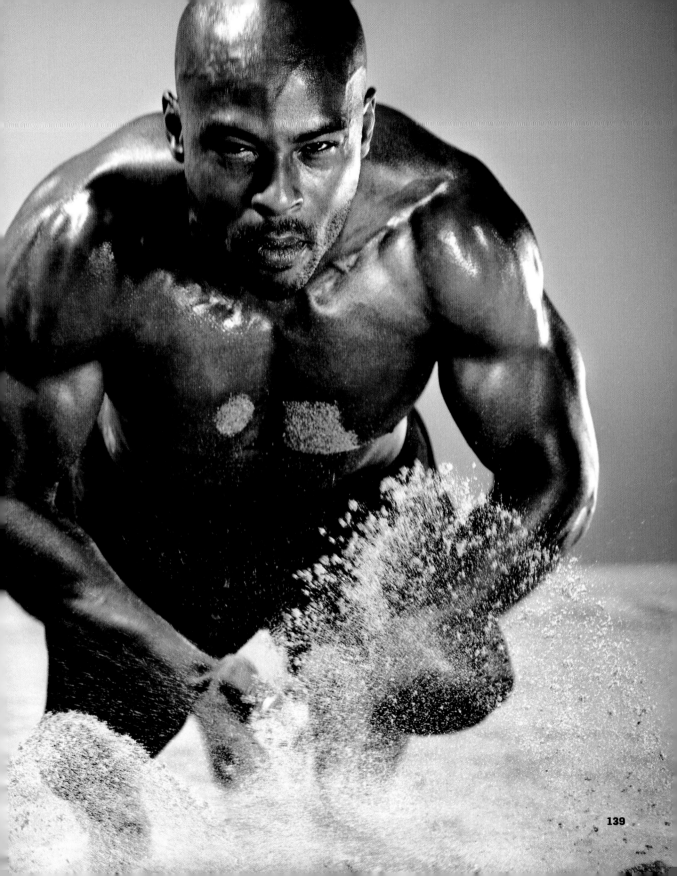

WORKOUT A

1

EXPLOSIVE PUSHUP

Assume a pushup position. Your body should form a straight line from your head to your ankles. Bend your elbows and lower your body until your chest nearly touches the floor. Then push up with enough force for your hands to come off the floor. Land and repeat.

WEEK 1: 2 SETS OF 8 REPS
WEEK 2: 3 SETS OF 8 REPS
WEEK 3: 2 SETS OF 10 REPS
WEEK 4: 4 SETS OF 10 REPS

REST: 90 SECONDS TO 2 MINUTES BETWEEN SETS

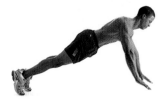

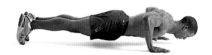

2

BARBELL SQUAT

Hold a barbell across your back using an overhand grip. Keeping your head up and chest high, push your hips back, bend your knees, and lower your body until your thighs are at least parallel to the floor. Push back to the starting position.

WEEK 1: 2 SETS OF 4 TO 6 REPS
WEEK 2: 3 SETS OF 3 TO 5 REPS
WEEK 3: 2 SETS OF 2 TO 3 REPS
WEEK 4: 3 SETS OF 2 TO 3 REPS

REST: 2 TO 3 MINUTES BETWEEN SETS

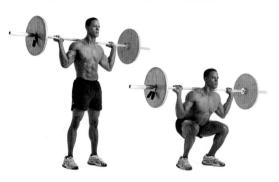

3A

BARBELL TEMPO SQUAT

Perform a barbell squat but take 2 full seconds to lower yourself and 2 full seconds to return to the starting position. Don't pause at the top or bottom.

WEEK 1: 2 SETS OF 10 TO 12 REPS
WEEK 2: 3 SETS OF 10 TO 12 REPS
WEEK 3: 4 SETS OF 10 TO 12 REPS
WEEK 4: 3 SETS OF 10 TO 12 REPS

REST: 1 MINUTE BETWEEN SETS

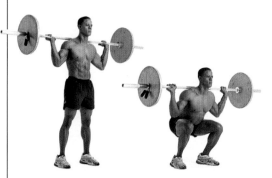

3B

TEMPO INVERTED ROW

Secure a barbell at about waist height. Using an overhand grip, hang under the bar with your arms extended; your body should form a straight line from head to ankles. Take 2 full seconds to pull your chest to the bar, and 2 seconds to lower yourself to the starting position. Don't pause at the top or bottom.

USE THE SAME SETS, REPS, AND REST AS IN EXERCISE 3A.

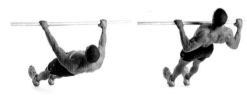

4A

BARBELL SHOULDER PRESS

Grab the bar overhand with your hands just beyond shoulder width, and hold it in front of your shoulders. Press the bar directly above your head until your arms are straight. Lower and repeat.

WEEKS 1 AND 2: 2 SETS OF 12 REPS
WEEKS 3 AND 4: 2 SETS OF 10 REPS
REST: 1 MINUTE BETWEEN SETS

4B

SINGLE-ARM LAT PULLDOWN

Attach a handle to the high pulley of a cable station. Grab the handle with one hand and sit in front of the weight stack. Without rotating your torso, pull the handle to the side of your chest. Do all your reps, switch hands, and repeat.

USE THE SAME SETS, REPS, AND REST AS IN EXERCISE 4A.

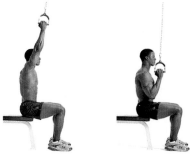

5

KETTLEBELL JUMP

Grab a kettlebell (you can also use a dumbbell) with both hands and hold it against your chest. Squat and jump as many times as you can in 15 seconds. Rest 45 seconds. That's one round.

WEEKS 1 AND 2: 8 ROUNDS
WEEKS 3 AND 4: 10 ROUNDS

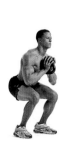
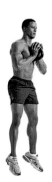

WORKOUT B

BOX JUMP

With your feet shoulder-width apart, dip down and then jump onto a step or box. Step down and repeat. Start with a box that's 18 to 24 inches high, and then use a higher box for weeks 3 and 4.

WEEK 1: 2 SETS OF 10 REPS
WEEK 2: 3 SETS OF 10 REPS
WEEK 3: 2 SETS OF 8 REPS
WEEK 4: 4 SETS OF 8 REPS
REST: 90 SECONDS TO 2 MINUTES BETWEEN SETS

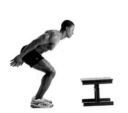

2
BARBELL BENCH PRESS

Grab a barbell and lie on a bench. Using an overhand grip that's just beyond shoulder width, hold the bar above your sternum, keeping your arms straight. Lower the bar to your chest, and then push it back to the starting position.

WEEK 1: 2 SETS OF 4 TO 6 REPS
WEEK 2: 3 SETS OF 3 TO 5 REPS
WEEK 3: 2 SETS OF 2 TO 3 REPS
WEEK 4: 4 SETS OF 2 TO 3 REPS
REST: 2 TO 3 MINUTES BETWEEN SETS

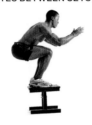 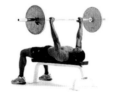 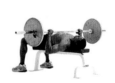

3A
TEMPO PUSHUP

Assume a pushup position. Take 2 full seconds to lower yourself to the floor and 2 full seconds to push back up. Don't pause at the top or bottom.

WEEK 1: 2 SETS OF 10 TO 12 REPS
WEEK 2: 3 SETS OF 10 TO 12 REPS
WEEK 3: 4 SETS OF 10 TO 12 REPS
WEEK 4: 3 SETS OF 10 TO 12 REPS
REST: 1 MINUTE BETWEEN SETS

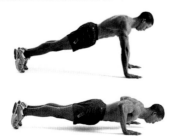

3B
BARBELL STRAIGHT-LEG DEADLIFT

Using an overhand grip, your hands just beyond shoulder width, grab a bar and hold it at arm's length in front of your thighs. Push your hips back and lower your torso until it's nearly parallel to the floor. Reverse the movement to return to the starting position.

USE THE SAME SETS, REPS, AND REST AS IN EXERCISE 3A.

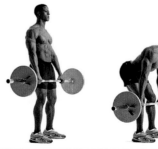

4A

DUMBBELL STEPUP

Grab a pair of dumbbells and place your right foot on a box or step. Push through your right heel until your right leg is straight. Lower yourself back down. Do all your reps with your right leg, and repeat with your left.

WEEKS 1 AND 2: 2 SETS OF 12 REPS
WEEKS 3 AND 4: 2 SETS OF 10 REPS
REST: 1 MINUTE BETWEEN SETS

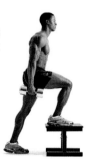
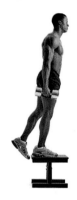

4B

FACE PULL

Attach a rope to the high pulley of a cable station. Grab the ends of the rope with your palms facing each other. Starting with your arms straight, pull the middle of the rope toward your nose (flare your elbows). Pause, and repeat.

USE THE SAME SETS, REPS, AND REST AS IN EXERCISE 4A.

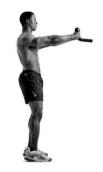
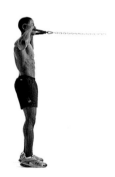

5

KETTLEBELL SWING

Without rounding your lower back, push your hips back and swing a kettlebell between your legs. Thrust your hips forward and let the weight swing to shoulder level. Start the clock, do 10 swings, and rest; when you hit the 60-second mark, repeat.

WEEKS 1 AND 2: GO FOR 8 MINUTES
WEEKS 3 AND 4: GO FOR 10 MINUTES

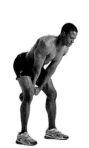
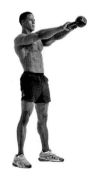

GSP: The Evolution of the Ultimate Fighter

Georges St-Pierre is one of the best fighters in the world. But to stay on top, he treats himself like a white belt.

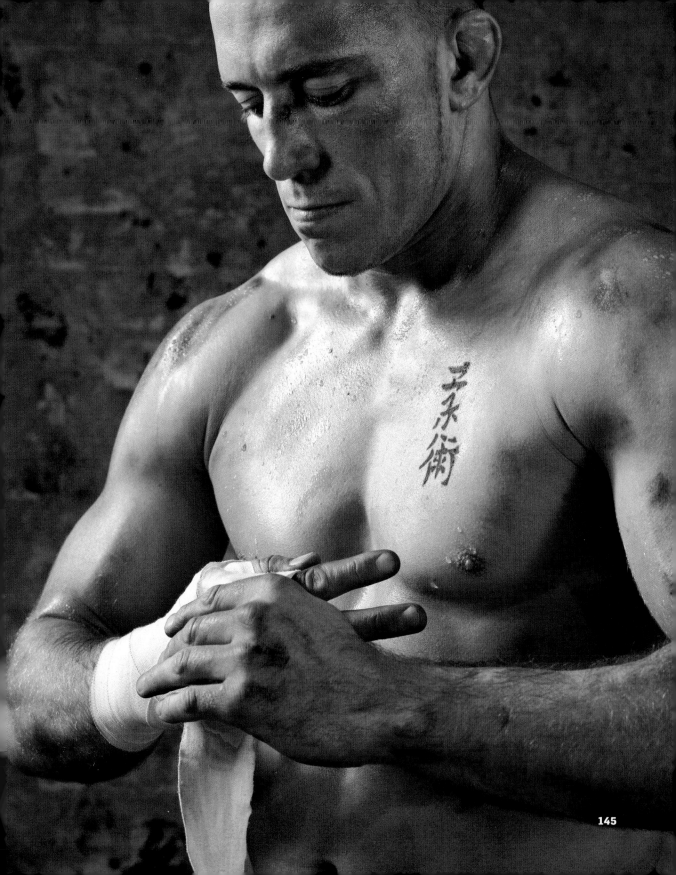

Georges St-Pierre knows an unusual amount about the megalodon, terror of the ancient seas. He speaks of it with grave importance; he wants to make clear that 2 million years ago, this predator, a shark larger than a city bus, went extinct. Poof.

As did the American lion, the short-faced bear, and several other giants whose Latin names sound musical in his Quebecois accent.

And why does he care so much about this?

"In fighting, in evolution, in life, efficiency is the key," says St-Pierre, who hopes to one day return to school to study paleontology. "It's not the most powerful animal that survives. It's the most efficient."

Paraphrasing Darwin is a neat trick for a guy who's paid to cut off the blood supply to people's brains. But St-Pierre isn't your typical fighter. He's arguably the best mixed martial artist in the world, a 5-foot-11-inch, 190-pound destroyer who drops 20 pounds for bouts. St-Pierre has cleaned out his division and could go down as the greatest champion in UFC history. He's faster than other fighters. More efficient. More fit, in the truest Darwinian sense.

"There is a difference between a fighter and a martial artist," St-Pierre says. "A fighter is training for a purpose: He has a fight. I'm a martial artist. I don't train for a fight. I train for myself. I'm training all the time. My goal is perfection. But I will never reach perfection."

The Only Constant Is Change

So why bother? Because evolution must be constant. He is never a master, complete in his studies. Rather, he is a trainer, a learner, as humble as a white belt. And he reminds himself of this by surrounding himself with smart people—all experts at something he wants to master—who can teach and challenge him.

He has coaches for every fighting discipline, and his main coaches work together to come up with the right strategies and to prepare him for individual opponents. But he also has a talent agent, who pushes him toward the kind of salesmanship and glad-handing that doesn't tend to come naturally to a fighter. That's led to promotional deals with Gatorade, Affliction Clothing, and Under Armour.

Understandably, St-Pierre's goals are lofty—and prioritized. For later: He wants to marry and have five kids. For now: He's single and aiming to become the best pound-for-pound mixed martial artist of all time, the man who crescent-kicks a fringe sport into the mainstream. Too bold? No.

"The danger is not to set your goal too high and fail to reach it," St-Pierre says,

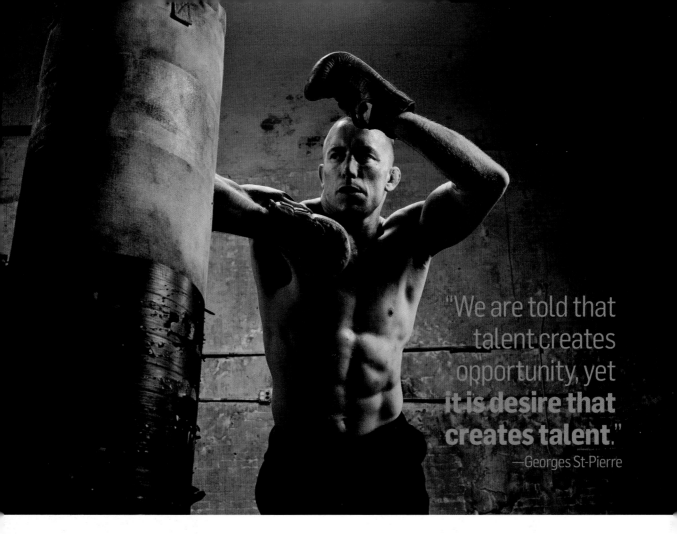

"We are told that talent creates opportunity, yet **it is desire that creates talent.**"

—Georges St-Pierre

now channeling Michelangelo. "It's to set your goal too low and reach it."

St-Pierre's first fight took place at around age 7. He reached the top of the hill during a schoolyard game, and an older kid punched him in the nose. More hits would come during his childhood in Saint-Isidore, a parish just outside Montreal, population 2,500.

"I was bullied," says St-Pierre, once a nerdy, studious boy who competed in chess tournaments. "I was not very popular."

To protect himself, he learned Kyokushin karate from his father. That gave him the striking base he still uses today,

he says. He discovered the importance of looking up to other experts when, at 15, he watched Royce Gracie, a skinny Brazilian jujitsu master, tap out oversize foes in the early days of the UFC.

"I asked myself, 'How can this happen? How can this small guy beat all these monsters?'" he says.

And now St-Pierre has the answer.

"Because of the knowledge that every war is won by the strongest weapon," he says. "Royce Gracie had the knowledge. The next day I started looking for a trainer."

By 2001, St-Pierre was competing

professionally. He'd remade himself as an expert in submission grappling. To pay for his training and kinesiology classes at a local college, he held three jobs: resurfacing floors, picking up garbage, and bouncing at a rowdy club called Fuzzy Brossard. In 2004, the UFC offered him a title shot against Matt Hughes. The opportunity was too good to pass up. He dropped out of school. Then he lost to Hughes. Once again, St-Pierre had climbed to the top of the hill only to be punched in the nose.

A lesser man might have been discouraged. St-Pierre grew more committed. Two years later, he fought Hughes again and TKO'd him to win the championship. Since then, St-Pierre has become a collector of people: those who help him in person, and those whose philosophies inspire him. He learned Muay Thai with the help of an elite trainer. Ditto boxing, Brazilian jujitsu, wrestling, strength conditioning, sports psychology. He can cite the 10,000-hour rule popularized by Malcolm Gladwell: You achieve success after that much practice. He might even turn profound and paraphrase Bruce Lee: "We are told that talent creates opportunity, yet it is desire that creates talent."

Desire creates talent. Let that concept linger. How many of us are brave enough to pursue a passion at any cost, as St-Pierre has? If the UFC didn't exist and there weren't a cent to be made in the sport, he says, he'd still be training twice a day for 90 minutes at a clip. He'd still be learning to punch on unstable surfaces in order to activate hidden muscles and increase his power. He'd be studying gymnastics and walking over obstacles on

his hands. It's about mastering himself.

"I don't do this for the fame," he says. "I do this for the love."

Maybe that explains St-Pierre's behavior when he ran into one of his childhood tormentors at a mall some time ago—and simply, casually nodded. Not to scare the guy. Just to say hi. To let him know that he'd moved past any place where revenge mattered. (The bully was scared nonetheless.)

"I don't have anger toward this guy anymore," St-Pierre says. "I don't want to fill up my heart with anger."

Ready for Success

On a mid-December night, and a holiday soiree is in full swing in the lower lobby of the Montreal Marriott Chateau Champlain. Guests arrive in expensive suits and shimmering gowns. As it happens, the lobby is also the muster point for undercard fighters at tonight's UFC 124, which creates a surreal scene: cauliflower-eared athletes and tipsy socialites appraising one another, unsure of who is more dangerous.

High above the clamor, St-Pierre sits silently in a suite on the 34th floor. The hours before a fight swell with tension, and the best way to deal with it is to move. But St-Pierre has been taught exactly when to start moving. Too soon and he wastes energy. He must stay calm as he is bundled into an SUV and transported to the Bell Centre, where, backstage, he will wait some more as the muffled thunder of the crowd oscillates through the walls: G-S-P! G-S-P! G-S-P!

At the arena, his focus is total. He tapes a simple handwritten sign, in

French, to his dressing room wall. Translation: "On December 11 in Montreal, I will destroy Josh Koscheck and remain world champion." An attainable goal. He makes a sign for each fight. "Every time I wake up in the morning," he says, "I put that up so I see it when I brush my teeth."

St-Pierre begins his warmup: trunk twists, crab steps, hamstring kicks, triangle submission drills, arm bar drills, guillotine chokes, superman punches, combination strikes on pads, breathing exercises with arms upraised against the wall, hands opening and closing methodically. Every movement is precise, efficient. His trainers go over his game plan. He is ready.

Time to move. St-Pierre runs out of his dressing room. He runs to the cage. The fight begins. "Watch how he controls the pace and rhythm," says Greg Jackson, one of St-Pierre's coaches. "Human brains are looking for a pattern. Establishing that pattern and then breaking it can be very powerful."

In the first round, St-Pierre establishes a rhythm, and then breaks it on Josh Koscheck's face. Over and over. St-Pierre's left jab is a trip hammer. He seems to have shattered Koscheck's orbital bone within minutes and begins attacking his opponent's leg with lead kicks.

The next four rounds mimic the first, with Koscheck looking increasingly battered and desperate. St-Pierre circles out of the range of Koscheck's looping, obvious right hand. When Koscheck lunges wildly, St-Pierre sidesteps him like a matador and taps him on the head. The crowd laughs. Actually laughs. Koscheck may be a four-time Division I All-American wrestler, but tonight he looks like an

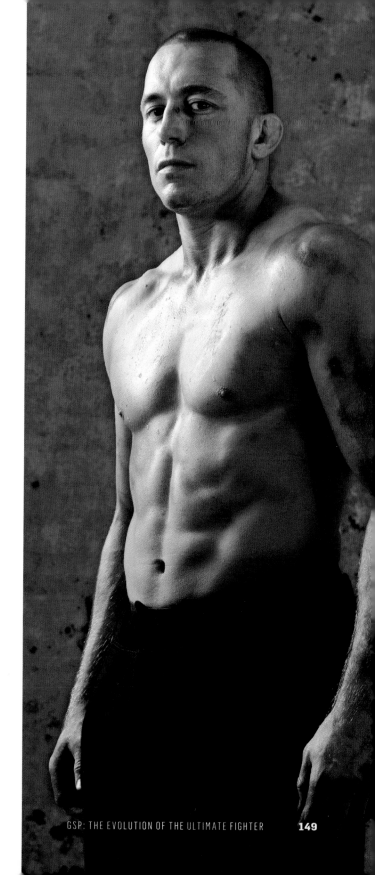

earlier model of fighter. Obsolete. Homo habilis. He keeps trying to slug it out with St-Pierre, who is superior on his feet and happy to oblige.

("Never interrupt your enemy when he's making a mistake," St-Pierre will say later, quoting Napoleon.) St-Pierre easily wins every round. He lands 136 strikes to Koscheck's 30.

And what is GSP doing moments later in his dressing room after defending his title in front of a hometown crowd? He's on a mat, rolling with a coach, training, taking pointers about what he did wrong, about how he could have used a move called the "head snapdown" when he had Koscheck on the ground at one point. He does this after every fight, always training, always learning. Desire creates talent.

"It's like life," St-Pierre says. "The more knowledge you get, the more questions you ask. The smarter you get, the more you realize that everything can be possible."

Behold evolution in real time.

Georges St-Pierre's Kick-Ass Workout

Learn the training secrets that helped build the most famous six-pack in sports.

Gym rats often debate the ideal number of workouts a week it takes to build muscle and look like someone who lifts. You can find good arguments for any number from three to six. But two workouts a week? You'd be laughed out of the weight room— unless you happened to be the toughest guy in the place, which UFC champion Georges St-Pierre most definitely is. He built his famously chiseled physique with just two weight workouts every 7 days. The plan allowed St-Pierre to increase his strength and explosive power and pack on muscle without adding any fat. Fair warning: This workout combines Olympic movements with body-weight exercises, cranking up your metabolism to slam whatever fat you have to the canvas.

Prepare like St-Pierre

Georges St-Pierre's impressive physique wouldn't exist if he spent all of his time recovering from injuries. The UFC champ protects his body by performing a fast-paced routine before he starts each training session.

"A warmup is essential because it activates all your muscles and improves bloodflow to help prevent injury, while also preparing your body to increase its performance," says Erik Owings, one of St-Pierre's trainers and the owner of Mushin Mixed Martial Arts in New York City.

Before your next workout, try this full-body igniter. It should take less than 5 minutes. Perform each exercise for 60 seconds, then move to the next without any rest.

3-WAY LUNGES

Do a forward lunge, a backward lunge, and a side lunge. Repeat, starting with the opposite leg. Continue in this pattern until the time is up.

SQUATS

Do traditional squats, using only your body weight.

WALKOUT PUSHUPS

Stand tall, and then squat and put your hands on the floor. Walk your hands forward until your body is in pushup position. Do a pushup, and then walk your hands back to the squat position and stand up. That's 1 rep. Repeat until the time is up.

THE PROGRAM

Perform this total-body workout twice a week. The workout is separated into three phases: power, strength, and fat loss. Make sure you finish all the exercises in each phase, using the directions below, before moving on to the next one.

POWER PHASE

Do the exercises in the order shown, completing the prescribed number of sets of each exercise before moving on to the next. Rest 2 minutes between each set.

1

DUMBBELL CLEAN

Grab a pair of dumbbells, push your hips back, and flex your knees as shown. Pull the dumbbells up and "catch" them at shoulder height as you rise to a standing position; keep your knees slightly bent. Return to the starting position. Do 1 set of 5 reps, and 1 set of 3 reps.

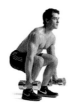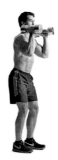

2

DUMBBELL PUSH PRESS

Hold a pair of dumbbells just outside your shoulders as shown. Dip your knees, and then push up with your legs as you press the dumbbells overhead. Lower the dumbbells back to the starting position. Do 1 set of 5 reps, and 1 set of 3 reps.

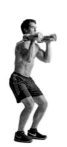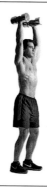

3

DUMBBELL CLEAN AND PRESS

Hold a pair of dumbbells below your knees as shown. Pull the dumbbells up and "catch" them at shoulder height. Then press them overhead, keeping your knees slightly bent. Return to the starting position. Perform 3 sets of 3 reps.

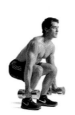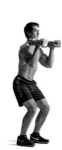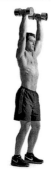

STRENGTH PHASE

Perform the exercises in succession as a circuit, resting 30 to 60 seconds between each. Do 3 reps of every exercise, and complete a total of 3 circuits.

1 GETUP

Lie faceup with your right leg bent and your left leg flat on the floor. Holding a dumbbell, raise your right arm straight overhead. Roll onto your left side and prop yourself up. Then raise your hips, squeeze your glutes, and straighten your left arm. Pause, and slide your right leg behind your body as shown. Move into a kneeling position, and then stand up while keeping the dumbbell above you at all times. Once you're standing, step back with your left leg and perform the movement in reverse to return to the starting position. Complete 3 reps, switch sides, and repeat.

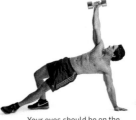
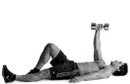
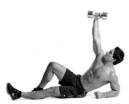

Keep the weight elevated and your elbow locked at all times.

Use your abs to help raise your body while keeping one leg flat on the floor.

Your eyes should be on the dumbbell at all times.

2 PULLUP

Hang at arm's length from a chinup bar, using an overhand grip that's slightly wider than your shoulders. Pull your chest up to the bar and squeeze your shoulder blades together. Pause, and slowly lower your body to the starting position.

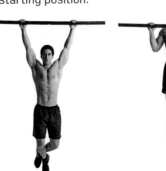

3 SWISS-BALL PUSHUP WITH FEET ON BENCH

Assume a pushup position, but with your feet on a bench or step and your hands on a Swiss ball. Slowly lower your body until your chest nearly touches the ball. Pause, and push back up to the starting position.

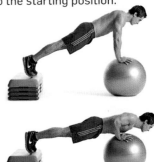

4
DUMBBELL FRONT SQUAT

Hold a pair of dumbbells with your palms facing, upper arms perpendicular to the floor, and one end of each dumbbell resting on the meatiest part of your shoulder. Push your hips back and lower your body into a squat, and push back up.

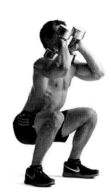
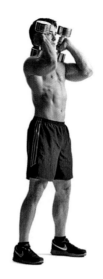

FAT-LOSS PHASE

Perform squat thrusts for 20 seconds, then rest 10 seconds. That's 1 set. Complete a total of 8 sets.

SQUAT THRUST

Stand with your feet hip-width apart. Lower your body until your palms rest on the floor about shoulder-width apart. Kick your legs backward to a pushup position. Perform a pushup, and then quickly reverse the movement and perform a jump as you stand up.

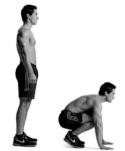
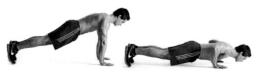
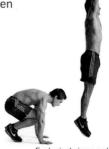

Drop into a squat and shift your weight onto your hands.

Your body should form a straight line from your ankles to your shoulders.

Explosively jump as high as you can. Reset, and then repeat the exercise.

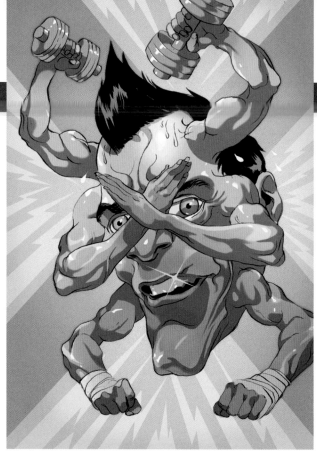

The Power of P90X

Tony Horton used to be a stand-up comedian. Now he's the frontman for P90X and a millionaire exercise guru. Is he an infomercial salesman? Or a fitness savior?

It's 11:30 p.m., and a man steps off the elevator in the Crowne Plaza Hotel in Valley Forge, Pennsylvania. Tony Horton enters the lobby wearing black shorts, a black sweater, and despite the hour, dark glasses. But two guys in their 30s, who just left the bar, recognize him.

"You're Tony Horton!" says one in disbelief.

"Dude!" is all the other can utter.

Both men tell him they're following his P90X workout program, which is sold relentlessly through infomercials across America. They boast of their results, showing off supposedly flatter guts and bigger biceps. One claims to have the DVDs in his hotel room at this very moment: "I use 'em when I'm on the road!"

By the time Horton finally breaks away, he has signed autographs, mugged for photos, struck his signature forearm-crossed "X-Man" pose, and even done a handstand by the front desk. Finally he exits the hotel and settles into the back-seat of a private car that's been waiting to take him to QVC headquarters, in nearby West Chester.

That's right. Horton is heading to QVC—the network darling of little old ladies in quilted housedresses—to sell his P90X workout program. ("Just two easy payments of $64.95, plus $9.43 shipping and handling.") He'll do an hourlong taping at 1 a.m. (right after Joan Rivers sells jewelry), grab a few hours of sleep in a back room, and then do more tapings at 6 a.m., 6 p.m., and 10 p.m.

It's hustle like this that has enabled Horton to hawk a reported 3 million P90X

DVD sets, in addition to his fitness accessories, nutritional supplements, and other workout programs. Not bad for a fiftysomething former stand-up comedian and theater major who lacks a college degree or, for that matter, any type of fitness credentials.

"Hey, George Bush became president. What was his experience?" asks Horton. "A lot of trainers are certified up the yin-yang and live in rent-controlled apartments out behind convalescent homes because they can't make a buck. Sorry I have a sense of humor, sorry I'm not certified, but my philosophy is based on 25 years of training everyone from moms to Bruce Springsteen."

Indeed, what Horton and the company behind him, known as Beachbody, do exceptionally well is excite people. Meet Horton in a hotel lobby or watch his infomercial, and you'll start to believe—in him, in his program, and most important, in your own potential to transform yourself. It happens that quickly. QVC alone has sold more than 135,000 units since P90X debuted on the network in 2008. That equates to more than $17.5 million shelled out by customers.

Beyond the compelling marketing, there are two reasons why P90X is so popular. First, Horton is the perfect frontman. At 5 foot 10 inches and 180 pounds, with 9 percent body fat, he is genuinely ripped. He says he can consecutively do 110 pushups, 80 dips, 35 pullups, and eight 260-pound lat pulls. Plus, he can hold a handstand for a minute and even do a backflip off a wall. To prove it, he often drops to the floor and pumps out a few reps of whatever exercise he's talking about. His motto, which he wears on the back of his shirt, is "Bring It!" Along with the brawn, he has a full head of hair and—even under the harsh QVC makeup lights—no telltale signs of any nips or tucks.

Always be open to new things. Your muscles won't know what hit 'em.

But second, and most important, P90X—unlike the garbage heap of other "miracle" infomercial products—can deliver results. That's because it's built on such proven fitness principles as consistency, intensity, and variety, and you don't need special gadgets—just a pullup bar and dumbbells (or resistance bands). Simply pop a disc into your DVD player, move the couch out of the way, and follow along with Tony and his gang. In fact, Horton's critics claim there's nothing new in his workouts; if you do anything 6 days a week for 90 days, you'll lose weight and build muscle at any age.

Horton says with a shrug, "You can't reinvent the pushup. Plyometrics has been around forever, yoga has been around for even longer, and Kenpo karate is nothing I invented . . . but the sequence, the pace, and the variety of my workouts is something that never existed before. P90X is hard. But do your best and forget the rest. If you're in trouble, hit the Pause button. If you can't do this move, here are two ways to modify it. I just want you to show up, man. That's all I want you to do."

Regardless of whether you ever pick up the phone ("Two easy payments, nothing to lose, give us a call!"), the chief elements of Tony Horton's exercise philosophy can be incorporated into any workout. Here's how.

P90X Principle 1

Bewilder your body.

Horton claims to have "exercise bipolar disorder," which means that although he works out regularly, the specifics of what he does each day depend on how he feels. So he may swap speed drills for strength work, chest for back, or even karate for Pilates. He often doesn't decide until 10 minutes beforehand, or improvises on the fly. He calls this approach "muscle confusion."

"Look at all the people who've been going to gyms for years and still look the same, or those who tried exercising and quit," he says.

"That's because they're doing mundane, myopic routines, and they're bored. Let's break the mold."

For More Info . . .

For information on Tony Horton's new book, *Bring It! The Revolutionary Fitness Plan for All Levels That Burns Fat, Builds Muscle, and Shreds Inches,* visit MensHealth.com/horton.

Bring It!

In Tony Horton's new book, *Bring It! The Revolutionary Fitness Plan for All Levels That Burns Fat, Builds Muscle, and Shreds Inches,* he uses a variety of circuits to help burn fat. Try this one: Do 20 reps of each exercise, rest 30 seconds, and repeat.

BURN

PIVOT PUNCHES

Stand with your feet shoulder-width apart and knees slightly bent. Bend your elbows as shown. Twist your torso to the left by pivoting on your right foot, and throw a punch with your right hand. Then twist to your right and punch with your left hand.

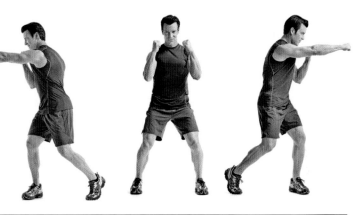

BLAST

LATERAL SHUFFLE

Stand in an athletic stance. Shuffle to your left by moving one foot and then the other. Do this four times, and shuffle back to the starting position. Then repeat the shuffle to your right.

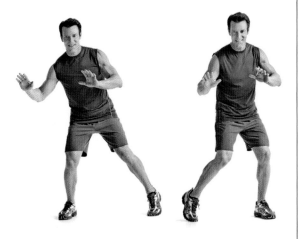

BLITZ

FRONT KICKS

Assume a staggered stance, with your feet about 12 inches apart. Balance on your front leg, and then kick forward with your back leg to about hip height. Do 10 reps, switch legs, and repeat. Try to keep your leg nearly straight as you kick it up.

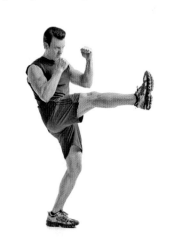

Before Horton became a celebrity himself, he trained lots of celebrities in Los Angeles. He says one of his clients, Billy Idol, nicknamed him "Muscle Confucius" because of his varied approach to fitness. And there is wisdom in it. If you're training for life rather than a specific event, mixing it up will help you burn more calories, protect yourself from injury, achieve a balanced physique, and keep motivated.

Your body doesn't respond to repetition, Horton says. It responds to novelty.

P90X AT YOUR PLACE

Schedule your workouts a month in advance, reserving exact times for each. (Horton blocks out 20 on his desk calendar at the start of every month.) Pencil in cardio, strength, speed, and flexibility days, but stop there. Let your mood determine your specific workout when each day arrives. Always be open to new things. If it's a cardio day, hop onto a different machine or into a kickboxing class. If it's a strength day, try using free weights instead of a Nautilus machine. "Your muscles shouldn't know what hit 'em," says Horton.

P90X Principle 2

Work your weaknesses.

Here's some more Muscle Confucius: The more you dread doing something, the more value it holds for you. So if you hate stretching or intervals, that's probably because flexibility and speed are your weaknesses. Since no man likes to feel inferior, we avoid dealing with our weaknesses and end up training our strengths. Wrong move.

"The only reason I'm as fit as I am," says Horton, who used to be a spokesman for NordicTrack, "is because I kept doing things that were hard and that I couldn't do well."

P90X AT YOUR PLACE

Select one exercise or facet of fitness that you struggle with, and commit to improving it. Schedule an occasional "weakness day." Once you overcome the initial aversion, your improvement will be dramatic, and the success will motivate you to take on more of your weaknesses.

P90X Principle 3

Find (and flirt) with the Line.

The Line is your discomfort threshold. It's the one pushup beyond what you think you can do. It's that extra agonizing rep after you've finished a set. But it's not just the effort that's important; it's the desire to want to go there again and again. That's the secret to becoming fit.

And it's the reason Horton scoffs at walking, riding an exercise bike while reading, or doing any mild form of cardio as a sole means of fitness.

"Walking is just a waste of time for most people," he says. "We're primates and we walk—that's what we do. And even though it's better than doing nothing, it's not enough. You have to find that Line in whatever you're doing and continually push it out."

P90X AT YOUR PLACE

Use Horton's discomfort scale to gauge where you are during your workout.

10 = so brutal, so awful, you're miserable.

9 = just short of the above.

7 or 8 = really hard, but you're maintaining form and hanging in there.

6 = it's not a 7 or 8, but you're working as hard as you can today.

5 = you can do more . . . but you're not.

1 to 4 = unless it's a recovery day, you're wasting your time.

The Line is at 6, 7, or 8 on the scale.

P90X Principle 4

Train resiliency, not vanity.

Horton says that if a law were passed that limited him to one type of exercise, he'd pick yoga. And for once he's not joking.

"Yoga is resistance, it's balance, it's coordination, it's stamina, it's even cardiovascular, depending on how you do it. . . . I can turn yoga into anything, and it's the reason I can do this"—he drops to the floor for clap pushups—"and this"—he hops back up for high leg kicks. "Ever see a 65-year-old guy run? That should be incentive enough."

Indeed, as you age, you lose your flexibility. That means by age 65, you'll practically be prepping for rigor mortis.

"I put off yoga for 4 years because I thought it was silly," says Horton.

P90X AT YOUR PLACE

Swallow your pride and enroll in a beginners' yoga class taught by an instructor with at least a 200-hour certification. Flowing vinyasa styles, such as ashtanga, are more rigorous. Once you know the basics, you'll be able to practice on your own. (There's a good chance you'll be the only guy in a class of very fit, flexible women, though, so you might not want to.)

Yoga has another advantage that's fundamental to Horton's exercise and life philosophies. Although it sounds contradictory coming from someone ironically nicknamed Tony Humble, he says that "externals," such as weight loss and muscle definition, should never be your primary motivators for working out.

"Focus instead on the internals," he says. Are you less fatigued? Do you have more energy? Are you sleeping better? Do you feel stronger? Are you happier? Yoga helps you become more aware and mindful of all these things, and they're what will keep you working out long-term.

It's 2:10 a.m. QVC is now featuring the Stan Herman Collection. And Horton is finally looking a little tired as he sits on the stage steps sipping a smoothie. It seems like a good time to ask him a philosophical question: Tell us, Tony, what's the one thing fitness still hasn't brought you?

After an uncharacteristically long pause, he says, "Honestly? Nothing. Fitness and healthy eating have changed my life from soup to nuts. There's no area that it hasn't given me confidence in—physical, mental, emotional. I feel blessed that in some weird way I've been given this opportunity to help people. . . . For me, fitness isn't about how long I'm going to live; it's about the quality of life right now. And let me tell you, man, I'm one happy dude."

PROVE IT

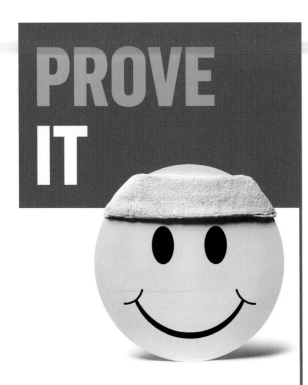

INCREASE YOUR SMILEAGE

If your motivation is lagging, consider this: Exercisers tend to underestimate how much they'll enjoy a workout, a Canadian study reports. That's because they focus on a session's beginning, which is often unpleasant, says study author Matthew Ruby, MA. The happiest people in the study scheduled their favorite exercises first. Just keep in mind that starting a workout with exercises that work multiple muscle groups can tire you out, making it harder for you to finish.

GET MOVING

Now's the perfect time to start!

If you're starting a workout program, here's some encouragement. Sedentary men who exercise just once a week can make sharp fitness gains, a study from Thailand reveals. The men performed a moderate-intensity cardio workout once a week for an hour. After 12 weeks, their average resting heart rate was down by 11 percent, and their VO2 max, which is a measure of aerobic capacity, was up by 24 percent. Get started: Schedule one workout on the same day each week, and make it a can't-miss appointment.

BOOST YOUR REPS

Protein isn't the only thing that'll help your muscle fibers. Citrulline malate—an amino acid—might boost the amount of weight you can handle, say researchers in Spain. When men consumed 8 grams of the supplement before a workout, they performed more reps than men who skipped the dose. That's because citrulline malate, which is similar to a compound found in watermelon, might buffer fatigue. But more research is needed to determine if eating the fruit would have a similar impact.

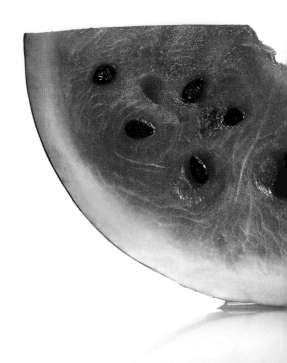

FISH FOR MUSCLES

What's good for your heart is also good for your biceps. Washington University in St. Louis scientists found that people who took a daily fish-oil supplement that contained 1.5 grams of docosahexaenoic acid (DHA) and 2 grams of eicosapentaenoic acid (EPA) doubled their ability to beef up compared with a group of placebo poppers. These omega-3 fats might help signal your body to start turning protein into muscle, says study author Bettina Mittendorfer, PhD.

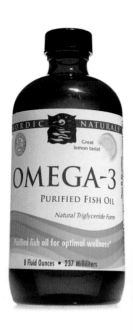

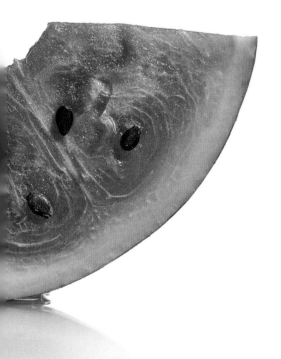

HARD TRUTH

36	The percentage of men who say they don't enjoy exercise but do it anyway for their health, according to Mintel

EAT THIS, LIFT MORE

Too much fructose can be bad for your health. But the right sugar ratio might boost your workout, a Spanish study reveals. Men who consumed fructose and glucose—sugars found in fruit—15 minutes before training cut their fatigue. This mix replenishes energy stores in your muscles and liver to help you last longer, says *MH* nutritionist Alan Aragon, MS. He suggests a piece of fruit before your workout.

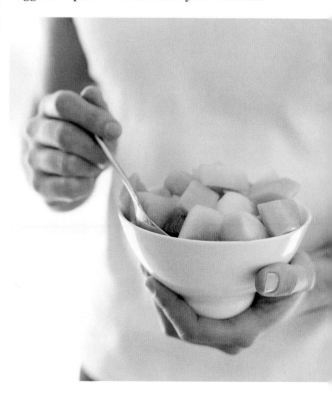

PROVE IT

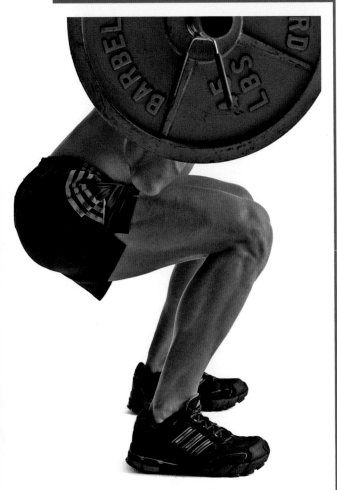

CHECK THE CLOCK

Want to build your biceps faster? The lowering portion of an exercise may build more muscle than the lifting phase does, according to a University of British Columbia review of 66 studies. "Taking 3 seconds to lower the weight adds size and strength," says Martin Rooney, PT, CSCS.

WEAR THIS VEST

An all-natural performance enhancer?

Wearing a weighted vest for your pregame warmup can help you run faster and jump higher during the game. But be careful: Researchers from Wichita State University found that guys didn't achieve this expected power boost when they warmed up with vests weighing 5 percent of their weight. Why? The vests were too heavy. Your fix: Warm up with bodyweight exercises for 6 to 8 weeks, then progress to a weighted vest that's about 2 percent of your body mass, says Mark Peterson, PhD, an exercise physiologist at the University of Michigan.

FREE YOURSELF

All squats are not equal

Machine squats might limit your gains. Canadian scientists say free weights work your muscles harder than the Smith machine, which

HARD TRUTH

43 Percentage increase in leg-muscle activation doing free-weight squats

is a squat station with a built-in bar that runs on guides.

"The Smith machine stabilizes the barbell, requiring your muscles to work less," says study author Phil Chilibeck, PhD. Free weights, like barbells or dumbbells, provide a better overall training effect by stressing more muscle fibers in your body.

GET ENERGY TO BURN

Scratch one more excuse: A low-carb diet still provides plenty of energy for exercise, Australian researchers say. In a study of 60 overweight or obese people, they found that the ability to exercise—as well as perceptions of fatigue and exertion—were consistent regardless of diet type. Subjects were assigned either low-carb, high-fat, or high-carb, low-fat plans. The low-carb group lost more weight than the low-fat gang, and burned more fat during exercise. Study author Grant Brinkworth, PhD, says the results show that aerobic exercise is not highly dependent on the availability of carbs. So cut your carb intake and don't skip workouts.

STOMACH IT

Strength in a bottle?

Digest this: A stomach enzyme could make you stronger. Protease, a digestive enzyme that helps your body break down proteins, appears to lessen muscle inflammation that occurs after resistance training, say Baylor University researchers. Faster recovery means you can lift more weight on subsequent trips to the gym. Study participants experienced benefits within 3 weeks of taking daily protease supplements.

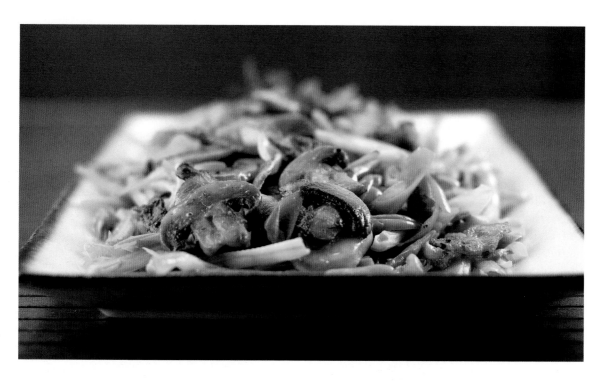

YOU ASKED

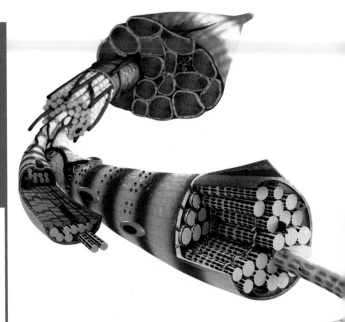

Q: How does my body build muscle?

A: Let's say you want your construction crew to erect bigger biceps. They'll rely mostly on two key building materials: myofibrils (ropelike strands made up of thinner protein filaments) and sarcoplasm (a gel-like fuel that surrounds the myofibrils). Now, if you lift low reps of heavy weights, the crew will mainly thicken your myofibrils, increasing size and strength. If, on the other hand, you lift high reps of medium weights, those hard hats will primarily boost the volume of your sarcoplasm, building size and endurance.

"Both kinds of growth require stressing your muscles beyond what they're used to, and the way you train dictates which kind of growth you emphasize," says Alexander Koch, PhD, CSCS, an associate professor of exercise science at Lenoir-Rhyne University in North Carolina. That's why he recommends cycling through weights that are moderately heavy (8 to 12 reps), heavy (4 to 6 reps), and maximally heavy (1 to 3 reps) over a period of several weeks.

SWELL

When you do a high number of reps with a moderate weight, some myofibril growth occurs (see "Shred"), but your body also sends a signal to increase the size and number of mitochondria, the mini motors inside all your cells. As your mitochondria multiply to handle the endurance demands of a high-rep workout, your supply of sarcoplasm also increases to make your muscles function more efficiently. Sarcoplasm is made up of adenosine triphosphate, creatine phosphate, glycogen, and water—a combination that not only transports energy to your muscles but also adds volume to your myofibrils.

SHRED

A workout of heavy weights and low reps causes microtears in your myofibrils. These tears trigger your immune system to send white blood cells to clear away damaged cell fragments, preparing the site for rebuilding. At the same time, your body experiences a boost in human growth hormone, which has a twofold effect: The extra HGH activates dormant stem cells and makes it easier for your body to use the amino acids in protein. Those newly awakened stem cells flock to your injured muscle. There, with the help of the amino acids, they may grow new filaments or fuse with the existing filaments, making your myofibrils denser, larger, and stronger.

Q: What's the best way to build powerful muscle?

A: Plyometrics

"Focus on your fast-twitch muscle fibers," says Todd Durkin, author of *The Impact! Body Plan.* "Plyometric exercises, which involve explosive action, are the best way." Do 2 sets of 10 reps of plyo-pushups (after you lower your body, blast upward so your hands leave the ground) and squat jumps (dip your knees, squat, and then launch up).

Q: What easy-to-learn whole-body exercise can I add to my regular workout?

A: Few moves offer a more practical payoff than the suitcase carry, says Dan John, an elite strength trainer based in Burlingame, California.

"It will help you lift any heavy load more easily, whether you're schlepping groceries, shoveling snow, or lugging your bags through an airport." The suitcase carry not only helps you build balanced strength but also forces your core to stabilize your body, giving you an ab blast to boot.

To do it, grab a heavy dumbbell using an overhand grip, and hold it at your side like a suitcase. Now slowly walk 50 yards. Switch hands and walk back. That's 1 repetition. (In tight quarters, find about 5 yards and walk back and forth until you reach your distance.) Do 5 reps, resting about a minute between reps, three times a week.

Q: Does it make a difference whether I use dumbbells, barbells, or machines when I exercise?

A: The numbers on the weight plates may be the same, but your body can tell the difference.

"When you use dumbbells, you have to lift and balance two objects—so your smaller stabilizing muscles have to work harder," says Bill Hartman, PT, CSCS, co-owner of Indianapolis Fitness and Sports Training. Machines are at the other end of the stability spectrum. When you use, say, a chest press, it keeps the weight steady for you, which makes it possible for you to activate more of your larger muscles and lift many more pounds than you would be able to with free weights—and therefore bulk up faster.

But don't let those bigger numbers seduce you; if you train using only machines, your smaller stabilizers will be neglected, and that can lead to injuries. Instead, sculpt your muscles by using all three options. You don't have to hit all three every session, but if you do, always progress from least to most stable, says Hartman. For instance, if it's a chest day, go from the dumbbell bench press to the barbell bench press, and finish with the machine chest press.

HARD TRUTH

60 The number of myofibrils—the strands that make up your muscle fibers—equal to the diameter of a human hair, according to *Gray's Anatomy.*

YOU ASKED

Q: I want to try kettlebells. How many should I buy and how heavy?

A: You'll ultimately need three of these bombs in your muscle-building arsenal—and you should start big.

"Many kettlebell exercises, such as swings and cleans, are easier to learn using a heavier bell because your body needs something to push against," says Jason C. Brown, head trainer at Kettlebell Athletics in Roslyn, Pennsylvania. He advises that most men start with a 16-kilogram (35-pound) bell ($60 and up, performbetter.com) and use it to master four exercises: the swing, squat, clean and press, and snatch. (For videos, see MensHealth.com/kettlebell.)

These moves can help you relieve tightness in your hips, a common problem area. They also prepare your muscles for the heavier weights: 20 kilos (44 pounds) and 24 kilos (52.8 pounds) if your strength is about average. Stronger men can move up to 32 kilos (70 pounds).

"You don't need to go over 32 kilos, because kettlebells are designed to build strength and endurance," says Brown. "Once you can handle these big boys, you can just add reps."

Q: Women love firm butts. Which exercise best activates the glutes?

A: Step up your workouts—literally. Doing the eccentric dumbbell stepup makes your glutes work overtime because it focuses on the lowering part of the exercise and not the lifting, says B.J. Gaddour, CSCS, fitness director of WorkoutMuse.com. "Your muscles can handle more weight during that phase, which can lead to greater muscle gains." Besides the cosmetic benefit of shaping your glutes, you're also activating the biggest muscle in your body, so you're boosting your metabolism as well. For the fastest results, do it barefoot, says Gaddour. Start with 3 sets of 6 reps on each side, 3 days a week.

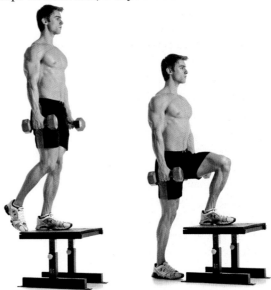

Place your left foot on a box or bench so your left leg is bent 90 degrees. Then step onto the bench. Your right leg should be dangling slightly.

Bend your left knee and very slowly lower your right foot to the floor. Once it touches, push back to the starting position. That's 1 rep.

Take 5 seconds to step down.

Q: What's the best way to avoid hamstring injuries?

A: Strengthen the muscles. If you're like most men, you emphasize leg exercises that build your quads, says Bill Hartman, PT, CSCS, co-owner of Indianapolis Fitness and Sports Training. "This can cause an imbalance that puts your hamstrings at risk when you accelerate or decelerate rapidly."

He recommends the Swiss-ball hip raise and leg curl to ensure that you avoid the DL. It's better than a hamstring curl on a machine because it trains your leg muscles in a more functional way, and also activates your lower-back and core muscles.

Lie faceup on the floor and place your calves on a Swiss ball.

Push your hips up so your body forms a straight line from shoulders to knees.

Without pausing, pull your heels toward you and roll the ball as close as possible to your butt.

Pause 2 seconds, and reverse the move until your body is in a straight line. Then lower your hips to the floor.

Do 2 sets of 10 repetitions, three times a week.

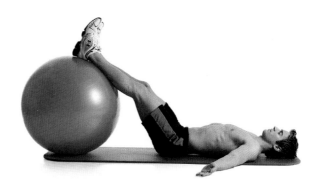

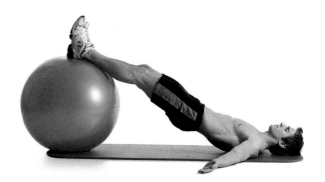

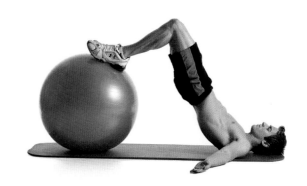

YOU ASKED

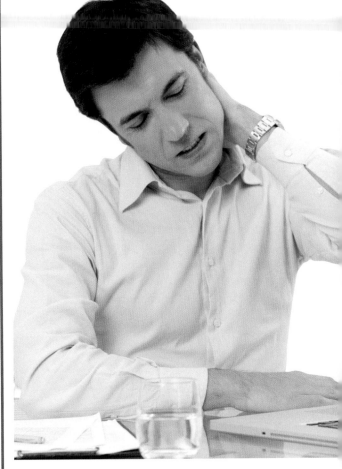

Q: I find planks boring. What's another great ab exercise?

A: Take an ab wheel for a spin.
"It turns out that ab-wheel rollouts train the exact same muscles in your core as planks do, except they hit them harder," says Mike Robertson, MS, CSCS, president of Robertson Training Systems and co-owner of Indianapolis Fitness and Sports Training. "Plus, you're moving, so it's not as boring."

To do an ab-wheel rollout, kneel on the floor with your shoulders over the wheel, and grab the handles using an overhand grip. Slowly roll the wheel forward, extending your body as far as you can without letting your hips sag. Stiffen your core and squeeze your glutes to keep your lower back from collapsing. Then use your core to pull the wheel back to your knees. That's 1 rep. Do 3 sets of 10 reps, three times a week.

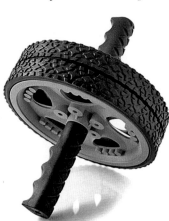

An ab wheel is inexpensive ($13 at performbetter.com), but to save money, you can use a barbell with a 10-pound plate on each side.

Q: My shoulders are so tight. How can I loosen them up?

A: Feel great instantly! To relieve shoulder tightness, do the swan dive stretch every time you exit your office. Raise your arms skyward, grab the top of the door frame, and lean forward as far as you can. Hold for 30 seconds, says Nicholas A. DiNubile, MD, an orthopedic surgeon at the Hospital of the University of Pennsylvania and the author of *FrameWork for the Lower Back.*

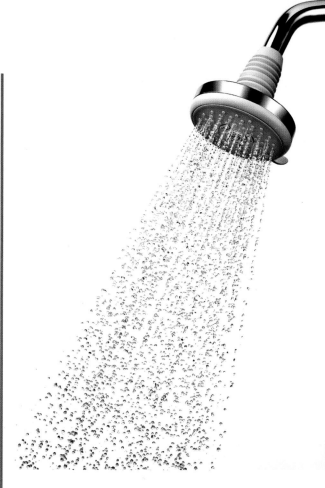

Q: What's the fastest way to eliminate a crick in my neck?

A: Get hot under the collar. "To relieve a crick—an involuntary neck muscle contraction—apply heat to the area and then stretch it," says Monica Rho, MD, a physician at the Rehabilitation Institute of Chicago. Her Rx: Take a shower. Position the showerhead toward your neck, and stand under it for 15 minutes. Next, tilt your head toward your shoulder (as if you're cradling a phone in the crook of your neck) and away from the side that hurts. If the pain is on your right side, stretch your head to the left; grab the top of your head with your left hand and gently pull, holding for 10 seconds. Keep your right hand at your side and reach for the floor, holding the position for 5 more seconds. Then slowly swing your head around to the other side and repeat the move. That should help speed your recovery. To quell any lingering pain, pop an anti-inflammatory, such as ibuprofen, says Dr. Rho.

Q: My knees stiffen up after I run. How can I get back on track?

A: By staying off the track. Take a 6-week break to give your joints time to recover. You'll also need to build up some key muscles, says Bill Hartman, PT, CSCS, co-owner of Indianapolis Fitness and Sports Training and coauthor of *Muscle Imbalances Revealed*. His diagnosis is that you've probably pounded the pavement too much. The resulting weakness in your hips and loss of knee flexibility caused your fascia, tendons, and ligaments to become stiff.

Do this test to see if Hartman's right: (1) Sit on the floor with your legs straight. (2) Roll up a small towel and place it under your heels just high enough for the back of your knees to clear the ground. (3) Flex your thigh muscles and press the back of your knees to the floor. You should be able to touch equally well on both sides.

If you can't, do this test as an exercise: 2 sets of 15 reps (each rep is flexing your thigh for 5 seconds) four times a day until your knees match. If they don't match after 2 weeks, see an orthopedist. If the test is easy but it still feels like you have cement in your knees, then see an orthopedist. For more leg-strengthening tips, check out Hartman's program for runners on *MH*'s Web site at blogs.MensHealth.com/muscle-guy.

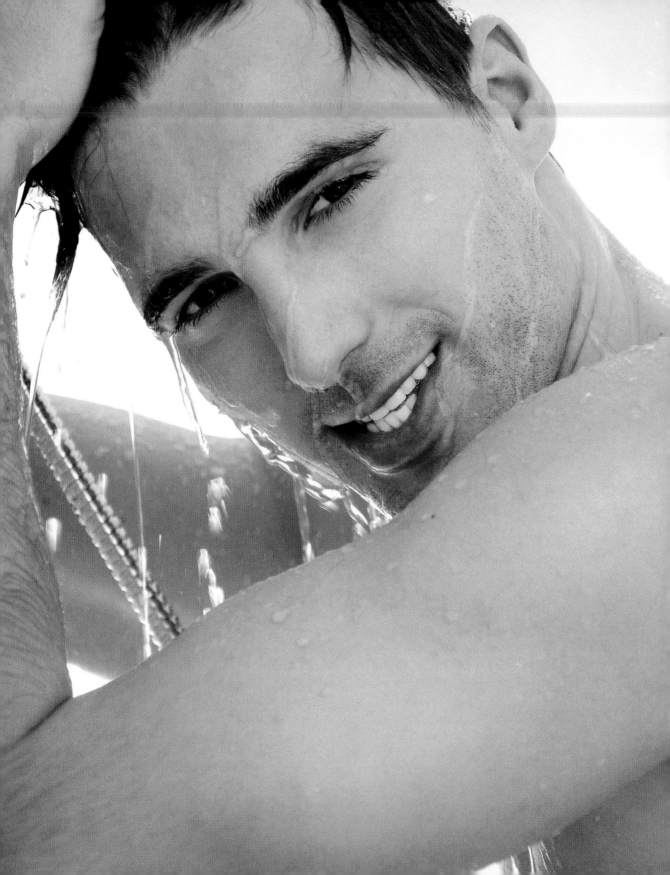

Look Better Instantly

Style: Now and Then

A smart wardrobe combines timeless essentials with timely trends.

With our simple style tips, you can mix the best styles of the past with the top current trends.

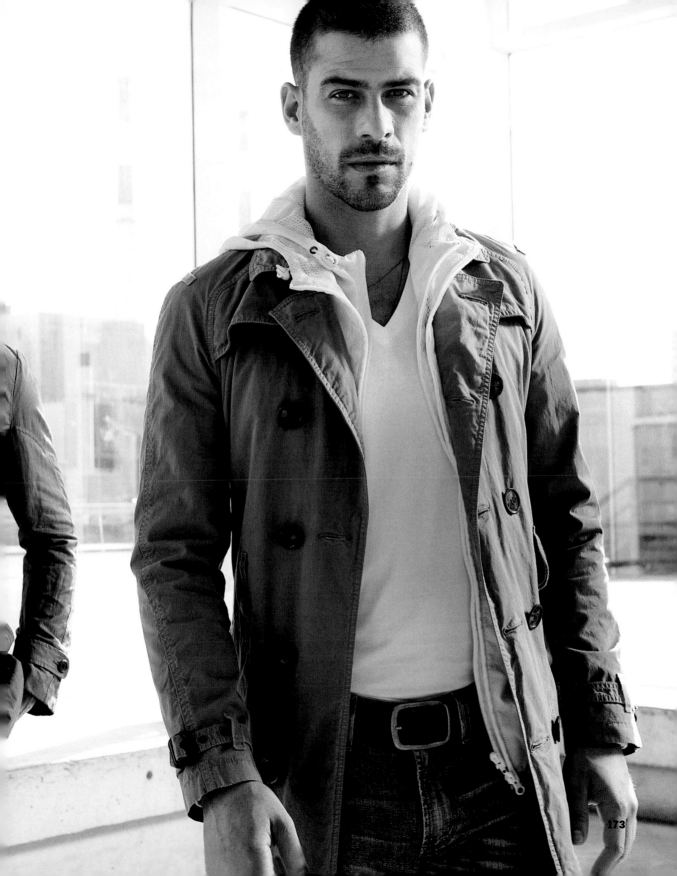

Essential: Trench Coat

This classic can look contemporary with new color options and a shorter, stream-lined silhouette. Combine it with your weekend wear and it'll look as sharp with a suit as it does with jeans and a hoodie.

TREND: BRIGHT COLOR

Warmer days are your signal to lighten up your wardrobe, and not just in fabric weight. A bright splash of citrus tells the world you're looking ahead to spring and leaving winter behind. Too bold? Then layer it underneath to reveal an unex-pected pop of color. Wearing a bright hue with a light neutral, like tan or gray, takes the intensity down a notch.

Essential: Polo

Men cannot live by T- shirts alone. A polo is vital to any warm-weather wardrobe; it's relaxed enough for shorts but cleans up nicely under a jacket. Throw it into your weekend bag and wear it from beach to bar.

Essential: Denim Jacket

Some things never change. A medium-wash denim jacket remains a guy's go-to spring element. Layer it under a coat on cooler days, or add it as your final touch on top of a T-shirt. You can even wear it with your favorite jeans, as long as the washes are at least two shades apart.

TREND: MILITARY PATTERNS

Maybe it's nostalgia for G.I. Joe action figures, but camouflage seems to work in

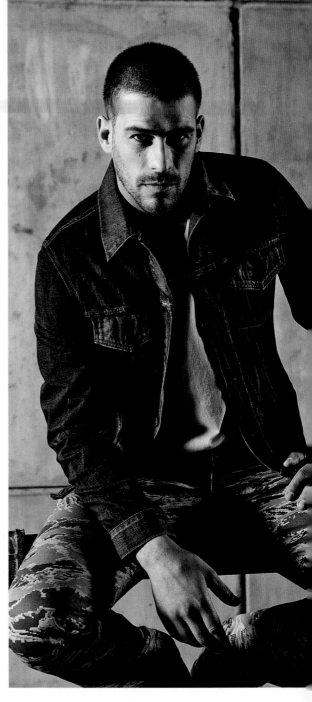

almost any man's wardrobe, no matter what his style. Avoid the oversize army-surplus look and opt for fitted pieces and new pattern interpretations in unique colors and shapes.

The Revealing Details

Los Angeles—land of spray tans and designer denim—might seem an unlikely locus for a resurgence in tailored clothing. But Greg Sato, who together with Annie Imamura cofounded the accessory brand Gentry, begs to differ. L.A.'s past— think Bogart as Marlowe—is a source of design inspiration, and of hope that modern men can recover the lost art of dressing. Here, Greg Sato reflects on what today's gentleman can learn from America's stylish past.

TIES TO THE PAST. My grandfather dressed really well. I grew up admiring his tie collection, cuff links, tie bars, pocket watches, money clips, and tie pins. When he passed away, around the time I was 20, my grandma gave me his collection. I sat down and really looked at all these things, and I was overwhelmed and enthralled.

STANDING OUT. I started wearing ties in college. People would ask, "Oh, where are you going?" Now if I wear a tie and tie bar, I don't hear that as much. A great part of the style renaissance is that wearing a shirt and tie or even a suit doesn't require a reason.

LOST BEAUTY. People look back and feel nostalgic about the golden era of American menswear. It was really refined in the 1950s and 1960s. The style was so well put together, and men paid so much attention to the details. In this casual era, we look back and realize what a beautiful time that was.

REFINED DETAILS. Tie bars, pocket squares, and tie pins are finishing touches that take your look from average to classic. But wear these items in moderation: Two will do.

LOVE OF THE HUNT. I love scouring flea markets and garage sales. America is the biggest junk-collecting society in the world. We don't throw anything away! As a result, you can often find many beautiful, unique pieces.

THE BOX. Being a man is about more than knowing how to fix things. It's also about presenting yourself to the world. Our box set (left) can help. It has the pieces a man needs for an evening, whether it's a business meeting or a date. Everything is there.

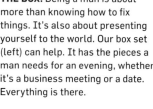

"A man's best accessory is **confidence**."
—Designer Greg Sato

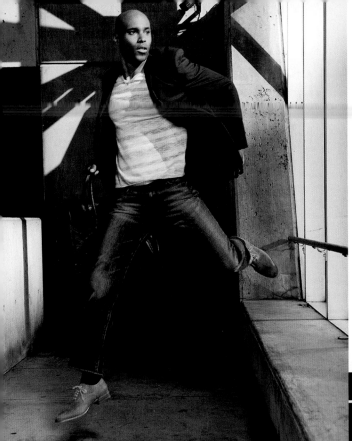

Those pleated, puffy chinos? Out of the closet and off to Goodwill. Sleek flat-fronts, cool shades, worn-in fabrics, and slimmer cuts are what you want. Wear them as you would jeans and they'll quickly become your favorite off-work pants.

TREND: SEASIDE

Notice we didn't say "nautical." An anchor on a navy-and-white striped shirt isn't the look. Evoke the sea with a masculine cable-knit sweater like this one; you're master and commander of your own style.

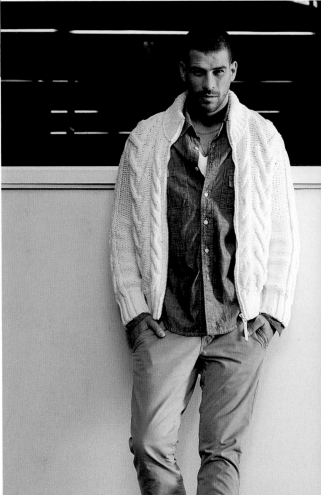

Essential: Navy Blazer

Knock the prep-school starch out of this classic by combining it with denim and a knit shirt. Treat it as an all-purpose jacket, not just a trousers-and-tie option. Stay away from shiny brass buttons; you're not in uniform.

TREND: RELAXED-FIT DENIM

Good news: Your legs are free to move again. The slimmer denim fits of the last few seasons have loosened up in favor of more relaxed looks. No, we don't mean bulky, sloppy, droopy denim, but cuts like these, which mimic the ease of trousers.

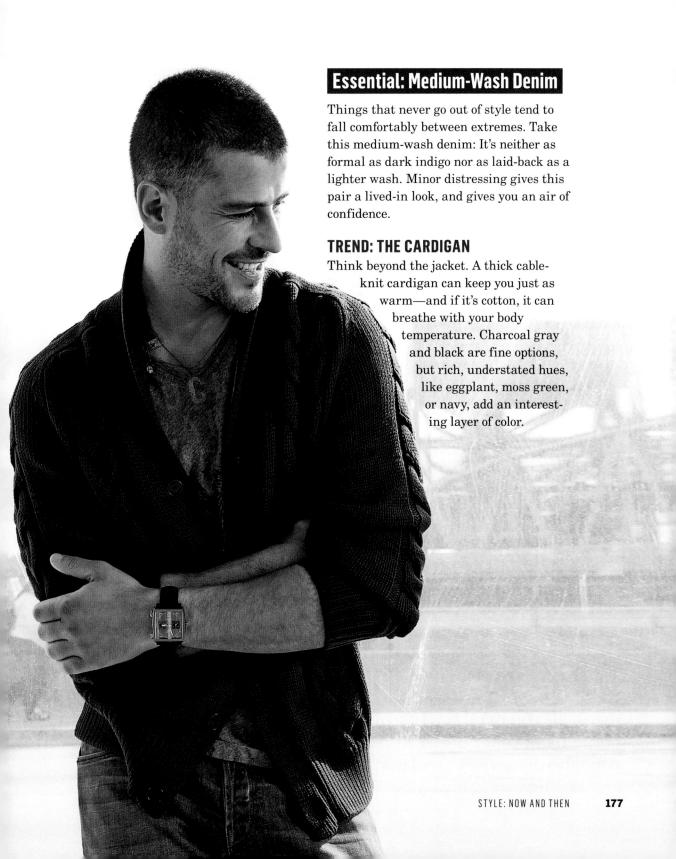

Essential: Medium-Wash Denim

Things that never go out of style tend to
fall comfortably between extremes. Take
this medium-wash denim: It's neither as
formal as dark indigo nor as laid-back as a
lighter wash. Minor distressing gives this
pair a lived-in look, and gives you an air of
confidence.

TREND: THE CARDIGAN

Think beyond the jacket. A thick cable-
knit cardigan can keep you just as
warm—and if it's cotton, it can
breathe with your body
temperature. Charcoal gray
and black are fine options,
but rich, understated hues,
like eggplant, moss green,
or navy, add an interest-
ing layer of color.

The Right Stuff

You want to look sharper, cleaner, and sleeker—and every year, hundreds of new grooming products promise to help you do just that. Here are the best, along with expert tips on how to make the most of them.

You could call it all goop, but that would miss the point. Grooming products are carefully designed tools—and next to TP, they're the most useful things in your bathroom. They clean you. Soften your skin. Help you smell good. You might think all you need is a bar of soap and the shampoo you brought home from that hotel, but we guarantee there's a woman near you who disagrees. And don't worry, she'll speak up.

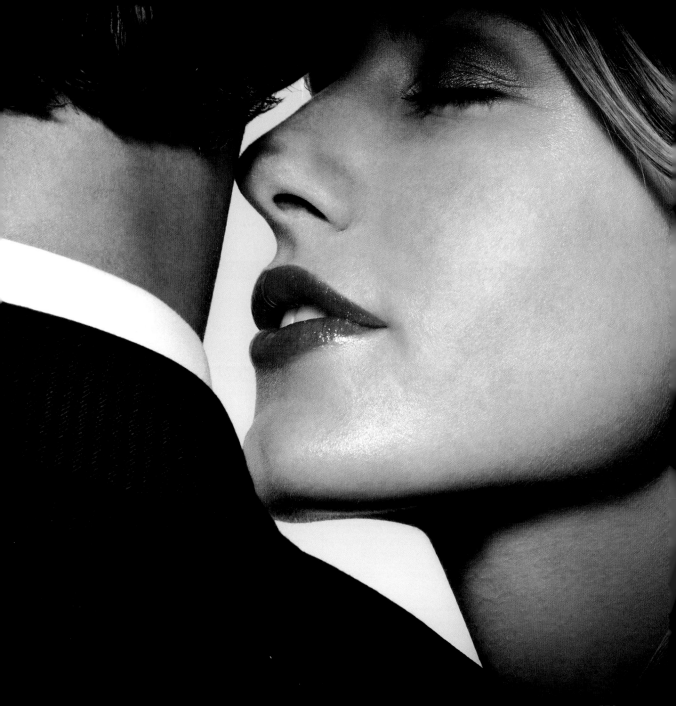

179

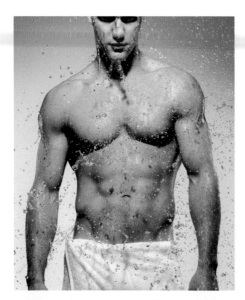

That's why we prepare our roundup of the best new products. We also asked hundreds of readers and trusted grooming experts to tell us about their longtime favorite products, and included their selections along with ours. Pick out a few and try them. You'll be hooked.

Body

The farther down your body you go, the more you need to attend to it. That's because bloodflow slows as you go lower—making, say, your legs drier (and potentially worse-looking) than your arms. The lesson: Attend to individual parts, and you'll have a whole body worth showing off.

Can You Smell Me Now?

Cologne makers say scents smell different on different men. True? Many sprays later, we found out.

THE TEST:

For 3 days, three cologne-wearing *MH* guys were sniffed by a panel of *Women's Health* staffers. But the gals weren't told they were smelling the same three products, each day on a new guy.

THE RESULTS:

Each woman described the same cologne differently, depending on who wore it. Sometimes she loved it, sometimes she hated it. This chart summarizes what the women had to say.

		On Andrew	On Clint	On Jemal
CREED AVENTUS		*"Really sweet and floral— too floral for a guy."*	*"It's like a sunburned cowboy–raw and sexy."*	*"I smell Christmas. Licorice. Pies. He's a walking holiday!"*
PURE NAUTICA		*"A little artificial. It reminds me of furniture polish."*	*"Is this soap? No? Then I'm pretty sure this is deodorant."*	*"Clean and crisp—like a man who has his shirts pressed."*
ODIN 04 PETRANA		*"It makes me think of someone who likes guns but doesn't like hunting."*	*"This is what movie stars wear. Very aggressive and fancy."*	*"Whoa! Intense. I picture a man who wears shiny shirts."*

HOW YOU SHOULD CHOOSE:

Your skin type, health, diet, and the medications you take all play a role in how a cologne smells on you. So instead of buying a scent because your buddy uses it, bring a woman to the store with you. Try a few on, give the scents a few minutes to mix with your own smell, and then let her weigh in. Trust us—she'll pick a favorite.

Scent

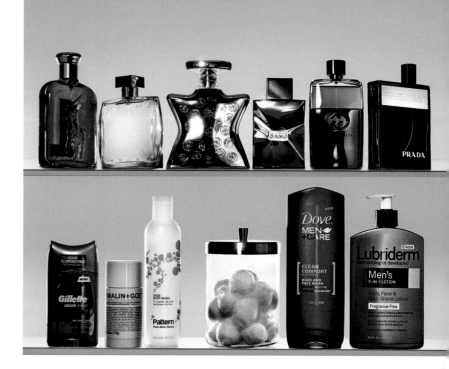

Sometimes the benefit of a good cologne has nothing to do with smell at all. When men wore cologne, women said they looked more confident, a 2009 study from the University of Liverpool found. And that's the big key to winning her over; smelling great is just a bonus.

ON THE SHELF

Everyday cologne:
Ralph Lauren Big Pony Fragrance Collection, #1: A morning mist of this light, refreshing grapefruit-and-lime scent wakes you faster than coffee. $65 (125 ml), bigponyfragrances.com

Classic scent:
Azzaro Chrome: It's woodsy, clean, and modern, an instant favorite. $70 (3.4 oz), macys.com

Statement scent:
Bond No. 9 Cooper Square: Hints of cognac, patchouli, and lavender earn you the right sort of attention. $230 (100 ml), bondno9.com

Spicy scent:
Marc Jacobs: Bang: The black, white, and pink peppercorns provide a bang indeed. $75 (3.4 oz), bloomingdales.com

Fresh scent:
Gucci Guilty for Him: The zing of lemon and mandarin mellows to a mix of sandalwood and cedar. $75 (90 ml), bloomingdales.com

"Women have a better sense of smell than men, so **she'll pick up scents you don't**."

—Alan R. Hirsch, MD, smell researcher

Evening scent:
Prada Amber Pour Homme Intense: This assertive infusion of myrrh, patchouli, and vanilla (with subtle citrus) is best worn after dark. $75 (3.4 oz), nordstrom.com

Antiperspirant:
Gillette Odor Shield: When your pits are really cooking, this is your best weapon. It's stronger than most, and its fresh scent sticks around. $4.50 (2.6 oz), gillette.com

Deodorant:
Malin+Goetz Eucalyptus: Use eucalyptus (with no aluminum, alcohol, or parabens) to smell great. $18 (2.6 oz), malinandgoetz.com

Body wash:
Pattern Sage Body Wash: Soaps can strip your skin of natural oils. This pH-balanced liquid protects pores with vitamin E. $20 (8.1 oz), patternbodywash.com

Reader's choice body wash:
Dove Men+Care Clean Comfort: At this price, nothing softens or cleans your face and body better. $5 (13.5 oz), dove.us

Moisturizer:
Lubriderm Men's 3-in-1 Fragrance-Free Lotion: What it doesn't have: fancy scents or oily films. What you'll love it for: smooth aloe that quenches dry skin. $8 (16 oz), lubriderm.com

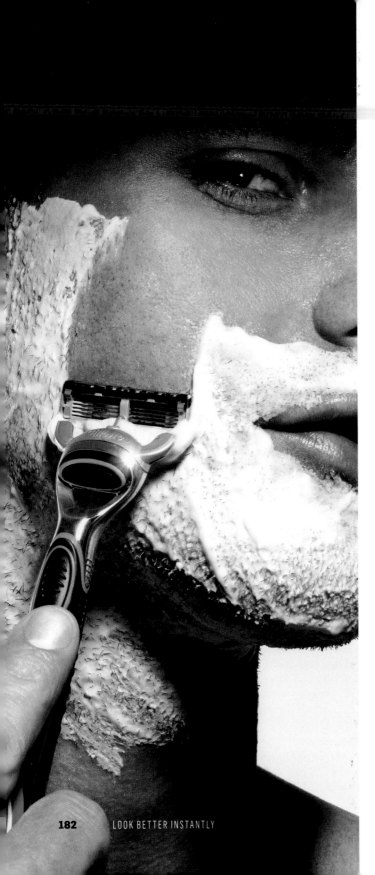

Razor commercials promote fast, sharp blades, as if shaving is a process in need of speed. Don't listen to them. A close shave requires time—for hot water to open your pores, for you to scrub your face clean and remove dirt that can snag the razor, and for the oils of your preshave lotion to make your skin smoother. Come on, your face is worth the 10 minutes.

GROOM YOURSELF FOR A JOB

We asked dozens of hiring managers and experts in nine fields if certain facial-hair choices would affect an applicant's chances of landing a gig. This is what they found acceptable. Make sure your face matches a future boss's expectations. Use this key to the chart (at right).

When flirting at a bar, **most women prefer guys with a day's scruff**. But they say they'd rather kiss a clean-shaven man. (Offer to shave at her place!)

—*MH* survey

+ = Yes — = No	Food service	Teacher	Office worker	Retail	Creative media	White collar	I.T.	Construction	Barber
CLEAN SHAVEN	+	+	+	+	+	+	+	+	+
5 O'CLOCK SHADOW	−	−	−	−	+	−	−	+	+
LONG SIDEBURNS	−	−	−	+	+	+	−	+	+
FULL MUSTACHE	+	+	+	+	+	−	+	+	+
PENCIL MUSTACHE	−	−	−	+	−	−	+	+	+
SHORT BEARD	+	+	+	+	+	+	+	+	+
FULL BEARD	−	−	−	+	+	−	−	+	+
CHIN SCRUFF	−	−	−	−	+	−	−	+	−
FULL GOATEE	+	+	+	+	+	−	+	+	+
SOUL PATCH	−	−	+	−	+	−	−	+	+
FU MANCHU	−	−	−	−	−	−	−	+	−
ZZ TOP	−	−	−	−	−	−	−	+	−

A man's good grooming habits **can lead 8 out of 10 women to overlook his weight gain.**

—MH survey

ON THE SHELF

Shave cream:
Aveda Men Pure-Formance Shave Cream: The seaweed, licorice root, and natural oils help your razor glide, quashing any potential skin rebellion. $18 (5 oz), aveda.com

Razor:
Gillette Fusion ProGlide Power: Its superfine blades have a low-resistance coating, so they move with ease. $13, gillette.com

Beard trimmer:
Conair for Men i-Stubble: Control your stubble down to the millimeter with this high-tech beard trimmer's 15 different settings. $50, conair.com

Preshave oil:
eshave Orange Sandalwood: If you're prone to razor burn, start your shave with this blend of oils. It tones, hydrates, and can protect your skin with antioxidants. $20 (2 oz), eshave.com

Brush:
Art of Shaving: The oscillating motion of this first-of-its-kind brush lifts your whiskers and creates a thick, moisturizing lather—fast. $125, theartofshaving.com

Postshave:
Kyoku SKN-FC 911, Razor Repair Balm: Essential oils from Japanese herbs help fight irritation. Witch hazel, chamomile, and aloe help your skin recover from the scraping. $35 (1.7 oz), barneys.com

Experts' choice shave cream:
Jack Black Beard Lube: It's a preshave oil, shave cream, and skin treatment in one. $16 (6 oz), getjackblack.com

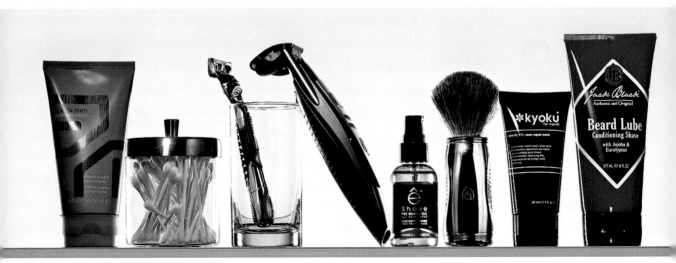

Hair

On average, a man's scalp produces more than twice the volume of oil that a woman's does (thanks in part to pores that are double the size of hers). So we have to be especially mindful of scalp acne, eczema, and other dermatological issues. A simple first line of defense: Wash your hair every other day.

MANAGE YOUR MUSS

It's a great styling irony: The most casual look requires precise prep.

Texture: Medium to thick hair is the easiest type to form into a mess; you'll need more product if you have finer hair.

Cut: Ask your barber for short sides and a texturized top. The key is to avoid being square on top. You want it choppy, and you need enough length to be able to move it around—2 to $2\frac{1}{2}$ inches is good.

Product: Use a dime- to nickel-size dab of a matte paste to hold the mess in place.

Style: Heed these styling tips from Theodore Leaf, Suave Professionals celebrity hairstylist.

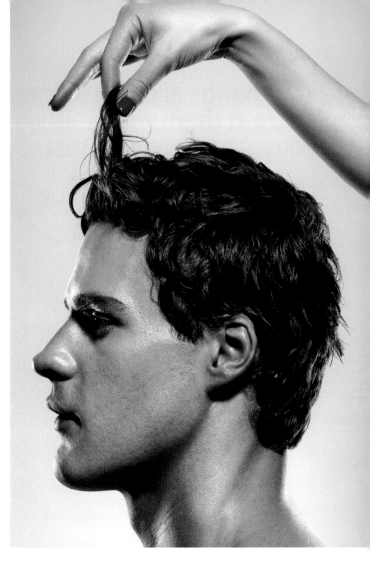

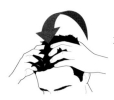

1. Hair is thickest in the back, so start there, massaging the product in. Then move your hands to the front.

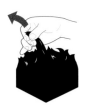

2. Grasp the ends of your hair and pull pieces to create definition. Pull to the right and left.

3. One direction will naturally look better than the other. That's cool. Just don't go straight up.

4. Once your hair is well mussed, don't pat it down; it'll settle naturally. It shouldn't look too shiny, styled, or perfect.

5. If you have fine hair, blast it for a few seconds with a blow-dryer to make the gel disappear. Or let it air-dry and then move your hands over your hair to erase the gel's wet look.

Your hands are thin-skinned on top, so treat them well. You don't want them to show signs of age before the rest of your body does.

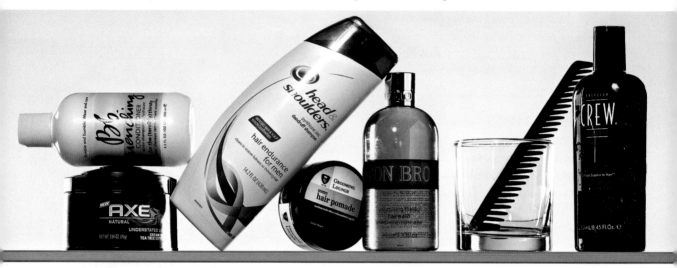

ON THE SHELF

Conditioner
Bumble and Bumble Quenching Conditioner: A dab replenishes moisture that was lost to shampoo. $32 (8.5 oz), bumbleandbumble.com

Styling cream
Axe Understated Look Cream with Tea Tree Extract: Gain sheen without looking too styled. $8 (2.64 oz), theaxeeffect.com

Dandruff shampoo
Head and Shoulders Hair Endurance for Men: It conditions your scalp as it cleans, leaving you flake-free. $8 (23.7 oz), headandshoulders.com

Pomade
Grooming Lounge Some Hair Pomade: This water-based product delivers light to medium hold, and rinses clean. $18 (2.5 oz), groominglounge.com

Shampoo
Molton Brown Volumising Thekku Hairwash: The thekku bark extract coats and restores your hair. $28 (10 oz), moltonbrown.com

Styling gel
American Crew Classic Firm Hold: A low-pH formula helps your hair look thicker and shinier without flaking. $22 (8.45 oz), americancrew.com

Face

Your greatest foes are time and gravity, and both are gunning for your face. The proteins collagen and elastin, which help keep your skin taut, diminish as you age. Sun exposure only piles on the damage. Even smooshing your face into a pillow is bad.

That's why protecting your face is so important: You can't beat time, but if you're smart, you can delay its impact.

ON THE SHELF

Peel
Dr. Dennis Gross Extra Strength Alpha Beta Peel: Presoaked pads freshen your face and shrink pores. $35 (10 peels), dgskincare.com

Toner
Origins Zero Oil Pore Purifying Toner with Saw Palmetto and Mint: Reduces shine and makes skin look smooth. $19 (5 oz), origins.com

Face wash
Neutrogena for Men Invigorating Face Wash: This oil-free gel cools as it gently cleans. $6 (5.1 oz), neutrogena.com

Face moisturizer
Sisleÿum for Men Anti-Age Global Revitalizer: Use it as a shine reducer or a post-shave balm, or both. $265 (1.7 oz), bloomingdales.com

Acne treatment
Dermalogica Concealing Spot Treatment: Sulfur and zinc oxide help combat outbreaks, and the subtle tint works to camouflage redness. $25 (.33 oz), dermalog ica.com

Eye moisturizer
Kiehl's Facial Fuel Eye De-Puffer: Roll on caffeine and hibiscus tea to stimulate skin. $20 (.17 oz), kiehls.com

Serum
Lab Series Skincare for Men Max LS Overnight Renewal Serum: This nighttime product fosters cell regeneration and locks in moisture. $55 (1 oz), labseries.com

SPF moisturizer
Action Anthony for Men Daily Advanced Moisturizer: As it protects your skin, its peptides help keep away wrinkles. $40 (2.5 oz), beautybar.com

Mask
Dr. Brandt Detoxygen Experience: Unlike masks that dry up, this one foams and crackles, releasing oxygen to revitalize your tired skin. $75 (1.7), drbrandtskincare.com

Face scrub
EvolutionMan Wash and Buff: Scrub on vitamin E and microbeads to remove dirt. $19 (4.4 oz), evolutionman.com

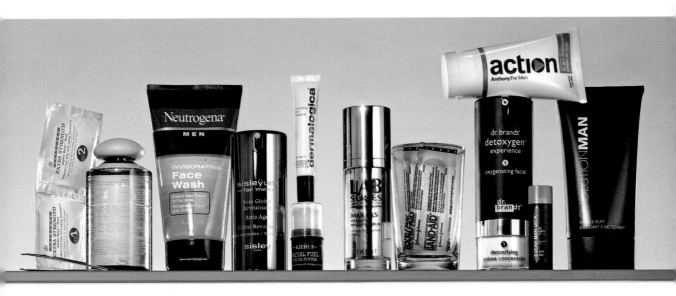

Build a Power Face

Looking for inspiration? We asked five guys in the spotlight what they use to look good.

Guy	A Sam Talbot chef and author of The Sweet Life: Diabetes Without Boundaries	B Ben Mezrich author of Sex on the Moon	C Troy Aikman lead analyst for NFL on FOX	D Doug Reinhardt former pro baseball player, CEO of Fugen Mobile	E Rudy Gay small forward with the Memphis Grizzlies
Why	"I love Anthony Logistics for Men Algae Facial Cleanser. I need something soothing after the kitchen oils set in after a long day."	"Panasonic's Es8043 Pro-Curve Pivot Action Linear Wet/Dry Shaver is the only one that doesn't make my face look like I fought a casino supervisor."	"I've used Crest toothpaste since as far back as I can remember. Same goes for Scope mouthwash. Why? They both work just fine."	"I'm a very active guy, and Kiehl's Facial Fuel No-Shine Moisturizing Lip Balm keeps my lips moisturized all day."	"I like Moroccan oil products because I am half American, half Irish, and half Moroccan. Wait, is that math right?"

A B C D E

Teeth

Everyone seems obsessed with having white teeth. Here's what you should be more concerned about: clean teeth. (They're related, sure, but even blindingly white teeth can have cavities.) If you don't brush and floss, plaque forms within 24 hours. Then it starts rotting away your teeth. Still smiling?

FIND THE RIGHT TOOTHPASTE

Dozens of new toothpastes come out each year. Ridiculous! Ignore the flood and use this guide.

Start here: "Despite all the marketing, there aren't many types of toothpastes," says Matthew J. Messina, DDS, of the American Dental Association.

What flavor? Pick any. "The only reason flavor matters is because you might not brush for long enough if you don't like the taste," says Dr. Messina.

Gel or paste? "There's no functional difference," says Dr. Messina. Just use the one you prefer.

Any teeth issues?

I have lots of tartar buildup: Use a tartar-control toothpaste that contains sodium pyrophosphate, which bonds with tartar and dissolves it.

My teeth hurt when I drink cold water: Use a sensitivity toothpaste with potassium nitrate. It helps fill in tiny holes on your teeth that cause the discomfort.

That's it, except: Use a fluoride paste with the American Dental Association seal, which shows that the product has been independently tested.

People who brush their teeth less than twice a day have a 70 percent **greater risk of having a heart attack or stroke** than those who brush twice daily.

—2010 *British Medical Journal* study

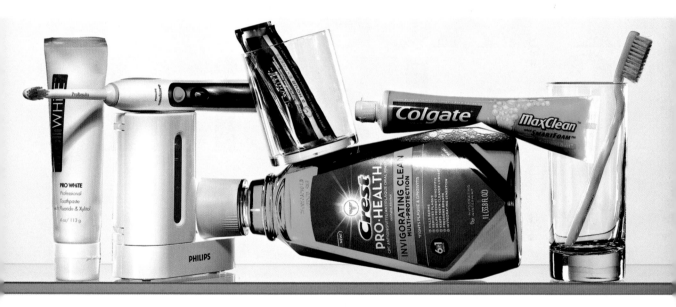

ON THE SHELF

Whitening toothpaste
IntelliWhite Pro White Professional: Low-abrasion, gentle on enamel. $23 (4 oz), rxbright.com

Toothbrush
Philips Sonicare FlexCare+: Its sanitizer kills bacteria. $190, sonicare.com

Whitener
Crest 3D White 2-Hour Express: No-slip strips. $55 (four treatments), 3dwhite.com

Mouthwash
Crest Pro-Health Invigorating Clean Multi-Protection: Kill germs as your mouth tingles. $6 (1 liter), crestprohealth.com

Toothpaste
Colgate Max Clean Smartfoam: It's the king of foamy toothpastes—with the magic ingredient, fluoride. $3.50 (6 oz), colgate.com

Easy Fixes for Facial Flaws

Late nights, fast foods, and fights with your boss will eventually take a toll on your face. Pair up home remedies and helpful products to save it.

What's that on your face? An uneven shave, chapped lips, and acne are just some of the facial faux pas to avoid. Here's how.

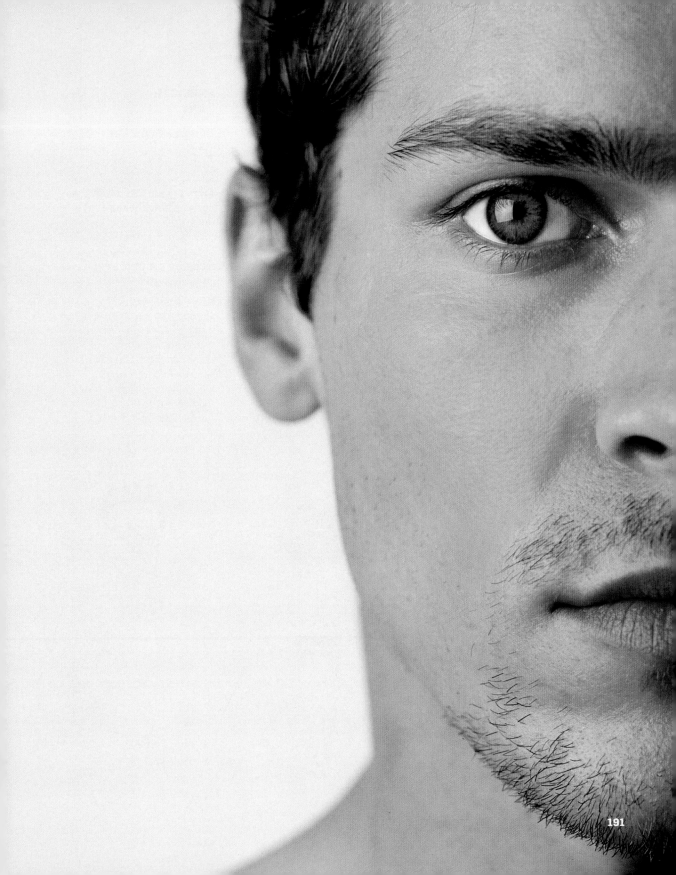

PROBLEM:
UNEVEN SHAVE

Home remedy: A good scrub

An exfoliating face wash is great for your skin, and you can use it to prep your beard for a closer shave.

"Move your fingers in a circular, upward motion to make your beard stand up," says grooming expert Pirooz Sarshar. Do that for 3 minutes, then rinse and shave.

From the store:

Need a new face wash? We like Gillette Fusion ProSeries Thermal Face Scrub. $9, gillette.com

PROBLEM:
CHAPPED LIPS

Home remedy: Water and vitamins

Scaly smackers might signal dehydration—or worse, a vitamin deficiency, says *Men's Health* medical columnist Travis Stork, MD. Eat healthy, vitamin-rich foods and drink plenty of fluids over the next few days, and avoid licking your lips, he suggests.

From the store:

Follow up with petroleum jelly or a balm that has natural ingredients. A good one is Jack Black's Therapy Lip Balm SPF 25 with Vanilla and Lavender, which contains shea butter and avocado oil. $8, getjack black.com

PROBLEM:
ACNE

Home remedy: Less sugar

When you eat sweets and carbs with high glycemic loads, your skin produces more sebum (the stuff that creates blackheads), says dermatologist Ariel Ostad, MD. This can make dead skin cells stick together, clogging your pores and causing acne.

From the store:

If you're prone to zits, help keep your skin clear with a 2 percent salicylic acid face wash, such as Bliss No Zit Sherlock Purifying Cleanser and Toner. The acid removes oils and opens pores. $22, blissworld.com

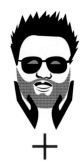

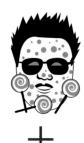

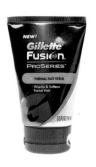

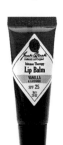

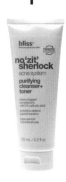

PROBLEM:
SHINY SKIN

Home remedy: Reduced stress

Ever notice that your face feels fried after your boss chews you out? Well, stress can trigger oil production.

"This is a protective action by the skin to increase its function as a barrier against pathogens," says Shawn M. Talbott, PhD, a nutritional biochemist.

From the store:

When stress can't be avoided, don't let them see you shine. Try the cooling Anti-Shine Refresher matifying gel from Shiseido Men. $33, shiseido.com

PROBLEM:
YELLOW TEETH

Home remedy: Crunchy fruits and vegetables

"Chewing apples, celery, raw carrots, broccoli, and other crunchy produce creates a natural scrubbing action," says Jennifer Jablow, DDS, a dentist in New York City. Apples also contain malic acid, which removes the film that forms on teeth.

From the store:

Amp up the effects of your good snacking with a blast from an at-home whitening kit, such as Supersmile's Professional Whitening Toothpaste and Professional Activating Rods. $21 (toothpaste), $32 (16 rods); supersmile.com

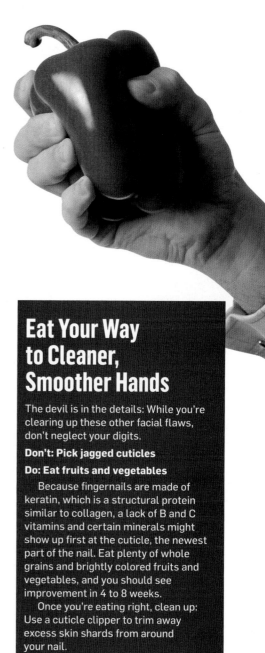

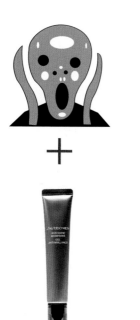

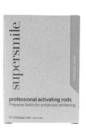

SPF 411

Test your sunscreen savvy.

Is a higher SPF all that much better for me than a lower SPF?

Above SPF 15 you're not missing out on much protection. Just apply something.

Should I reapply waterproof sunscreen after swimming?

Yes. It's not totally waterproof. Reapply it immediately after swimming or perspiring, and every 2 hours otherwise.

Which ingredients provide the best protection?

Look for products with avobenzone, ecamsule (a.k.a. Mexoryl SX), titanium dioxide, or zinc oxide. All of these stop most UVA and UVB rays.

Is a bottle of sunscreen good for more than a year?

Most are good for 2 to 3 years. If you haven't used it for a while, shake the bottle to remix the ingredients, which can separate over time.

Source: American Cancer Society

This model is 87 years old. He's been using sunscreen since 1947.

The Sun Also Fries Us

Not a beach guy? Doesn't matter. If you don't use UV protection, even brief intervals of sun exposure—a walk here, sitting by a window there—can damage your skin, says Neal Schultz, MD, a Manhattan dermatologist. Protect your most vulnerable areas, and block a burn with these smart skin-saving products.

SCALP

The crown of your head is a prime sunburn zone. But typical sunscreens turn your hair into a greasy mess.
TRY: Axe Buzzed Look Cream with SPF 15, which works easily into your hair: $6, theaxeeffect.com

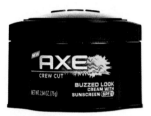

HANDS

Sleeves cover your arms, but your hands are left out there all alone. Some sunscreens need 30 minutes of skin contact before they start to work, so apply it before you leave the house.
TRY: Lubriderm Daily Moisture Lotion with SPF 15: $8 lubriderm.com

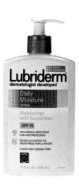

EYES

The skin under your eyes is the thinnest on your body, so that's where your Clint Eastwood squint starts to look alarmingly realistic. Sunglasses with UVA/UVB filters are good, but you're not always wearing them.
TRY: Shiseido Sun Protection Eye Cream SPF 32 PA+++: $33, shiseido.com

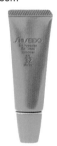

LIPS

Women's lipsticks and balms may help protect their lips, which may be one reason a 2010 study in the *British Journal of Dermatology* found that men are at a higher risk of lip cancer than women.
TRY: Every Man Jack Lip Balm with SPF 15: $5, everymanjack.com

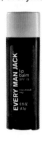

EARS

A study published in the *Skin Cancer Foundation Journal* found that cancer on the ears was more prevalent in men than women. So swab them down.
TRY: Dr. Dennis Gross Powerful Sun Protection SPF 30 oil-free towelettes: $18, dgskincare.com

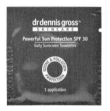

FULL FACE

A blob the size of a quarter gives full protection, says Dr. Schultz. Using less may save money, but you're also reducing the cream's effectiveness by up to half.
TRY: Neutrogena Men Active Protect Face Lotion SPF 50+: $11, neutrogena.com

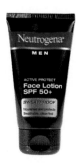

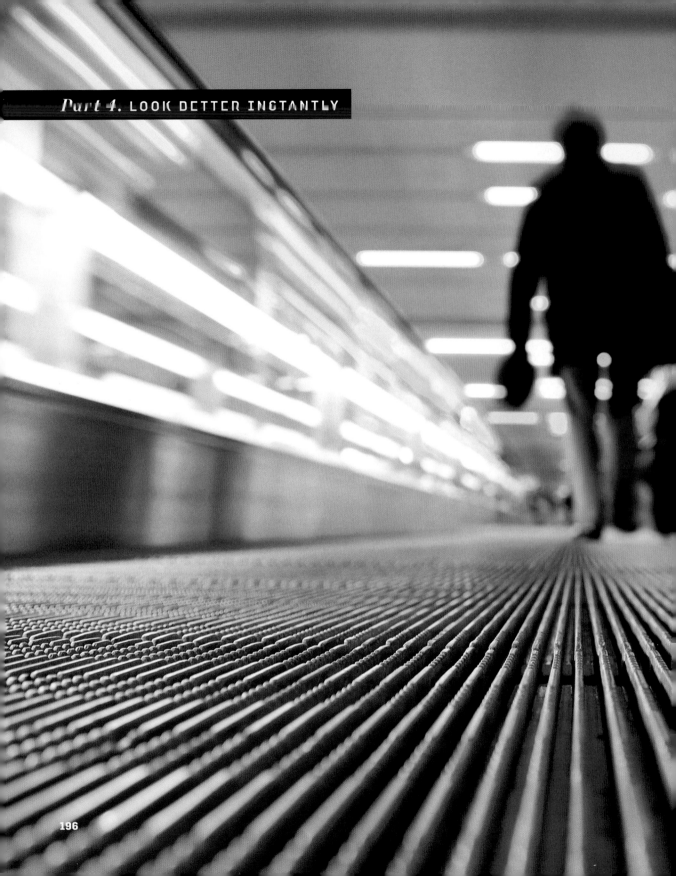

Your Style— To Go

So you need to take your show on the road? Here's how to pack it—with style.

Travel is plenty stressful enough without worrying you look like you flew in your suitcase in the luggage compartment. With these simple tips, you can keep it all together.

Travel Smart

Some of your favorite grooming brands are now in TSA-friendly sizes. Peter Greenberg, CBS News travel editor, shows how to go in style—and we add our travel-size picks.

Moisturize before boarding

Cabin air can seriously dry your skin and lips. Here's the fix.

Air Repair Rescue Balm ($10), which soothes lips and craggy cuticles.

If you're prone to eye wrinkles, try Anthony for Men Eye Cream ($28). It keeps lines where they belong—at the security gate.

Pack twofers

That hair-washing experiment with bar soap didn't succeed when you were a kid, because you weren't using the right soap.

A squirt of Jack Black All-Over Wash ($9) can tackle your skin and hair, and saves you carry-on space.

Bring your own stuff

Sure, hotel soaps are free and plentiful, but they're laced with irritating perfumes that can dry your face. (And even if they don't, who wants to smell like honeysuckle?)

Billy Jealousy White Knight Gentle Daily Facial Cleanser ($6) cleans and moisturizes your face without the tacky scent.

Remember the sunscreen

Don't forgo sun protection because of lack

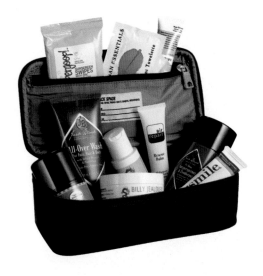

of space. A wipe with Supergoop SPF 30+ Sunscreen Swipes ($10) has you covered. It's not considered a fluid, so you don't have to wedge it into a clear plastic bag at the security line.

Debug that tray

A 2007 study from the University of Arizona found that 60 percent of airplane trays tested positive for MRSA. So if you touch one, use an antibacterial wipe like Herban Essentials Towelettes ($15/bag) to clean your hands before you pop open the pretzels.

Keep your smile bright

Drugstores rarely carry more than a few basic travel-size options, which almost never include a whitening toothpaste. So grab a 1.75-ounce tube of Supersmile Original Mint Whitening Toothpaste ($13) before you go.

Also pictured: The Art of Shaving Shaving Cream Pump ($15), Billy Jealousy Cool Medium Hair Gel ($16), Jack Black Pit Boss Antiperspirant and Deodorant ($16). Grooming products featured are available at 3floz.com.

Know the Rules

The TSA's rules may be familiar, but they're still confusing. Here we grill TSA spokesman Kawika Riley for answers.

TSA signs say 3 ounces is the limit for liquids, but I hear 3.4. Which is it?

"Our 3-1-1 campaign [containers 3 ounces or smaller, in 1 quart-size clear plastic bag, and 1 bag per traveler] is easy to remember. But our European and multinational counterparts don't use ounces, so we settled on 100 milliliters—which is 3.4 fluid ounces."

If my toothpaste tube is too big, can I just squeeze gel into a baggie and travel with that?

"Both gels and liquids need to be in a container at or below the 3.4-ounce limit. So if something strays from that, it will probably be stopped."

Pack Your Suitcase like an Engineer

Use what computer scientists call "best-fit decreasing order." We just like to call it the "cram more stuff in" technique.

1. **Line up your stuff.**
   Arrange what you'd like to pack from largest to smallest.
2. **Roll soft items.**
   Cylindrical objects fit into tight spaces better than squares or rectangles do.
3. **Start packing.**
   Working from the perimeter and moving inward, place large items in first and work down to the smaller ones. Wedge soft items, such as rolled T-shirts, in the remaining gaps. Instead of compartmentalizing, you optimize space by using the entire suitcase.

Source: Richard Korf, PhD, optimization researcher and professor of computer science, University of California at Los Angeles

---

But at some airports, they're more lax about checking. Why?

"Screeners use their discretion based on the intelligence they receive on an ongoing basis. It's up to them to assess whether any item may be prohibited."

Just the Essentials

Pack your toiletries in a bag as sleek as you are.

Jack Spade ($145), jackspade.com

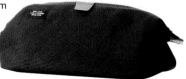

L.L. Bean ($20), llbean.com

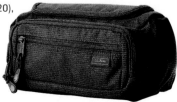

Pack Strategically

You don't need lots of clothes for a trip; you just need items that travel well together.

"Figure out what you can wear multiple times and what can transition from day to night if you add a layer," says Chris Cox, creative director of Nautica and a very frequent flier.

Take this jacket for example. The interior moisture-wicking technology on this Nautica True Travel blazer keeps you cool and dry. Lightweight, wrinkle-resistant wool, with natural stretch, is ideal for travel. A secure inside chest pocket protects your PDA and travel documents.

Here are three simple travel guidelines.

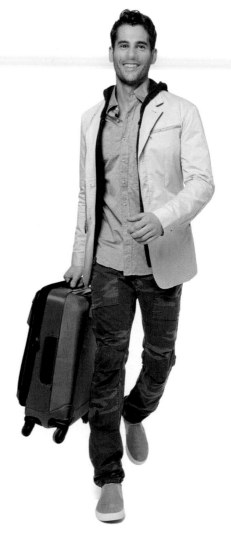

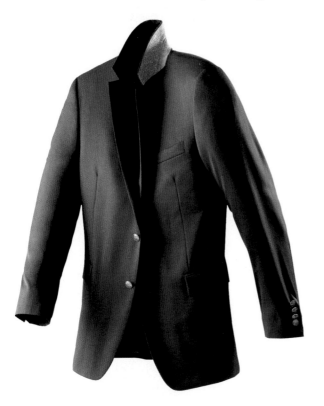

Keep colors consistent.

A suitcase full of neutrals gives you plenty of mileage, because the items all match up. "Everything I pack is navy, white, gray heather, or black," says Cox.

Travel with a jacket that has lots of zippered or Velcro pockets, as this one does. Your gadgets will stay connected—and won't spill out at the security check. Take three pairs of shoes on a business trip: loafers or deck shoes, plain oxfords for dressing up, and slip-on sneakers (like these) for the airport.

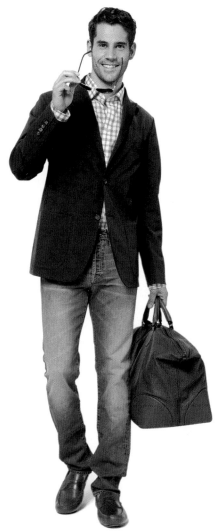

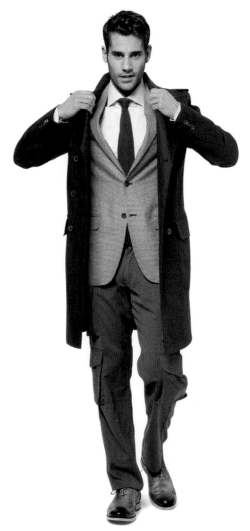

Add a crisp layer.

A sport coat that's wrinkle-resistant can work for any occasion; you can pair it with jeans or wool trousers. But stay simple. Coats with shiny nylon fabrics and giant zippers don't dress up well, Cox says.

After days of wearing those solid neutrals we've told you to pack, you might look and feel a bit bland. Bring a colorful patterned shirt to brighten things up.

Cox prefers wearing jeans whenever he can, but even denim has degrees. "I pack a lighter pair for daytime and a crisp, clean, dark wash for evening," he says.

Warm up.

The most functional outerwear is light-weight and relaxed. This three-quarter length is sporty enough for dressing down and long enough to cover a blazer.

A solid shirt is a blank canvas, so add personality with a colorful tie. To pack one, just roll it (and your socks and underwear) into those shoes you brought.

Jacket pockets shouldn't have to bear the entire burden of your essentials. Sleek cargo pants, like these, distribute the bulk and never show it.

What Every Woman Wants

Do you know what women desire? We went out and asked 1,400 women in their 20s, 30s, and 40s about their deepest dating and sex secrets. All you have to do is listen.

Ask a group of ladies what they look for in a man, and buzzwords fly. Confidence. Independence. Humor. Kindness. Looks. It's as if women are all seeking the exact same guy. (Hot damn—lucky dude.)

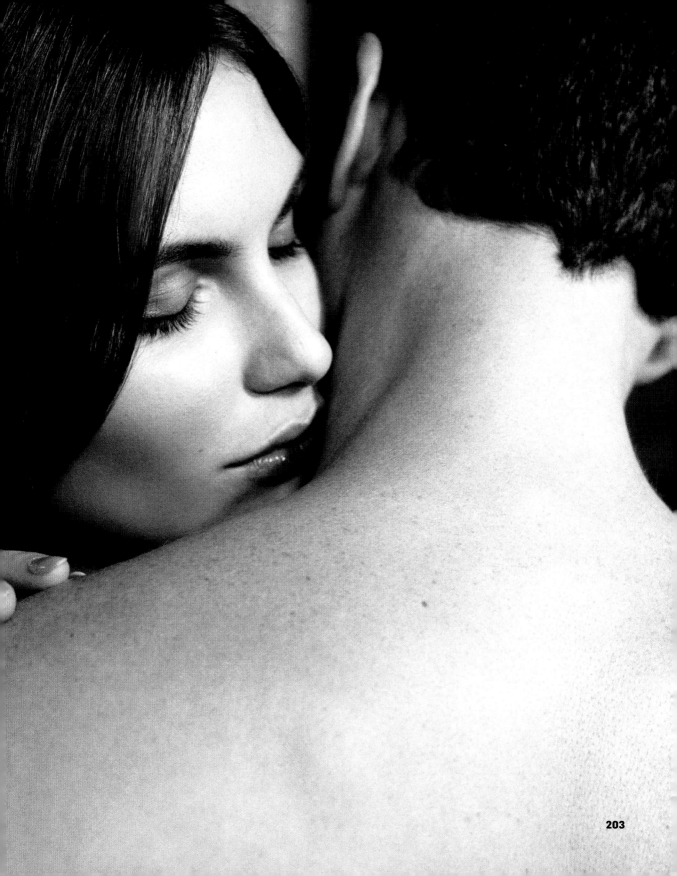

But here's the rub: They reorder these priorities depending on where they are in their lives.

"What a woman looks for in a partner changes as she ages," says Helen Fisher, PhD, a professor of anthropology at Rutgers University and a relationship expert, whose most recent book is *Why Him? Why Her? Finding Real Love by Understanding Your Personality Type*.

So if you want a decent shot at success, you have to recognize what she values at this stage of her life—and know what to expect if you plan to stay with her. A woman who once prioritized, say, grinding to Lil' Wayne on the dance floor will eventually start to prefer intimate conversation accompanied by a glass of Barolo and a plate of homemade Bolognese.

These changes extend into the bedroom too. Very few women become set in their sexual ways. Quite the opposite: A *Men's Health* exclusive survey of nearly 1,400 women found that sexual tastes shift with the passing years. To be specific (and the women we asked were very specific), two-thirds of the women in their 30s and almost half of the women in their 40s revealed that their sexual palates had evolved in the past decade.

For example, a woman who once avoided being on top because she worried about how her double D's looked might eventually become sexually confident, knowing exactly what she wants, how she wants it, and how to guide you there. Sex becomes more of an adventure with age, it appears.

But that doesn't mean you have to wait. Whether the woman you're dating or living with is in her 20s, 30s, or 40s, here's your guide to hitting her hot spots.

20s

With youth comes beauty, ambition, and energy, but also inexperience (and its annoying sister, insecurity). Our survey revealed that trying to label women in this decade of discovery is about as easy as predicting what getup Lady Gaga will wear to her next awards show.

- 17 percent are up for sex on the first date if there's chemistry.
- 1 in 5 have had intercourse with only one partner.
- Kindness was the highest-ranked quality in a long-term partner.
- 9 in 10 have talked dirty during sex.
- 38 percent had two or more orgasms during their most recent sexual encounter.
- 27 percent didn't reach orgasm during their most recent sexual encounter.
- 30 percent say they want more oral sex performed on them.
- 33 percent keep their pubic area bare.

HER DATING PROFILE

A woman in her 20s has three priorities, says Nina K. Thomas, PhD, a psychologist based in New York City. She wants a career, a personal identity, and a relationship. There's also a good shot that she'll walk down the aisle: The average American woman marries when she's 26, according to the U.S. Census. But whether she's husband hunting or taking aim at the glass ceiling (or both), expect her to be a social butterfly.

"Coming out of their teen years, they

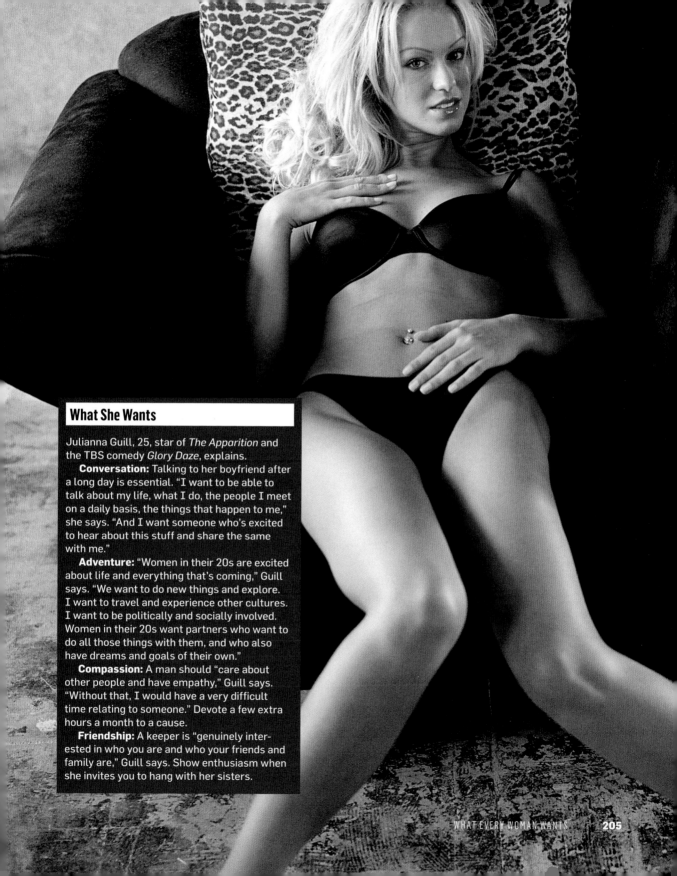

What She Wants

Julianna Guill, 25, star of *The Apparition* and the TBS comedy *Glory Daze*, explains.

Conversation: Talking to her boyfriend after a long day is essential. "I want to be able to talk about my life, what I do, the people I meet on a daily basis, the things that happen to me," she says. "And I want someone who's excited to hear about this stuff and share the same with me."

Adventure: "Women in their 20s are excited about life and everything that's coming," Guill says. "We want to do new things and explore. I want to travel and experience other cultures. I want to be politically and socially involved. Women in their 20s want partners who want to do all those things with them, and who also have dreams and goals of their own."

Compassion: A man should "care about other people and have empathy," Guill says. "Without that, I would have a very difficult time relating to someone." Devote a few extra hours a month to a cause.

Friendship: A keeper is "genuinely interested in who you are and who your friends and family are," Guill says. Show enthusiasm when she invites you to hang with her sisters.

want excitement, they want to go to portion, they want an active lifestyle filled with adventure," says Robert Axel, PhD, a New York City psychologist.

Win her over: Befriend her friends. The math minds behind the online dating site OkCupid analyzed 3.2 million user profiles and found that the most common phrase straight women use is "my girl-friends." Also in the top 20: "close with my mother." "More than any other adult age group," Fisher says, "a woman in her 20s still has strong ties to her own family and strong ties to her girlfriends." So if you date a younger woman, you'll face the friend gauntlet. Be up for anything, especially if it offers a chance to bond with her besties—road trips, dance parties, brunches. Pay attention when she talks about her friends; remember names and stories.

"She's going to want you to fit in," Fisher says.

HER SEXUAL PROFILE

In our survey, women in their 20s were least likely among all the age groups to achieve orgasm during their most recent sexual encounter. And the National Survey of Sexual Health and Behavior (NSSHB) reports that they were also more likely to feel pain during that encounter than women in their 30s and 40s were.

One possible reason: They're fairly new at sex and eager to please—sometimes before they're fully lubricated.

"Women in their 20s tend to be trying every move in the book, and some positions are not as comfortable as others," says Debby Herbenick, PhD, the *Men's Health* relationships advisor and coauthor of the study.

Ignite her lust. Let there be light, says Herbenick. During sex, even a little light—like a candle—is better than total darkness, and not just because you can take in more of her lithe form.

"It allows you to see how she is reacting to what's going on," Herbenick explains. You'll be better able to gauge her pleasure (or pain).

Our survey backs this up. In response to the question "What makes a man good in bed?" Courtney, 20, says, "If he can pick up on subtle hints, changes in body movement or sounds, he's amazing. The more he makes it about me, the more I can make it about him." And when we asked for best-sex-ever stories, Jen, 22, said, "He kept telling me how sexy I was and how tight I felt." So pay attention, and speak up about your desires so she'll feel comfortable speaking up about hers.

She's bound to like variety: The NSSHB study found that the more acts you engage in during a sexual experience (manual, oral, and vaginal sex), the more likely she is to have an orgasm. So stretch out foreplay and mix it up. And keep in mind that in our survey, a plurality (45 percent) of the women in their 20s said the ideal time for penile-vaginal sex was 15 minutes or less.

30s

Obsessions with socializing and fitting in are on the wane. Women in their 30s are more interested in being happy. She may have a lot on her plate—career, friends, a home—but she's independent and ready to indulge her desires. Our survey revealed a sexual awakening: Women at this stage have learned to enjoy themselves.

- 28 percent are up for sex on the first date if there's chemistry.
- Sense of humor was the highest-ranked quality in a long-term partner.
- 48 percent had one orgasm during their most recent sexual encounter.
- 22 percent had two orgasms during their most recent sexual encounter.
- 2 in 3 have used pornography during sex.
- 60 percent have had more than five sex partners.
- 33 percent want more oral sex performed on them.
- 19 percent want more kissing.
- 14 percent used a vibrator during their last sexual encounter.
- 26 percent keep their pubic area mostly shaved or waxed.

HER DATING PROFILE

Many women at this age are starting to see themselves as mothers, says Thomas, the New York psychologist.

"Their selection process is much more guided by the idea of settling down and having children." That's good news! All you men who complain that women date only jerks, rejoice: The more serious a woman becomes about finding a life partner, the more likely she is to reconsider the nice guy she might have once overlooked. You'll enjoy a more fully formed individual too, Fisher says. "She'll be more economically stable and therefore able to express more of who she really is."

Win her over. A date with a woman in her 30s tends to be more intellectual and less social: visiting museums, cooking dinner together, with a lot more one-on-one time. Ask about her passions and tailor your date accordingly. Check out the lecture lineup at the local university, for instance. If any of her favorite authors are slated to speak, take her. Come up with ideas that'll give her something to witness, to think about, and to talk about afterward.

Warning from Axel: Women in this age bracket are "quick to break up with a man who isn't 'the one.'" To improve your odds, Fisher, the anthropologist and relationship expert, endorses online dating, where both parties can find exactly the kind of person they're looking for. Try Match.com or eHarmony (or other pay sites) to find women who are serious about finding a long-term partner.

HER SEXUAL PROFILE

There's another upside to all that buzz-killing biological-clock talk: Women in their 30s are having a lot of sex. And they want more—tonight! Researchers from the University of Texas at Austin surveyed 827 women between the ages of 18 and 65 about their sexual thoughts, fantasies, and behaviors. As expected,

What She Wants

Nadine Velazquez, 34, star of the FX show *The League*, dishes.

Action: I didn't care for sex in my 20s. But now I understand songs and movies about sex and why people are so sex-driven. It's like I turned 30 and suddenly, overnight, I became hungry!"

Maturity: My husband has had to adapt," Velazquez admits. The pair married 8 years ago, when she was 26 and he was 38. "Men who've dated women in their 20s and 30s have told me that women in their 20s are babies, just like I was. They are bratty, selfish, the whole nine yards. And women in their 30s are more balanced, more grounded, and better partners."

Honesty: Velazquez says she and her husband are more honest with each other than any other couple she knows. That has helped her develop into the woman she is today because she's not afraid to be herself. "It takes a lot of courage for a man to be that open," she says. "It's such a gem to be able to have a man who can both tell me what he's thinking and accept what I'm thinking."

Fun: When she was younger, Velazquez would go out because that's what everyone else was doing. "Now my attitude is, if it's interesting and there's a reason for me to be there, I'll be there." Her suggestion for a fun date night: "Spend a Friday night playing games—charades, Mafia, Words with Friends on my iPhone," she says. "I would never have wanted to do that in my 20s."

women with declining fertility (from 27 to 45) acted in ways that increased their odds of having babies (not necessarily consciously). These women thought more about sex, had more frequent sexual fantasies, had more instances of sexual intercourse, and were more likely to want to have sex with someone they'd known only a short time.

However, Fisher believes that the reproduction-expediting explanation might be too simplistic: "It could be that women in their 30s simply know their bodies better than women in their 20s do. They've figured out what they like, and they've figured out how to tell men what they like." Your mission, should you choose to accept it: Listen to her!

Ignite her lust. Among the age groups we surveyed, we found that women in their 30s are most open to using toys in bed. For instance, 14 percent indicated that they'd used a vibrator during their last sexual experience with a man, and 42 percent said they wished they'd used restraints (like handcuffs) the last time they had sex. For a set of restraints that won't hurt her wrists (or yours), try the Lelo Etherea Silk Cuffs ($50, lelo.com). Not sure if she's open to the idea? "Baby steps," says Gloria Brame, author of *Come Hither: A Commonsense Guide to Kinky Sex*. "First pin your girlfriend's wrists over her head while you fool around, and judge her reaction. If it makes her really hot, chances are you're with the kind of person who'd be interested in being restrained." Then casually ask her about it at another time—not while you're naked.

Another tip our survey fairly shouted:

Be more vocal. When we asked women what they wanted to hear in bed, women in their 30s said they wanted to hear how good it feels. "I like any sounds—I like to know he's into it as much as I am," says Miranda, 31. "I love to hear anything about how I make him feel, how I'm doing, or how I look, any dirty talk," says Tiffany, 30. And, "You are so sexy, I can't get enough of you" always works for Karla, 36.

40s

These women know what they want, and they're not afraid to ask for it. Maybe it's because they've done the marriage-and-kids thing, or maybe they're just successful, self-assured, and feel no pressure to settle down. Our survey revealed that a woman in her 40s might be demanding, but that has its upside: more adventure between the sheets.

- Kindness was the highest ranked quality in a long-term partner.
- 86 percent had one or more orgasms during their most recent sexual encounter.
- 68 percent reached orgasm before their partner did during their most recent sexual encounter.
- 28 percent want more oral sex.
- 38 percent have used a blindfold during sex.
- 69 percent have masturbated in front of a partner.
- 1 in 4 have had intercourse with 20 or more partners.
- 30 percent keep their pubic area mostly shaved or waxed.

HER DATING PROFILE

Expect 40ish women to be bold—in their relationships, in their careers, and in their approach to having fun. It's hormones, Fisher says: In their early 40s, estrogen and testosterone levels drop, but testosterone doesn't go down as much. "And so you see more expression of the testosterone system as women grow older," she says. What this means: "A woman in her 40s is going to be more direct, more decisive, more tough-minded, perhaps more daring and independent."

Win her over. Bring enough energy to match hers. "When she wants to go off and do something," Fisher says, "she'll want a man who's eager to jump up and do it with her." This can mean anything from hiking to gallery hopping. "They're not calling up their girlfriends to meet in the bar anymore," Fisher says. Don't worry—she isn't going to expect you to replace her girlfriends. Instead, she'll want someone who's able to enjoy the world with her. To impress her, check out some luxury bargains on jetsetter.com and sweep her off for a weekend getaway.

HER SEXUAL PROFILE

Women in their 40s love sex. In our survey, this was the age group most open to considering sex on a first date. These women were also the most likely to have had an orgasm during their most recent sexual encounter (86 percent). "A woman in her 40s is, for the most part, relieved of the worry of having babies, so she can be more relaxed about sex and have it more often," Fisher says.

Ignite her lust. When we asked women in their 40s how their attitudes had changed in the past 10 years, this was the refrain: "I want sex more often!" Norma, 42, says, "I've become bolder in expressing what I want and in suggesting new things for us to try." That's your cue!

Women of all ages in our survey said they want more oral sex performed on them. Some of their tips: "Use your fingers as well as your tongue," advises Rose, 41. Laina, 40, wants a delicate touch: "Nibble my thighs and be gentle on the clitoris." Larisa, 41, adds, "Clearly enjoy what you're doing. Being hesitant is a turnoff, a rejection of the most intimate part of me."

What She Wants

Elizabeth Mitchell, 42, who starred in the ABC hit show *V*, shares.

Attention: Mitchell has played both lesbian and straight characters. She jokes, "When I play a straight woman, I flatter, and when I play a gay woman, I listen." Take note: "Listen to what she's talking about—if she mentions something once, she's probably interested in it. Bring it up again later. She'll be so impressed!"

Appreciation: "My husband [of 9 years] tells me daily that he thinks I'm beautiful," Mitchell says. "As a result, I feel comfortable walking around naked in front of him. I feel that when he looks at me, he's unconditionally thinking I'm hot. I'm all for it."

Compliments: There's nothing sexier than really taking someone in—looking at everything, and not in a critical way," Mitchell says. Pay attention to all sensory details: "What do her lips taste like? What does she smell like? How does her hair feel? Take the time to pay attention to these details, and a woman is going to notice your effort."

Independence: Mitchell is not a fan of neediness. She's independent and strong, and pleased to be married to a man who's her match. "A man needs to know himself, have his own passions, likes, and interests, and he should want to talk about those passions with me," she says.

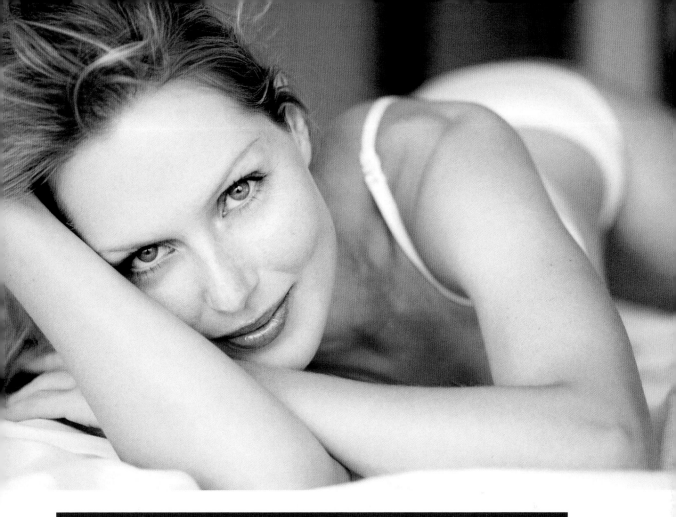

Essential Sex and Relationship Skills

Everything we know about relationships boils down to the following four simple steps.

SHOW HER KINDNESS. For their most desired trait in a long-term partner (out of 10 traits listed), 58 percent of our survey respondents picked kindness. "Showing kindness is as easy as bringing her a towel after sex, or glass of water or wine," says Joy Davidson, PhD, a sex therapist based in New York City. "The best form of kindness isn't forced; it's about giving special treatment to someone you care about."

LISTEN TO HER. Of the same 10 traits, 39 percent of our survey respondents picked listening skills as most desirable in a long-term partner. When she says she likes something, make a mental note and mention it later—that'll impress her, says Isadora Alman, MFT, a California-based sex therapist.

KEEP HER HAPPY. Forty percent of the women who took our survey indicated that they had two or more orgasms during their most recent sexual encounter. After you've reached orgasm, take a couple of minutes to regain your senses, says Davidson. Then challenge yourself to become a multiple threat by showing off your oral or vibrator skills. She will adore the continued attention, and also eventually you'll be ready for round two.

BRING HER A FRIEND. Fifty-six percent of our survey takers said they've used a vibrator, so toy shopping might not be as uncomfortable as you think. Embarrassment-free shopping is what the Web is all about (try babeland.com or mypleasure.com). There's no better time to break it out than after you've reached orgasm and she still wants more.

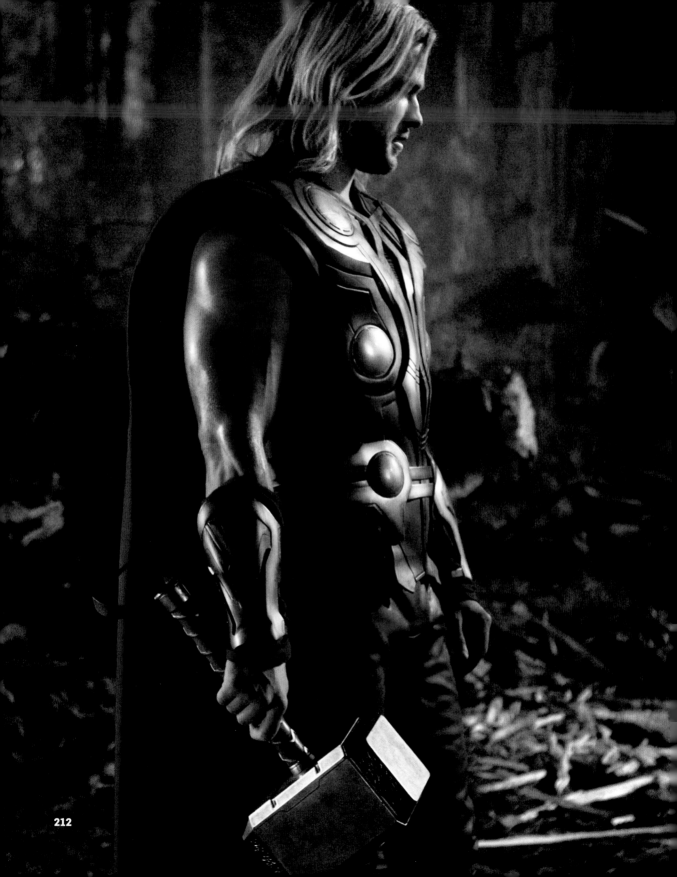

How to Build a Hero

Chris Hemsworth never lifted weights until he set out to become Thor. So if you've ever hit the gym, you're already one step ahead.

Chris Hemsworth first pushed his limits at age 7, while living in an Aboriginal community in the bush north of Melbourne, Australia. He was the rare white child, there because his parents herded buffalo and ran the local food store, which doubled as the post office. "We'd heard many Aboriginal spiritual beliefs about things. We'd been told there was a cave nearby that had spirits in it," he says.

What's a kid to do? This, naturally: "We built wooden swords and hammered nails into them, and we checked out the cave. My friends and I were convinced we'd meet some ghosts and devils."

All they found were craggy walls that echoed their deep breaths.

Hemsworth still dives into places that challenge him—but now, 20 years later, those spots are more likely to resemble the Santa Monica farmers' market where we've come to walk around. It's the sort of place that was crucial for a man who had to pack 20 pounds of muscle onto his 6-foot-3-inch frame so he could play the lead in the movie *Thor*.

Adding that much weight required a constant intake of food, most of which came from protein sources, vegetables, and fruit. "I feel as if I've been busy, but all I've been doing is eating all day," he says as we pass a farm stand brimming with organic broccoli. "Eating when you're not hungry and taking in that amount of food is exhausting."

But every bite was useful, because you can't rely on just protein shakes to help you grow. Sure, protein was Hemsworth's foundation. But nonprocessed carbohydrates, such as fruit, helped him rebuild muscle by slowing muscle protein breakdown. Fruits and vegetables provide fiber, which can strengthen cardiovascular health, and their antioxidants aid muscle recovery. He was strategic, eating for value. For example, he didn't bother with rice but scarfed quinoa.

"It's one of the few grains that actually has protein," he says. It also has healthy fats and fewer carbohydrates than most grains.

Food was only a third of the equation.

"Rest and exercise were equally as important," he says.

Sounds sensible enough. And it's a formula anyone can follow. Need proof? "It wasn't until *Thor* that I started lifting weights. It was all pretty new to me," he says. Before that, he'd built a foundation of fitness purely by playing sports. He surfed as if it were his religion; he boxed; and he even played Australian Rules Football, a

---

How Chris Hemsworth Ate to Grow

Here's how to eat like Thor.

Grow slowly. Don't just eat a ton. Use this formula: Your goal weight × (workout hours per week + 10) = calories to eat daily. If your weight doesn't change in 2 to 3 weeks, bump up your daily calories by 300 to 500.

Pack protein. To put on size, Chris Hemsworth ate more protein than he usually did. The reason: He was eating for the body he wanted, not the body he had. Every day, try to eat 1 gram of protein per pound of your goal weight.

Eat with awareness. Changing your diet isn't easy. Hemsworth was told to remind himself of what each meal was doing for his health. "I ask myself, 'Why am I eating this chicken? For protein. Why am I eating this broccoli? For vitamins and fiber. Why am I eating this Ho Ho?'" (Yeah, why are you eating that Ho Ho?)

Go red. Lean protein is great, but don't give up on steak. "It's a dense source of protein and helps your muscles repair," says one of Hemsworth's trainers, Duffy Gaver. A trimmed 3-ounce cut packs 27 grams of protein, as well as B vitamins, zinc, and iron—all of which can help you grow.

Fuel your workouts. Hemsworth made the most of his workouts by eating before and after them. Drink a protein shake within an hour of training, or eat a solid full-size meal up to 2 hours before you hit the gym, says Alan Aragon, MS, a *Men's Health* nutrition advisor. Within an hour after the workout, eat or drink the same amount.

"You can't obsess over every aspect of your life and career. **Allow yourself to take risks and a chance to fail**."

—Chris Hemsworth

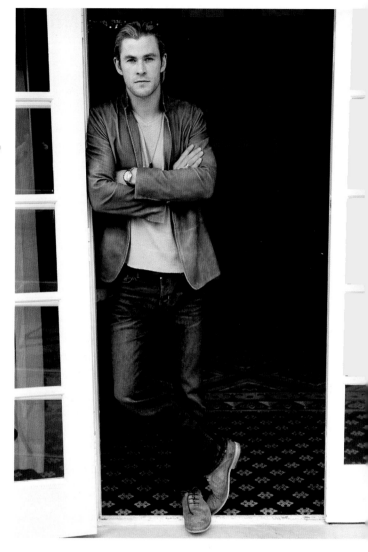

sport that's like the overstimulated love child of soccer and rugby.

But when he hit the gym, he needed to build dense muscle that would show on-screen. That meant dedicating himself to a regimen that incorporated ever-changing challenges. His trainers constantly forced him to vary weight, reps, and even speed so that his muscles never adjusted to workouts. Even minor changes, such as swapping hand placement on a pullup, can stimulate muscles in new ways. In fact, mixing things up is important no matter what kind of muscle gain you're looking for. When your usual workout starts to feel easier, it isn't benefiting you as much as it once did.

If you visit the gym regularly, eat right, and rest enough, how quickly will you see results? Consider this: Hemsworth trained hard for *Thor* while filming *Red Dawn*. If you watch that film closely enough, you will actually see the size of his neck change from scene to scene. (Who smells DVD bonus material?)

These days, with filming over, Hemsworth has dialed back the gym visits—but he hasn't left them entirely, and he's playing plenty of sports. After all, for any sequels he'd have to retain his size—which would disappear quickly if he didn't stay active and eat enough. He learned that the hard way, when he shrunk after only a 4-week vacation.

"My body doesn't sit at that weight," he says.

But with enough work, it will.

THE GOD OF THUNDER WORKOUT

After bulking up for the role, Chris Hemsworth was too big for his Thor costume. So he ate less and did metabolic circuits to burn calories without sacrificing muscle. A few weeks later, he was the right size—and still looked big.

You too can focus on muscle definition, not just size, with this Thor-inspired workout from Eric Cressey, MS, CSCS, the author of *Show and Go*.

Do this: Perform this circuit, rest 60 seconds, and repeat three more times.

SLEDGEHAMMER SLAM
8 reps each side

Stand about a foot from a tire, with your knees slightly bent. Rotate your upper back slightly to the right and raise a sledge above your right side. (Don't rotate your hips.) Brace your abs and swing the hammer down; aim for the tire's inside edge. Do all reps, and switch sides.

The power of the hammer: Thor's weapon of choice is his hammer, which is fitting: It's one of the best home workout tools. "Sledgehammer swings are not only an incredible way to

improve your upper-back mobility and core stability, but they also add upper-body power," says Cressey. What's more, if your legs are shot at the end of a workout, these offer a perfect cardio alternative to crank up your heart rate and pound away extra calories.

If you don't have a tire or a sledgehammer, you can reap similar benefits by doing overhead medicine-ball slams.

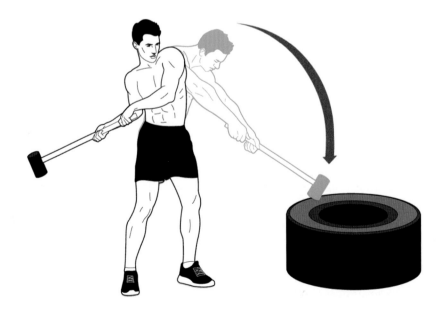

LATERAL HOP
8 reps each side

Stand with your chest up and hips back. Dip your knees slightly; explosively hop off your left leg and move horizontally to your right. Land on your right foot, and "stick" the landing so your body stops moving. Pause, and then immediately hop back off your right leg, landing on your left.

T-PUSHUP
8 reps each side

Assume a pushup position with your hands on hex dumbbells. Lower your body to the floor, and as you push yourself back up, rotate the right side of your body upward as you pull the right dumbbell toward your torso. Now straighten your arm so the dumbbell is above your right shoulder. Lower the dumbbell, and repeat on your left side.

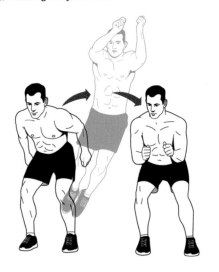

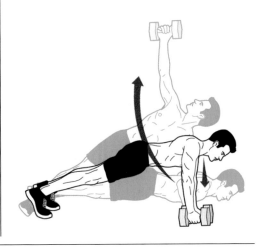

MOUNTAIN CLIMBER
15 reps each leg

Assume a pushup position, making sure your arms are straight. Lift your right foot off the floor and slowly raise your knee as close to your chest as you can. Touch the floor with your right foot. Return to the starting position. Repeat with your left leg. That's 1 rep.

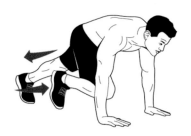

Farm Boy to Action Hero

Skinny farm kid Garrett Hedlund transformed himself into *Tron*'s hero. All it took was hard work and the threat of a skintight suit.

Other kids practiced to make the track team. Garrett Hedlund didn't have time for that, so he chased cows instead.

His family's 400-acre cattle farm in northern Minnesota was at the end of the bus route, 2 hours from school. When he arrived home, he spent his time plowing fields and mending fences. But Hedlund wanted to be the fastest kid in his grade school, so chasing wayward bovines during weekend cattle runs became his practice.

"Everybody else would drive a truck or a four-wheeler, but I'd go out in my boots," says Hedlund, the country lilt still in his voice despite 8 years of living in Los Angeles. "When a spooked cow took off, I'd run as fast as I could to chase him back to the herd."

Soon Hedlund was one of the best runners at his school. His speed propelled him into wrestling, football, and cross-country. These things tend to snowball: You prove to yourself that you can succeed at one endeavor, and that gives you the confidence to try another.

Perseverance became habit, and that habit kicked in when Hedlund made the leap to acting. He had to train heavily for supporting roles in *Troy* and *Friday Night Lights*. But then he reached leading-man territory with the big-budget *Tron: Legacy*, and all that prep just wasn't enough.

"When Garrett came in, he was a little skinny and a little soft," *Tron*'s lead training instructor Logan Hood says. Hedlund's character is a futuristic gladiator, a guy who's playing a video game from the inside as he hurls discs at opponents and competes in a vicious version of motorcycle roller derby. "We needed him to look more like an action hero—lean with muscle mass."

For men with competitive spirits, a challenge can be rousing in itself. But vanity is also a fine motivator, and Hedlund had reason to worry: He'd be wearing a skintight action-hero bodysuit throughout the movie.

"They do a body scan so they can formulate the suit around you. It's three-quarters of an inch of foam rubber that fits you like a glove," he says. "If you have a belly, your scan's going to have a belly." In other words, he needed to shape up. Fast.

Hedlund had been there before. His career sputtered for years because he was either too big or too small for the roles he wanted. At 160 pounds, he was passed over for the role of a soldier-type guy. Too thin. So he worked out and put on weight. But then he was too bulky for the skinny-intellectual part that came up next. Being able to quickly transform his body (and convince skeptical casting agents that he could do it) became a matter of survival.

There are easy ways to shape-shift, of course: You can starve yourself, or over-eat, or just do curls all day long. But Hedlund knew such tactics would be unsustainable and downright dangerous.

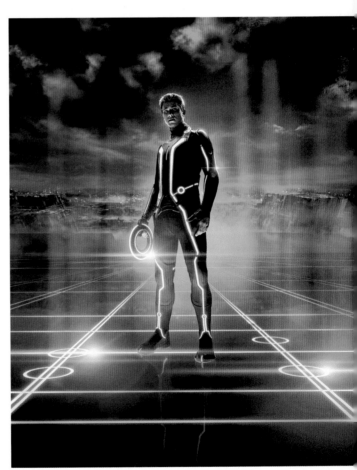

He'd be yo-yoing through cycles of muscle-imbalance injuries, plus giving in to the inevitable bounce-back binges that follow extreme dieting.

Real weight control requires commitment. Once you build a healthy foundation, your body will transform in whatever way you need it to. So during those lean years of his acting career, long before he could afford a gym membership, he regularly ran 2.2-mile loops around the reservoir near his L.A. apartment. Then he'd head home for what he calls "a living-room prison workout" of pushups, situps, pullups, squats, and squat thrusts.

But squat thrusts alone don't make an action hero. That's why Hedlund turned to Hood, a former Navy SEAL who had

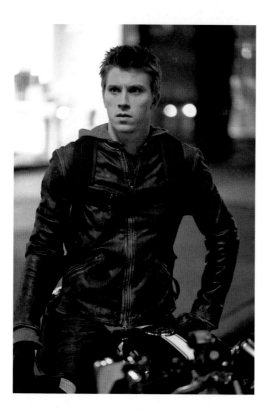

helped train the conspicuously toned cast of the movie 300. Hood had 9 weeks to do with Hedlund what normally would take 6 to 12 months. The plan: "Garrett didn't repeat any workouts, which helped keep him engaged," the trainer says. "If you don't know what you'll be doing when you walk into the gym, you don't fall into a rut."

Hood needed Hedlund to become leaner and more athletic while adding muscle mass, so part of his workouts involved circuits of farmer carries, bear crawls, tire drags, and box jumps—with no rest in between. Try it. A combination like this builds strength from all angles, and busting through at a fast pace keeps your heart rate up and burns fat.

Hedlund didn't love the work at first.

"But then he started to connect the dots: Doing stuff he didn't like was going to make him good at the things he does like," Hood says.

That's because these exercises help train your body for real-world movements. Not all exercises do. Take crunches: How often do you need to lift things while lying on the floor? But a ball slam is basically a crunch in a standing position. It mimics the way you move throughout the day, and how Hedlund had to move on-screen.

In addition to slimming Hedlund down and hardening him up, Hood focused on Hedlund's shoulders. Strength there is key for any physical demand, action sequences included. Without strong shoulders, you're more likely to injure yourself.

"We did a lot of overhead presses," Hood says. Most days he'd also squat heavy, deadlift heavy, or do heavy push presses—a version that should be part of any workout.

Hedlund started as a sloucher, but by the time filming began, he was walking into the gym with swagger. It wasn't just mental confidence showing, though; it was the result of stronger core and back muscles, which helped his posture and gave him a visible physical confidence.

"If he stands taller and pulls his shoulders back and down, he looks more imposing, more heroic," Hood says. "Body-fat percentage doesn't matter. It's really about how you look."

And how you feel.

"You might think the thinner version of yourself is going to be the most positive or confident, but that's not how it is for me," Hedlund says. "When I'm over 200 pounds, that's when I'm the most confident version of myself."

But he's also comfortable with a less sculpted self. Perfection is never what he strives for. That's an impossibility; being afraid to screw up only limits you. It's why Hedlund says he thinks of life as a new car—one you've already scratched. Now you no longer fear a ding or a dent.

There are many correct ways to do something, and a setback isn't the same as a failure. That singular insight is the source of his confidence, he says. It's what allowed him to overcome all the bumps a farm kid hits as he auditions and struggles and finally breaks through in Hollywood.

Where did he learn that? Maybe back home: When Hedlund was 10, his best pal was a steer he raised for competition. The animal won a blue ribbon.

"I came home from school one day and the steer was hanging from the tractor bucket," he says. It was a shock; he was so focused on nurturing it that he never

considered what came next. But after a good cry, he had no choice but to accept that dinner came from the backyard. "Now when somebody says, 'I saw a bird die when I was 3 years old and I don't eat meat,' I'm like, 'Are you kidding me?'" he says. "I eat steak. I eat everything."

You're slapped down, you learn, you adjust and move on.

Hedlund learned from an early age that there's an endless horizon when you live at the end of the road in Minnesota. There's also an endless yearning for forward progress. Garrett Hedlund is on his way.

The *Tron* Workout

Garrett Hedlund whipped himself into action-hero form by doing a variety of daily workouts, like this one from *Tron* trainer Logan Hood.

WARMUP
Rowing: 10 minutes, with your average wattage equal to your body weight.

Bag sprawl: Jump over a barrier, such as a heavy bag, and then drop and do a pushup. Stand back up and repeat in the other direction. Go for 40 seconds, rest 20 seconds, and repeat four times total.

WORKOUT
Pick up a barbell, and don't put it down until the circuit below is complete. Hedlund did 7 reps of an exercise before moving to the next, resting only after completing the circuit. That's a huge challenge, so begin by doing each exercise in the circuit one time. Rest as needed, and repeat for 15 minutes.

1. Deadlift
2. Row
3. Hang clean
4. Front squat
5. Push press
6. Good morning
7. Back squat

For instructions on all these exercises, visit http://www.menshealth.com/celebrity-fitness/garrett-hedlund-workout.

PROVE IT

DON'T MANSCAPE

Here's the naked truth. There's no need to feel pressured by porn's bare-down-there trend. Research reveals that even kinky women don't expect you to manscape. In a Boise State University survey of 456 women, those who watched porn were no more likely than non-watchers to expect their partners to shave below the belt, go commando, or dress sexily. That's because women tend to respond more to actions than appearances, says study author Elizabeth Morgan, PhD.

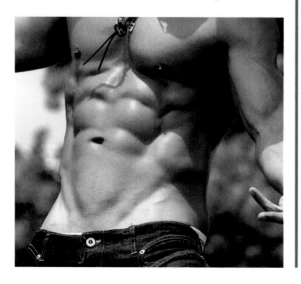

KEEP COOL

Get an unnatural advantage: Technical fabrics—typically sweat-wicking polyesters—are said to keep you drier and cooler. Now Lithuanian scientists confirm that polyester cools your body more effectively than cotton does. In the study, men who wore polyester T-shirts cooled off significantly faster after running in the heat than those who wore cotton ones. The less absorbent synthetic fiber spreads out sweat for fast evaporation, while cotton traps it. The runners wore tees of 93 percent polyester and 7 percent elastane, similar to the blend in Under Armour shirts.

TALK THIS WAY

Ben Stein, ladies' man? Men with monotone voices have more sex, a new study in the *Archives of Sexual Behavior* reports. Researchers told males they were competing with a man in another room for a date and then recorded them as they addressed him. The less a man's pitch varied, the more sex partners he reported.

A monotone might intimidate other men, giving you a better shot, says study author David Puts, PhD. "If you're scared, your voice wavers; if you're calm, you can maintain even pitch." Give yourself a pep talk. Confidence can steady your voice, the scientists say.

SAVE YOUR SKIN

Add about a tablespoon of flaxseed oil or ground flaxseed to your protein shake, yogurt, soup, or salad. It's packed with essential fatty acids that help your skin stay hydrated, say researchers in Germany.

LISTEN CLOSELY

Is she into you? She might say she's single, but listen closely so you can be sure.

If a woman says a breakup with her ex was mutual, that's good news, a recent study in the *Journal of Social Psychology* concludes. Calling a split mutual and dating others means a woman is less likely to go back to her former partner, researchers found.

"But if she has a hard time defining her relationship with her ex, she may be more likely to reunite with him," says study author René Dailey, PhD. Here's another warning sign: venting about their last fight. Frustration that stems from isolated events rather than the relationship itself may lead to impulsive—and temporary—breakups.

SKIP THESE SHOES

It's not the shoes! Besides being a sartorial felony, some "toning" shoes might be a waste of money. In a study at the University of Nevada at Las Vegas, walkers had their leg-muscle activity tested while wearing either regular kicks or sneakers with rocker-shaped soles.

"The rocker soles didn't make their legs do any more work than normal shoes," says lead researcher Jenevieve Roper, MS.

WEAR RED

Red alert: Before you head out tonight, remember, women are more attracted to men wearing red than to those wearing other colors, according to a recent University of Rochester study. When researchers asked 283 women to judge the attractiveness of a man shown in photographs wearing or sur-rounded by various colors, red always came out on top.

"Red is associated with power and status, and it catches women's attention," says study coauthor Markus Maier, PhD. Even better? You don't need to be wearing it—just being near the color can work.

FIND YOUR GROOVE

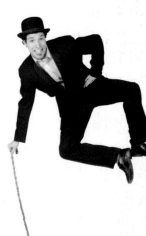

Does your "Thriller" thrill her? Women judge how hot you are by your dance moves, say researchers in Germany. Two groups of women watched men dance and scored them on either attractiveness or risk-taking propensity. The most adventurous men, the study found, were also rated the hottest.

Killer moves might signal desirable traits such as status and competitiveness, says study author Bernhard Fink, PhD. So bust out some signature steps with confidence. Imitating others is obvious—and unattractive.

PLAY HARD TO GET

Try to stay cool around a crush. Women are more attracted to men whose feelings about them are a mystery, the journal *Psychological Science* reveals. In a study using online profiles, women were told that men either liked them, rated them average, or had unknown feelings. The women rated the mysterious guys as most attractive. Being inscrutable makes her think about you more, the study authors say.

Q: Are those sunglasses with interchangeable lenses really worth the price?

A: It depends on how much of a control freak you are. An array of interchangeable lenses allows you to precisely match lens tint to the light conditions and your activity so you can make out certain sights more clearly, says Bill Harrison, OD, an optometrist who advises the Philadelphia Phillies.

Pictured here, the 0.9-ounce Rudy Project Rydon works with 28 different lenses (from $230, e-rudy.com). Our pick: the gray polarized photochromic option.

But a single pair of photochromic lenses, which can adjust to a range of light conditions,

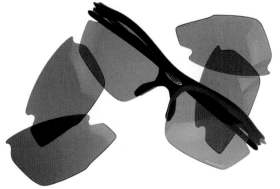

can be more practical. Use this guide to select the right shades for your needs.

Lens color: Gray keeps colors true while reducing glare. Red knocks out more blue light, creating a tint that improves depth perception, which is useful for runners and cyclists. Amber and green add to the contrast of objects on grass and against blue skies, helpful for tennis, golf, and softball.

Polarization: This lens filter works like window blinds to reduce horizontal glare, especially reflections off shiny surfaces like water.

Light transmission: This refers to the percentage of visible light that the lens allows through. (Also check that all UVA and UVB rays are blocked.) A 10 to 20 percent rating is best for bright conditions; 20 to 50 percent for semibright light, says Harrison. Photochromic lenses bridge the gap: They adjust utomatically to changes in brightness and typically have a 30 percent range, from 15 to 45 percent, for example.

Q: How can I instantly rev up my confidence?

A: Think about the happiest moment of your life. Feels great, right? Confidence isn't about saying the right things or using learned gestures. It's about focusing on a positive emotion and letting that generate positive body language, says Nick Morgan, PhD, a communications consultant who has advised politicians and Fortune 500 CEOs.

"Research from MIT shows that when people believe they'll be successful, their body language conveys confidence. You're channeling that same pathway."

Before a date, a dinner party, or an important meeting, take several minutes to think about a moment when you were truly successful. Engage all your senses, says Morgan. "Remember sounds, smells, tastes, colors, and feelings associated with that moment, whether it was the day you walked down the aisle or the day you earned your first promotion." Then have at it. You'll stand straighter, radiate energy, and wow everyone around you.

Q: If a soft-bristled toothbrush is best for my teeth, why do they still make the medium and firm kind?

A: To clean grout? Actually, it's because there's a perception—an incorrect one—that a firm toothbrush cleans teeth better, says Matthew J. Messina, DDS, of the American Dental Association (ADA). "So people ask for them and companies label them that way."

The bristles on soft brushes have finer, more flexible filaments that are gentler on your teeth and gums, yet still clean efficiently. In fact, researchers from Poland recently found that 37.5 percent more hard-brush fans than soft brushers suffer from receding gum lines.

Q: I'm in my 20s and already have some gray. Is this normal?

A: Check out the hair at your next family reunion. We're betting you blend right in. Scientists now believe that about 80 percent of graying is genetic, says Desmond Tobin, PhD, a professor of cell biology at the University of Bradford, England.

No one knows what actually drives hair to lose its ability to make natural pigment and turn gray, but Tobin's research has shown that oxidative stress can damage the pigment cells in hair follicles. To slow graying naturally, eat a diet rich in antioxidants and avoid environmental pollutants, especially cigarette smoke, says Tobin. Of course, there's always the dye option.

"Try a demipermanent color, which fades out and doesn't show a line as your hair grows," says Francine Nash, national technical director of John Allan's grooming clubs. "Dark-brown 'lowlighting' can give you a natural, smoky look."

Q: What's the best way to banish bad breath?

A: To slay this dragon, you have to attack it at night.

"While you're asleep, you produce less germ-killing saliva, allowing the bacteria that cause halitosis to flourish," says Kenneth Young, DDS, a Manhattan-based dentist and *Men's Health* dentistry advisor. You already brush (and should be flossing) before you go to bed, but you should also scrub your tongue: It's a haven for a large proportion of the bacteria in your mouth.

Pick up a tongue scraper—the low-profile kind, so you can reach the back of your mouth—and while you're at the drugstore, grab a bottle of mouth rinse containing cetylpyridinium chloride. Research from the University of Southern California shows that this antibacterial agent is the most effective bug killer you can buy over the counter.

Our pick? Crest Pro-Health Complete, because it doesn't contain any drying alcohol. As for your daytime strategy, it's simple: Try to brush and rinse after lunch. And to keep your saliva levels high and your bacteria levels low, opt for sugarless varieties of gum or candy.

YOU ASKED

Q: My washer smells kind of funky. Is there some trick to cleaning it?

A: Turns out your washing machine can clean your clothes but can't clean itself. Dirt, grease, bacteria, mildew, and skin cells form nose-wrinkling residues that stick to the outer tub, and the machine's normal wash cycle isn't really able to clean them away.

The only way to scrub this tub is by running it empty on the hottest cycle with a dose of washing-machine cleaner. Linda Cobb, a cleaning expert and owner of the Queen of Clean website (queenofclean.com), recommends citrus-based Smelly Washer ($17, smellywasher.com) because it can bust the crud without using any harsh or toxic chemicals. If your machine still stinks after the treatment, check the owner's manual for the location of the drain filter. Most washers have a filter in the back that you can unscrew. As much as a gallon of water could pour out, so keep several towels on hand. Once you've finished draining (and screwed the filter back in), do a final sniff test. All clear? Going forward, drain your washer annually, and make sure you always use the right amount of detergent when you wash your clothes, says Cobb. "If you use too much, that nasty residue builds up faster."

Q: My buddy is using his wife's eyelash thickener on his bald spot. Bad idea?

A: The stuff your buddy is siphoning is probably Latisse, which is an Rx treatment for women who want to grow fuller, longer eyelashes. Latisse binds to receptors to stop hair-follicle shrinkage. It also extends the hair's growth cycle and makes more hair sprout from each follicle.

But don't get too excited, says Robert M. Bernstein, MD, a clinical professor of dermatology at Columbia University. "We don't know if it's safe to apply over a large area where there's more potential for side effects."

The most current research from the manufacturer shows that only about 4 percent of women have experienced eye irritation and redness, and that skin darkening can also occur. But even if the side effects from a scalp-sized dose are innocuous, there's still the question of whether Latisse is worth its price: $120 for a month's supply. That's quadruple the price of Rogaine and almost double that of Propecia.

"Latisse would probably work better than Rogaine but not as well as Propecia," says Dr. Bernstein. "And it would be best used on thinning hair, not bald spots."

Our advice: For now, stick with the proven (and cheaper) ways to save your pate.

Q: What's the best way to lace my dress shoes?

A: Take your cue from the style maestros of the Old World and run the laces horizontally rather than crisscrossing them. The European pattern looks elegant, and it holds your foot securely on the inside, explains John Halton, ScD, a retired mathematician

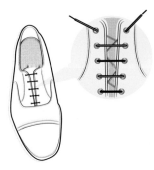

who has studied lacing techniques. Cap it off with a nonslip Cambridge knot, a variation of a surgeon's knot, and you'll never have to retie an unruly shoe again.

1. With your shoes facing you, feed one end of the lace down into the bottom-right eyelet and the other end down into the bottom-left eyelet. Then pull them through, making sure they're equal. You'll make a straight bar across the outside; the lace should be on the inside.

2. Thread the right-side lace up through the second-left eyelet, across the shoe, and down through the matching right-side eyelet. Do the same with the left-side lace in the third pair of eyelets, and then the right-side lace in the fourth pair.

3. Feed the ends of the laces up through the remaining eyelets.

4. Secure your shoe with a nonslip Cambridge knot. Make a half knot and then two bunny ears. Cross and pull the left loop through, but before you pull the two bunny ears tight, pass the left ear through the loop again and pull tight.

Q: Is it worth switching to an organic dry cleaner because of the cancer risk?

A: The dirty truth is that researchers don't know. After recently reviewing the EPA's assessment of the toxicology of perchloroethylene, or PERC—a solvent used by 80 percent of dry cleaners—the National Research Council (NRC) confirmed its conclusion that PERC is a likely human carcinogen.

"We didn't feel there were strong enough human studies to list it as a known human carcinogen, but many animal studies link PERC to cancer," says Ivan Rusyn, MD, PhD, a professor of environmental sciences and engineering at the University of North Carolina at Chapel Hill and a member of the NRC panel. "The problem is that it's very difficult to know how much exposure you receive from visiting a dry cleaner or being around the clothes, because no conclusive studies exist."

Until that research is done, it's prudent—and easy—to lower your exposure, he says. Keep your windows down in your car when you're bringing your clothes home. Then, to let the solvents dissipate, remove the plastic and leave the clothes in a room with good air circulation for a few hours instead of storing them in the closet right away. As for organic options, wet cleaning and carbon dioxide are the most ecofriendly, but few businesses use them; find one at nodryclean.com. A third option is liquid silicone, which is less green but more widely available; find a cleaner at greenearthcleaning.com.

Q: Everyone wears blue dress shirts. What's an alternative summer color that will make me stand out?

A: Pink. It works because it has a highly reflective quality, says Leatrice Eiseman, executive director of the Pantone Color Institute. "It gives a warm glow to your face no matter what your skin tone, boosting the appearance of well-being, which is an added bonus on days when you're not feeling so hot."

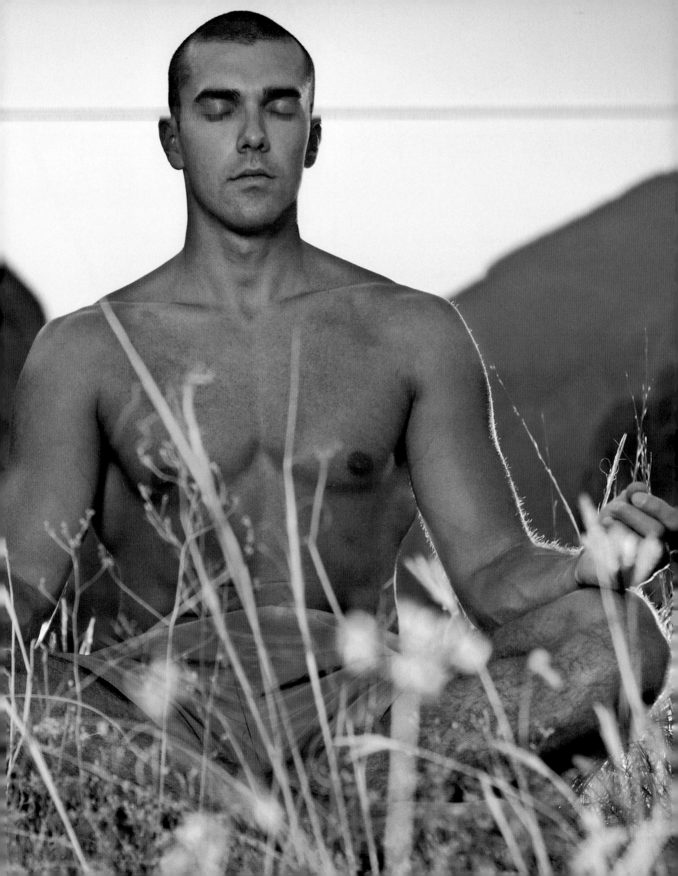

Live Longer, Live Better

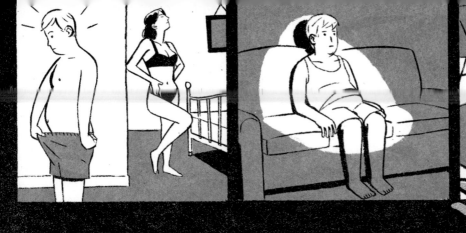

Your Healthiest Year Ever!

Check your vitals against the average guy's. Then remind yourself: It's not about making the cut. It's about setting the bar.

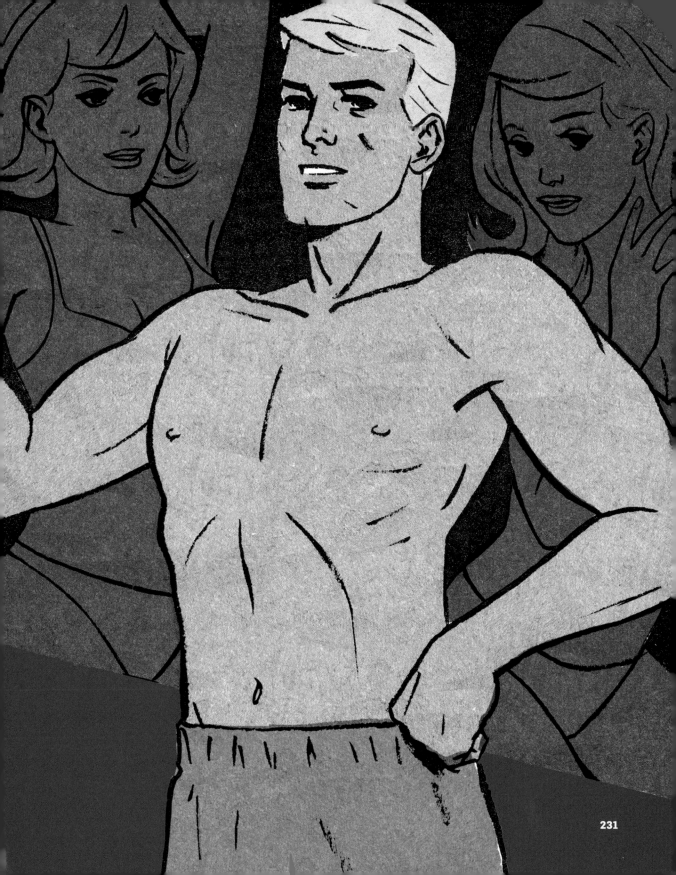

You wouldn't ask an average guy to stand beside you at your wedding. After all, you want someone you can call your best man. Nor would you brag to your buds about your amazingly average sex life. (Then again, maybe you'd be perfectly happy with seven or eight times a month.) And you probably wouldn't tell your boss that you put "just average" effort into that critical project—unless, of course, you have only an average aversion to unemployment.

Guess what? Settling for average health is an even dumber move. That's because in the past half century, "average" health has come to mean overweight, sedentary, and significantly more vulnerable to illness than men were a generation or two ago.

"Our bodies have changed over the years," says John Elefteriades, MD, chief of cardiothoracic surgery at Yale University's School of Medicine. "We've engineered physical exertion out of our lives, and we eat all day. It's time for our bodies to revert to the way they're supposed to function."

Fortunately, we're not average. We've scoured the latest research and talked to the nation's top docs to bring you two dozen strategies that can help you achieve chart-topping vitals. Follow our advice, and you'll reengineer your body for optimal performance—in the bedroom, at the gym, and most important, on the exam table.

So go ahead, dust off your tux. In a few months, you'll be your own best man.

Protect Against Heart Disease

- Odds that the average 40-year-old guy will develop heart disease in his lifetime: **1 in 2**
- Percentage of male heart-disease sufferers who never showed any symptoms before it killed them: **50**

Tame that temper. If you frequently find yourself flipping the finger at other drivers or yelling at the TV when your team tanks (um, Cowboys?), repeat this mantra: Lose my cool, lose my life. Accord-

YOUR MOST VITAL VITALS
Resting heart rate

AVERAGE GUY: 75 beats per minute (BPM)

TARGET: Less than or equal to 60 BPM

HELPS ASSESS: Cardiovascular fitness, heart disease risk, stroke risk

IMPROVE YOUR NUMBER: Speed it up to slow it down. During pickup games, volunteer to play guard rather than center. You'll raise your heart rate (and improve your cardiovascular fitness) more, according to a 2009 *Journal of Strength and Conditioning Research* study.

ing to a recent study review in the *Journal of the American College of Cardiology*, angry outbursts are more likely to cause heart disease in men than in women. While the reason for the gender difference isn't clear, the effect on your arteries is: chronic inflammation that can lead to a chest-clutching clog.

Can't manage your anger? Maurice Schweitzer, PhD, a psychology researcher at the University of Pennsylvania, recommends eliminating the little everyday irritants in your life—that leaky faucet, your cluttered desk at the office, those unanswered e-mails lingering in your in-box. This way, when the bigger triggers hit— and they will—your short fuse won't already be smoldering.

Lower your heart volume. Listen up: Is your work environment annoyingly noisy? In a 2010 study in the journal *Occupational and Environmental Medicine*, people who were chronically exposed to loud noises while on the job were twice as likely to have heart disease as those who toiled in blissful silence.

"Noise exposure may trigger the release of stress hormones, which can constrict coronary arteries and reduce blood supply to your heart," says study author Wenqi Gan, MD, PhD.

Interrupt the aural assault by taking periodic "quiet" breaks of 10 to 15 minutes: Wear noise-canceling headphones or go for a stroll to a less populated part of the building. Also consider turning off the ringer on your phone and muting your computer to eliminate the occasional shrill bursts of noise.

Improve Your Sexual Health

- Percentage of men who suffer from premature ejaculation: **18**
- Of those, percentage who haven't sought help from a doctor: **96**
- Length of time a man with PE lasts: **20 to 80 seconds**
- Time the average guy lasts: **7 minutes**

Flex your sex muscle. While your bulbo-cavernosus isn't the kind of muscle you can work in the gym (unless you want to be thrown out), it's worth training, especially if you suffer from premature ejaculation.

"When this muscle contracts, nerves send a signal up your spinal cord to suppress arousal and keep you going longer," says Darius Paduch, MD, PhD, an associate professor of urology at Cornell University.

YOUR MOST VITAL VITALS
Testosterone

AVERAGE GUY: 511 nanograms/deciliter (ng/dl)

TARGET: Greater than or equal to 650 ng/dl

HELPS DIAGNOSE: Decreased sex drive, erectile dysfunction, infertility

IMPROVE YOUR NUMBER: Exercise is already a natural T booster, but you can raise this hormone even higher by popping a piece of caffeinated gum before you start sweating. In a recent study from New Zealand, athletes who chewed Jolt gum prior to exercising had testosterone increases that were 12 percent greater than those of the gum-free guys.

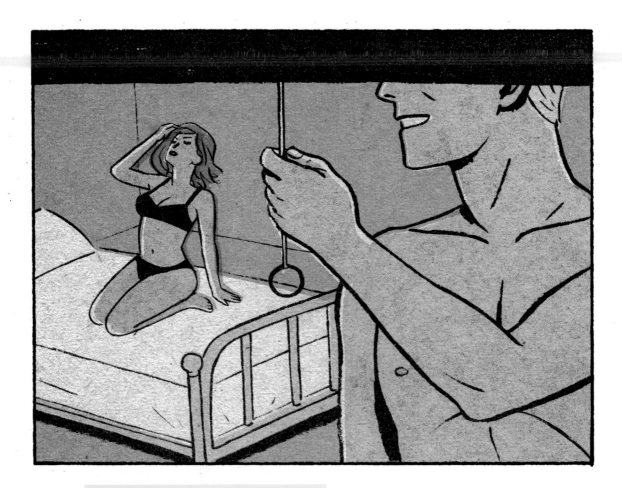

YOUR MOST VITAL VITALS
Sperm count

AVERAGE GUY: 89 million/milliliter (million/ml)

TARGET: Greater than 40 million/ml

HELPS DIAGNOSE: Infertility, celiac disease, infection, tumors

IMPROVE YOUR NUMBER Kick your Coke habit. Danish scientists recently found that men who guzzled more than a liter of cola a day had 40 percent less sperm than nondrinkers. Focus instead on finishing your salad: A 2009 Spanish study found that men with the highest sperm quality also ate the most lettuce and tomatoes.

To find the bulbocavernosus, place your fingers behind your scrotum and try to flex the muscle there. (If you feel your stomach contract, you're squeezing the wrong muscle.) Now move your hand to your stomach and, while keeping your abs relaxed, begin masturbating. When you're about to reach orgasm, flex your bulbocavernosus. Once you get the hang of it, flex during sex.

"This won't bring you from 2 minutes to 20 minutes, but you can definitely progress up to 5 to 7 minutes," says Dr. Paduch.

Practice makes perfect. Ejaculations don't just feel good—they're good for you. "I've seen men lose up to 2 inches off their erections because they didn't masturbate and have enough sex," Dr. Paduch says. "Your penis is basically a big muscle—it will atrophy if you don't use it." His Rx: Masturbate as often as you'd like to be having sex. "What really matters is having an adequate outlet. Your penis doesn't care whether that outlet is sex or masturbation."

Achieve Optimum Fitness

- Percentage of men who are sedentary: **37**
- Percentage of men who exercise to offset their unhealthy habits: **16**
- Number-one challenge the average guy faces when it comes to exercise: **Staying motivated**

Show her what she's missing. Before working out, flip through photos of a former flame who broke your heart. A 2010 study in the *Journal of Neurophysiology* found that viewing images of a woman who spurned you activates the areas of your brain that control motivation and reward.

"Rejection—that sense of loss—stimulates desire," says Christopher Proulx, MS, CSCS, an assistant professor of movement science at Westfield State University. "And this desire increases your level of adrenaline—the same chemical response that occurs in preparation for physical activity."

This might enhance your focus and overall performance.

Lift with the underdog. Believe it or not, seeing your buddy's scrawny biceps may be more motivating than seeing some other guy's anaconda arms coiled around a barbell. A 2010 study in the *Journal of Experimental Social Psychology* found that people work about 30 percent harder when they're competing against those they see as easily beatable.

"Men produce higher levels of testosterone when they're winning than when they're losing," says Proulx. Also a factor: The chance that your less fit friend will surpass you.

"Which is more embarrassing," Proulx asks, "being beaten by someone who's bigger than you or someone who's weaker?"

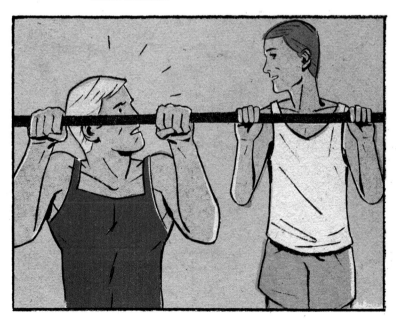

Stave Off Prostate Cancer

- Average man's risk of developing prostate cancer in his lifetime: **1 in 6**

- Percentage increase in your risk of developing the disease if you also have hypertension: **50**

Eat your chicken naked. Take hypertension out of the prostate-cancer equation by following our blood-pressure tips (see "Tame Your Blood Pressure," page 237), and then further manage your risk by skinning your favorite protein: chicken. In a 2010 study in the *American Journal of Clinical Nutrition*, prostate-cancer patients who ate the most skin-on chicken were more than twice as likely to face progression of their disease as those who consumed the least. By contrast, scarfing down any quantity of skinless chicken appears to be prostate-safe. Blame the fact that grilling or broiling poultry skin results in the

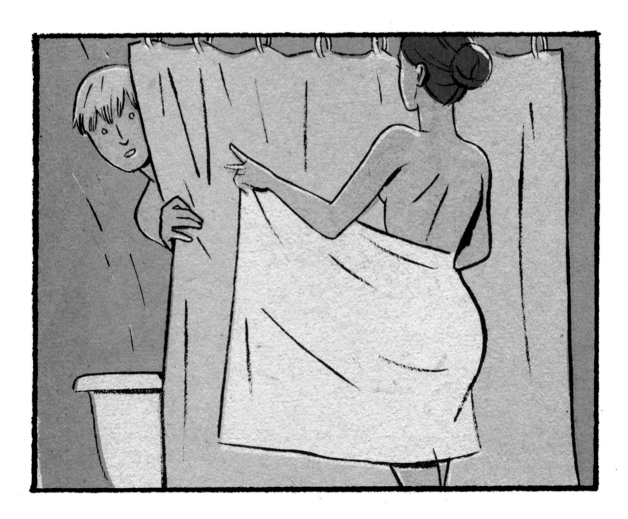

formation of heterocyclic amines, compounds shown to damage DNA in human prostate cells.

Recruit from the farm team. Almost everything in nature has a natural enemy, and for prostate cancer, it's cruciferous vegetables. A recent study in the *Journal of the National Cancer Institute* found that men who ate more than one weekly serving of broccoli or cauliflower had a 25 percent lower risk of developing aggressive prostate cancer. Credit a storehouse of antioxidants and glucosinolates, bitter-tasting compounds that shield your DNA from damage.

YOUR MOST VITAL VITALS
Blood pressure

AVERAGE GUY: 121/71 millimeters of mercury (mmHg)

TARGET: 120/80 mmHg

HELPS ASSESS: Heart-disease risk, stroke risk

IMPROVE YOUR NUMBER: Don't let revenge leave you cold. People who focus on blaming others when conflict arises face an increase in systolic blood pressure, according to a 2010 study in the *British Journal of Psychology.* Any time you feel you've been seriously slighted, reappraise the situation.

"Try to understand the aggressor and what circumstances may have triggered the behavior—stress, for instance," says Maurice Schweitzer, PhD, a psychology researcher at the University of Pennsylvania. "This gives you a richer context and better insight, and can help moderate your reaction to the outburst."

Tame Your Blood Pressure

- Odds that the average guy will have high BP when he's 35 to 44 years old: **1 in 5**
- Average number of years a 50-year-old man with normal blood pressure will outlive one with hypertension: **5**

Scale back your BP. Regular trips to the fish market don't just help your waistline. A seafood diet is also low in sodium and rich in magnesium and taurine, two compounds that can slash your risk of hypertension, according to Japanese researchers. Seek out seaweed, a natural source of magnesium that can be added to soups (it's also commonly found in sushi), and freshly harvested, taurine-rich shellfish, such as oysters and scallops. Going fresh helps you avoid an unwanted shot of sodium-laden preservatives.

Prevent Skin Cancer

- Number of sunscreen bottles the average guy uses in a year: **1.5**
- Number of 8-ounce bottles he'd go through if he applied the recommended amount of sunblock every day of the summer: **11**

Respect your enemy. A false sense of confidence can be fatal: People who use high-SPF sunscreens tend to go out in the sun when it's stronger and stay there longer, putting themselves at a greater risk of melanoma than those who slather on a low-SPF formula, according to recent French research.

"People mistakenly assume that if they put on high-SPF sunscreen, they're good to go the whole day," says David Leffell, MD, a professor of dermatology at the Yale School of Medicine. His advice, Stick with a photo-stabilized sunscreen, such as Neutrogena's Fresh Cooling Body Mist Sunblock ($10, neutrogena.com), and set your watch or smartphone to remind you to reapply every 2 hours. Also, wash your beach clothes with SunGuard to increase the UV rating to 30 ($2, sunguardsunprotection.com), and throw them in the dryer before you head out—the laundering will tighten the weave of the fabric, providing extra protection, say Henry Ford Hospital researchers.

Uncover a mole. Tell your wife or girlfriend you need to examine every inch of her body—doctor's orders. Jump in the shower together, lather up, and before you towel off, look her over for irregular, dark, or raised moles or sores that don't heal, says Dr. Leffell. Monthly self-examination may catch melanoma earlier, when it's easier to cure, he says.

Is she balking at the idea of you playing detective with her dermis? Tell her this: In a 2008 Northwestern University study, couples who were the most satisfied gave skin exams that were three times more effective than those of discontented duos.

Watch Your Body Weight

- Percentage of men who are overweight or obese: **70**

- Average number of years a man loses from his life span if he is obese at age 20: **13**

- Size of the average guy's waist: **40 inches**

- Maximum waist size that could fit into the escape pod used by the trapped Chilean miners: **35 inches**

Never assume "healthy" is healthy.
Beware the Subway diet: Diners grossly underestimate the calorie counts in "healthy" fast food, according to a recent study from Cornell University's Food and Brand Lab. When people ate a Subway meal with as many calories as a McDonald's meal, they misjudged the Subway meal's load by 21 percent (159 calories).

"Not only do you underestimate the amount you eat, but you end up indulging later because you thought you were so good at lunch," says study author Brian Wansink, PhD. His advice: Estimate the number of calories in your healthy fast-food meal, and double it. "You'll be a lot

YOUR MOST VITAL VITALS
Blood sugar

AVERAGE GUY: 104 milligrams/deciliter (mg/dl)

TARGET: 70 to 99 mg/dl

HELPS DIAGNOSE: Hyperglycemia, hypoglycemia, diabetes, prediabetes

IMPROVE YOUR NUMBER: In a 2010 University of Massachusetts study, researchers analyzed people's blood-sugar responses to seven snacks: half a glazed doughnut, skim milk, an apple, oatmeal, wrinkled peas, smooth peas, and walnuts. The least jarring bites? Wrinkled peas and walnut halves. Sprinkle the nuts with cinnamon (a blood-sugar tamer), and try the shriveled legumes instead of chickpeas in homemade hummus.

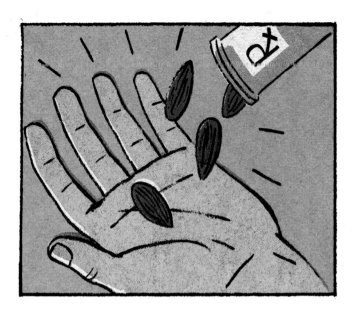

- Odds that the average guy will develop diabetes even if he's disease-free at age 40: **1 in 3**

- Increase in a man's risk of diabetes if he boosts his TV-watching time from less than an hour to 4 or more hours: **Twofold**

Go a little nuts. Eating almonds can help ward off insulin resistance (a red flag for diabetes), according to a 2010 study in the *Journal of the American College of Nutrition*. When people with prediabetes ate 2 ounces of almonds (about two handfuls) each day for 16 weeks, they experienced a 23 percent drop in fasting insulin levels, while those who said no to nuts saw a 19 percent increase. The credit goes to oleic acid, a fat that triggers the release of GLP-1, a peptide that can improve insulin sensitivity.

Look forward to commercials. Some health threats can be beaten using brute strength: A recent UCLA study found that lean people with low muscle mass are 67 percent more likely to be insulin resistant than their more buff counterparts. Having a sculpted physique may help your body use insulin to regulate blood sugar, the researchers say. Our advice: Cut your TV time to an hour a day, and during commercials, crank out a few sets of body-weight squats, lunges, or pushups.

Find body-weight exercises at MensHealth.com/fitness/body-weight-exercises-1.

more accurate," he says. And, of course, use our own 2013 edition of *Eat This, Not That!* as a guide: Go to eatthisnotthatbook.com.

Calculate your grains. Exercise won't offset the waist-inflating effect of white bread, according to a new study in the *American Journal of Clinical Nutrition*. Among exercisers, those who ate refined grains daily had 12 percent more visceral fat—the most dangerous kind—than those who consumed the least amount of the processed stuff. The researchers also found that people who ate the most whole grains had 17 percent less belly flab than those who consumed the least. The catch: Continuing to consume refined grains offsets the fat-blasting effect of whole grains. Pasta, English muffins, white bread, and pizza are your primary offenders. Cut these carbs, and replace them with at least three servings of whole grains a day.

Lower Your Cholesterol

- Percentage of men concerned about their heart health who limit their dietary cholesterol intake: **25**

- Percentage increase in HDL (good) cholesterol in men who started eating three eggs a day: **20**

Pop a pistachio. Eggs aren't the only shells you should be cracking. In a Penn State study, people who ate two servings of pistachios a day slashed their LDL (bad) cholesterol by an average of 13 percent.

"Phytosterols in nuts act almost like a drug. They bind cholesterol in the GI tract and block its absorption," says Paul Ziajka, MD, PhD, a clinical lipidologist with the Southeast Lipid Association.

YOUR MOST VITAL VITALS
LDL cholesterol

AVERAGE GUY: 126 milligrams per deciliter (mg/dl)

TARGET: <100 mg/dl

HELPS ASSESS: Heart-disease risk

IMPROVE YOUR NUMBER: Here's one more reason to skip fast food. In a new study in the *Archives of Pediatrics and Adolescent Medicine*, teens with high blood concentrations of perfluoroalkyl acids—chemicals found in such grease-resistant packaging as Chinese food containers, pizza boxes, and burger wrappers—also had high LDL. Researchers aren't sure why the link exists, but they're confident the problem isn't limited to teens.

"The control of cholesterol is uniform throughout our lives," says Yale cardiologist John Elefteriades, MD. "So this would likely translate to adults."

Why pistachios? They pack a higher concentration of phytosterols than any other nut, according to a 2005 study from Virginia Tech.

Beat Depression

- Percentage of men who suffer from depression: **4.4**

- Percentage of men who take antidepressants: **6.7**

Watch your diagnosis. Why are so many more men being medicated for depression than actually suffer from it? Part of the disparity is due to the fact that SSRIs (the most commonly prescribed antidepressants) help treat other problems, including premature ejaculation and migraines. But that still doesn't account for all the scrips being written, says Michael Addis, PhD, director of the Men's Coping Project at Clark University in Worcester, Massachusetts.

"There's a lack of knowledge about what these drugs are appropriate for—and many illnesses have symptoms that mimic depression, including thyroid disorders and celiac disease," he says.

Compounding the problem is the fact that a third of primary-care docs say that they won't ask about mental health at all, and half say that assessing psychological issues causes them to lose time and money, reports a study by University of Cincinnati researchers. That disinterest may prompt a lot of knee-jerk prescription writing.

"Don't let them jump to a quick diagnosis," Addis says. And if you have any doubts about whether your blues are truly depression-related or instead a symptom

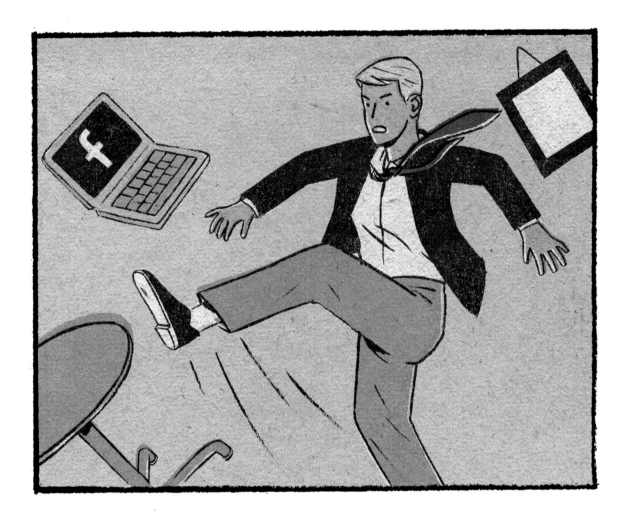

of something else, seek a second opinion—from a psychiatrist or psychologist.

Un-friend depression. Facebook might actually be the antisocial network. British scientists recently found that Internet addiction is linked to a greater risk of depression and is often characterized by overuse of social media sites.

"People make positive, sound bite–caliber posts on Facebook—'the changing leaves are beautiful,' 'I just heard an awesome song,' and so on," says Addis.

"The discrepancy between what you're feeling and what you think everyone else is feeling can make depression worse. You can develop a pretty stilted view of the world."

Consider "hiding" your most Pollyanna-ish pals, and then strive for perspective by bumping up your real-time interactions.

"Facebook needs to be supplemented by face time and phone conversations so the unscripted truth can unfold more completely," Addis says.

Why Our Health-Care System Is Hurting

The French helped us win the American Revolution. They gave us the Statue of Liberty. Writer Tom McGrath speculates: Maybe it's time to turn 'em loose on our health-care system.

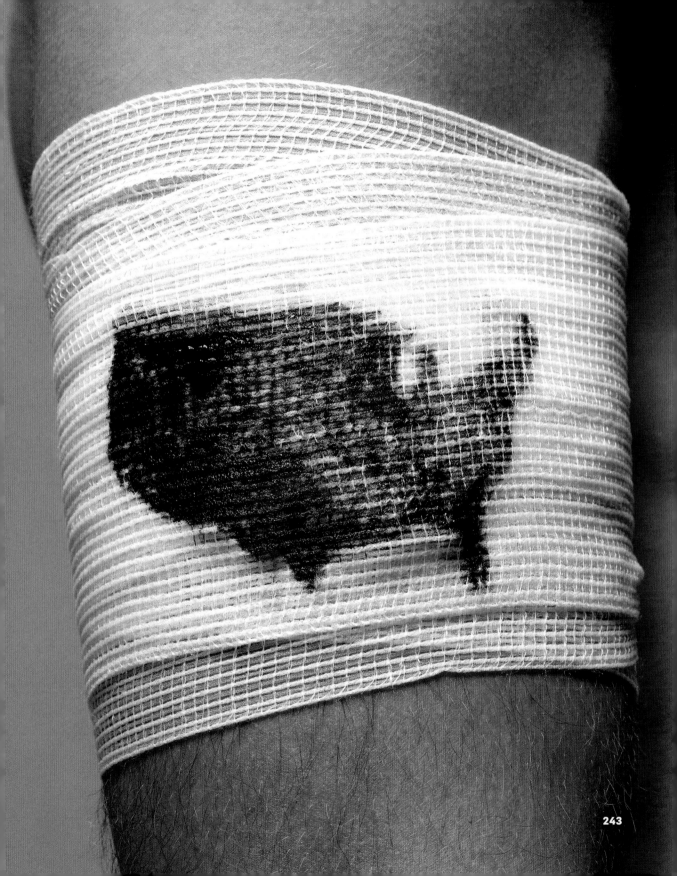

On a gray winter day, I'm sitting in an emergency room in Center City Philadelphia, staring at a guy with a surgical mask on his face and a cane in his hand.

It is, I'll admit, a strange time to be dreaming of Paris. But I am.

"Latoya Jones," the nurse calls out, holding a clipboard with paperwork on it. The masked man—a fellow in his 30s with vaguely Middle Eastern coloring and a look in his dark eyes that says, "Dude, I am seriously not feeling good"—slumps lower into his seat. Not his turn yet.

If you're looking for a microcosm of everything that's wrong with the U.S. health-care system, a big-city emergency room is the place to go. For starters, as has been frequently noted, the ER is the only option for people who don't have health insurance. It's the place you go when you're sick enough that you have to go someplace. A message keeps flashing on the big flat-screen TV monitor: "No health insurance? Unable to pay your hospital bill? You may qualify for charity care for medically necessary services."

Of course, as I can attest to firsthand, an ER is no treat even if you do have health insurance. Twice in the past couple of years, my wife and I rushed our now-8-year-old daughter to an emergency room. The first time it was for what turned out to be appendicitis. (I'd been telling her for days to suck it up, that she just had "gas.") The second time was after a sledding accident that left her with a fractured skull. (I figured she'd miss the tree in the middle of the hill; I figured wrong.) I'm thankful that, despite my best efforts, my

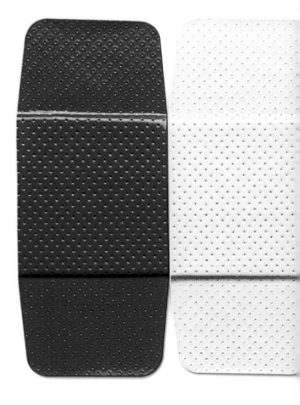

daughter is fine. But the total bill for both visits was $41,000, more than $8,000 of which, thanks to my company's stellar health plan, I paid out of my own pocket.

Still, the full suckiness of America's health-care setup didn't really dawn on me until recently, when I traveled to France—specifically, when I toured the Hôtel-Dieu, a nearly 1,400-year-old hospital around the corner from the Notre-Dame cathedral in the center of Paris. As I was led through the ER by the hospital's director, François Crémieux—whose spiky hair, black jeans, and black T-shirt made him look a little like a roadie for Abba—he explained the way the system works. Unlike people in the United States, he said, no one in France needs to go to an ER for basic medical care, because everyone in France has health insurance. If you're sick, you just call your doctor and go. What's more, if you do require emergency care, well, a trip to the ER won't wipe out your kids' college fund. When I mentioned the $41,000 in charges for Sarah's maladies, Crémieux gave me that look the French frequently give Americans.

"The basic charge for treatment in an emergency room is 22 euros," he said. Then he stopped and thought for a moment. "Actually, that is not correct . . . because the national health insurance will reimburse 70 percent of that." Actual cost to the patient: about $9.

That memory of Paris comes back to me as I watch the masked man in Philadelphia. There was a period when we all had hope that our national leaders would solve some of the problems plaguing the U.S. health system, when it appeared we might be able to elevate it to its rightful place as the best in the world. But we all know how that's turned out.

The nurse comes out again, holding a clipboard. "James Wilson," she calls out. The guy with the surgical mask rests his head back again. Keep waiting, chief, I want to tell him. Just like fixing the health-care system, they'll call your name—eventually. Probably. Or not.

So. How are you enjoying health-care reform so far?

No matter which side of the street you walk on politically, you'll undoubtedly agree with me when I say that few events in recent memory have made me want to jab a hypodermic needle in my eye more than the so-called debate on health care in Congress. Partisanship! Grandstanding! Backroom deals! Rank lies! About the only way this process could have been more loathsome would be if it had been emceed by Larry Craig and Eric Massa.

The tragedy, of course, is that while the politicians have bickered, the insecurity the average guy feels about his health insurance has risen to Defcon 1. Thanks to the recession, the number of people in America without health insurance climbed to 49.9 million as of 2010—and it has surely risen even higher since then. Meanwhile, millions more are suddenly forced to buy insurance on their own, which is like paying protection money to the Mafia, only less effective. The other option: Go without. And even if you still have a job with benefits, I'm betting that you, like me, have spent a few anxious nights during the past year wondering how you'd cope with a health disaster if a pink slip came your way or your company went into Chapter 7. (Note to Wall Street investment bankers: "Anxiety" is an emotion humans feel when they don't have a government bailout or a seven-figure bonus to fall back on.)

And the U.S. health-care system was no great shakes even before the double whammy of recession and overwrought political interest hit it. Indeed, one of the things I was hoping to see in the health-care debate—I mean, aside from Senate leaders Harry Reid and Mitch McConnell being beaten with their own shoes—was an acknowledgement of how un-American the American health-care system has become in the past several decades. Now, by "un-American" I don't mean commie pinko or socialist. I mean, purely apoliti-cally, that given all the money we spend (a staggering 17.9 percent of our GDP, easily the highest in the developed world), we get lousy results. Seventy-five years ago, the United States was near the top of the heap in life expectancy. Today, we rank . . . drumroll, please . . . 50th! And it's not just that the poor and uninsured are pulling down our average. As Jean de Ker-vasdoué, a French health economist, noted, "The poorest third of the population in England or France live longer than the richest third in the United States."

Somewhere, the so-called Greatest Generation just felt a great pain.

Fortunately, I believe I have found the solution to our woes, a blueprint we might follow to take our health-care system where it needs to go: All we have to do is imitate the French.

Okay, I can hear you grumbling already. The French? Really? Is suicide not an option? Granted, Americans have always had, shall we say, a complex relationship with France. On the one hand, we frequently find the French baffling or annoying, what with their government-mandated 30 days of annual paid vacation and general predilection for folding like a cheap tent when it comes to defending their liberty. On the other hand . . .

Look, I'm pretty sure there's another hand. I just can't think of it right now.

But really, if there's an area in which we might actually want to pay attention to what the French are doing, it's health care. Twice in the past decade, the French system has been ranked best in the world. In 2000 the World Health Organization lauded the French for the high quality of their care, for covering every person in the country, and for doing it all relatively inexpensively—or at least more cheaply than we do it. (The United States was 37th.) When a 2008 study of developed nations by U.K. researchers ranked 19 nations on their mortality rates due to treatable conditions, the United States came in dead last. France topped the list—and it spends only about 11 percent of its GDP on health.

What's intriguing is that in many ways the French system isn't really all that different from the one we're stuck with. While there is a government-run health-insurance program (a sort of public option on steroids) and a strong network of public hospitals, France has few other hallmarks of the dreaded socialized medicine. French citizens have more or less complete freedom to choose their doctors and the hospitals they prefer.

And given where we are in our own efforts to tinker with our system, maybe the most important thing to note about the French is that they didn't invent their system overnight. It evolved over time, piece by piece, and they're constantly tinkering with it. True, this might be because the French work, like, only 22 minutes a week, and so it took them six decades to pull off what any halfway industrious country could have done in about a day and a half. Still, there might be some magic to doing things the French way.

My first close-up look at France's health system—or, more accurately, how the French feel about their health system—came one day as I stood outside one of Paris's busiest train stations, the Gare de Lyon, talking with a fellow named Geoffrey. Tall and lean, Geoffrey was 38 and worked for an international aerospace company. He struck me as typically French in two ways. First, he was quite satisfied with his country's health system. "Yes, yes, it is good," he said. "Expensive, but good." The last time he went to the doctor? "Uh, about 1 year ago." He took a drag on his cigarette and then pointed to his nose. "Allergies," he said. Then he exhaled.

Ah, yes, the cigarettes. That's the other way Geoffrey was typically French—he smoked more than a roomful of Rastafarians. A couple of years ago the French government banned smoking inside all public buildings. However, judging from the hordes outside the station and the cloud of smoke hovering above them, that ban didn't appear to have done much to cut down on smoking. I asked Geoffrey if

he wanted to quit. He shrugged. "Eh."

Back to the health care: So how does this system that Geoffrey and, judging from surveys, most of his fellow Frenchmen love so much actually work? Let's start with the money. As in the United States, the insurance system in France is funded by contributions from employers and employees. "Nineteen percent of my salary" is what Geoffrey told me that he

The French are skeptical of letting the market control health care. **"Health is a common good,"** one Frenchman told me smugly. **"It is not Pepsi-Cola."**

and his employer pay toward the French social security system. This might seem like a lot, but that payment isn't just for medical insurance; it also includes contributions to Geoffrey's retirement pension, unemployment insurance, disability insurance, and a number of other coverages that fall under the umbrella of French social security. Total up what the average American pays for that stuff—plus health care—and you end up with a number that's not much different.

So what does Geoffrey get for his money? For starters, he, like every resident of France, has a government-issued carte vitale—the green health-insurance card—that he can use at pretty much every health-care provider in France. The carte vitale isn't a payment card (one of the peculiarities of the French system is that patients are expected to pay for health-care services out of their own pockets, on the spot), but it does expedite reimbursement. Indeed, within 5 days of visiting a doctor, one of the health-care funds that form the backbone of the French system reimburses 70 percent of a patient's cost right into his or her checking account. As for the remaining 30 percent? Most people in France carry what's called mutuelle insurance—a second policy that covers deductibles as well as things like supplemental dental and eye-care costs.

What's really cool about this insurance setup is that Geoffrey's coverage will stay with him if he ever switches jobs—no angst, no waiting period, no hassle over preexisting conditions. So unlike the U.S. system, France's plan is perfectly built for the realities of a 21st-century economy in which people switch jobs jillions of times over the course of their lives. Geoffrey's coverage also stays with him if he loses his job. In 2000, in what was more or less the final step in a decades-long march toward universal health coverage in France, the government created a program that provides exactly the same health insurance to everyone, regardless of a citizen's ability to pay.

Now, I should probably clarify something I said earlier about reimbursement. As with all health-insurance plans, there is fine print that a savvy consumer needs to be aware of. In France, if you are unlucky enough to have a really serious condition—cancer, heart disease, or a stroke, for example—insurance will not reimburse you 70 percent of your costs.

It will reimburse you 100 percent.

"There is a list of diseases, perhaps 30 or so, in which 100 percent of the care is paid for," said Fabien Calvo, MD, PhD, the associate director of the French National Cancer Institute, whom I interviewed one morning in his office in a Paris suburb. The concept is simple enough: The sicker you are, the better your coverage—which, Dr. Calvo says, is the point of having insurance in the first place.

From a practical standpoint, offering uncapped catastrophic coverage has ramifications. First, it means high-quality care is available not just to people who can afford it, but to everyone.

"When people are sick, they believe that they have paid for that. So they should have access to the best care," Dr. Calvo said.

The other ramification is that, for the patient, financial stress is out of the equation—if you're sick, you don't worry about paying for treatment. When I met with another doctor, Jacques Milliez, MD, I mentioned that one of the problems U.S. families face is underinsurance, or not having enough coverage to pay for hospital bills that can run into the six or seven figures for a grave illness. It's one reason that more than half of bankruptcies in America cite out-of-pocket medical costs as a factor.

Dr. Milliez, a severe-looking man whose obstetrics career has taken him from New York to North Africa to Paris's St. Antoine's hospital, nodded. He said such a thing would never happen in France. Then he smiled wryly. "If you are young and healthy, then the American system is good," he said. "But if you're sick, it is not so good, right?"

I mentioned that the French could be annoying, right?

The French are well known for their socialist leanings—virtually free education, onerous work rules for employers, a willingness to strike and take to the streets if a politician even suggests messing with any of that. And yet it wasn't that long ago that the social safety net in France was similar to the one in the United States. Back in the 1920s, there wasn't yet a French welfare state, and the country's health insurance was handled the same way as ours—mostly through trade unions and other nongovernment federations.

That began to change in earnest in 1946 with the creation of the French social security system. If you're American, two things about this are a little bit galling: First, the French wouldn't have had a society to secure if we hadn't essentially saved their behinds in World War II. Second, their system basically mimicked ours. The only real difference was that their social security arrangement included health insurance as part of the deal. As the French penned in the preamble to their Constitution of 1946, "[The Nation] guarantees to all . . . health protection, material security, rest and recreation. Every human being who, because of his age, physical or mental, economic situation, is unable to work has the right to obtain from the community suitable means of existence."

Pretty big talk, though it's worth noting that France didn't live up to that fancy rhetoric right away. At the outset, only industrial and commercial workers were covered. It wasn't until the 1960s that farmworkers and then independent professionals were brought into the

The French Food Connection

Only 49 percent of French adults are obese or overweight, compared with 63 percent of American adults. "They break all the rules we're taught will keep us thin," says Will Clower, PhD, the author of *The French Don't Diet Plan*. Here's how to start a French revolution at your dinner table.

BEFRIEND FAT

The French perspective: "The French don't shun saturated fat," says Clower, "and incidentally, their heart-disease rates are lower than ours." In fact, 37 percent more American men than Frenchmen per 100,000 died of cardiovascular disease in 2004, a World Health Organization survey found.

Your move: The link between saturated fat and heart disease is ill-founded, an *American Journal of Clinical Nutrition* review revealed. In fact, ditching saturated fat may even be harmful. That's because we tend to replace it with unhealthy refined carbs. So go ahead and eat full-fat foods, but watch your portions, says Clower. For example, stick to a French-size portion of full-fat yogurt, which is about half of a standard American yogurt cup, according to a University of Pennsylvania study.

DRINK UP

The French perspective: In 2006, the average French citizen consumed more than 50 liters of wine, compared with only 9 liters for Americans, according to the Wine Institute. Even so, 77 percent fewer Frenchmen than American men reported drinking heavily (5 or more drinks in a sitting) over a 2-week period, according to the Institute of Alcohol Studies. The likely reason? Americans view vino as an intoxicant rather than a food, Clower says.

Your move: Consider wine a side dish to a well-orchestrated meal. (Who wants five servings of green beans?) In moderation, it's also a treat for your heart. Drink a glass or two with dinner. Many studies tout the resveratrol in red wine, but a recent Italian study found that white wine produced by an ancient Tuscan method is also loaded with antioxidants.

DON'T CLEAN YOUR PLATE

The French perspective: Parisians are 35 percent more likely than Chicagoans to use internal cues to drop the fork, notes a recent study in the journal *Obesity*. The French stop eating when they feel full or when food no longer tastes good, while Americans rely on external cues, like the end of a TV show or an empty plate, says study author Brian Wansink, PhD.

Your move: Add courses, including dessert. The trick: Slow down your meal. The average American fast-food diner eats in 14 minutes, but the French take 22, according to University of Pennsylvania researchers. It takes 15 to 20 minutes to feel full, Clower says. Adjust your pace, and you'll feel satisfied with a small sugary bite or a piece of fruit.

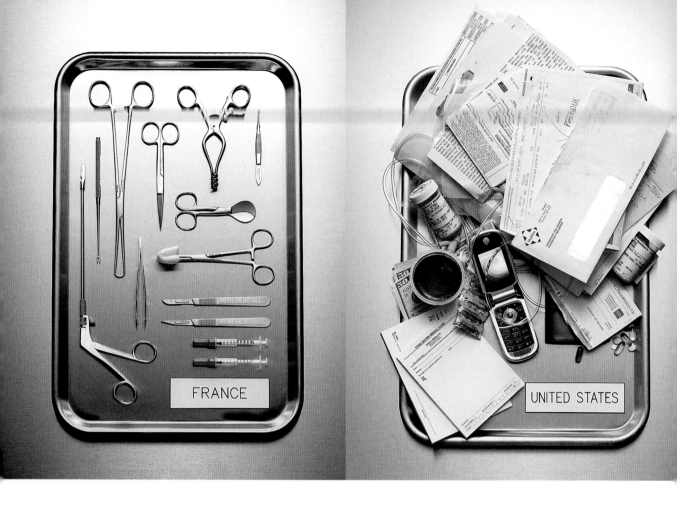

FRANCE

UNITED STATES

health-insurance system, and it wasn't until 2000 that coverage was extended to every resident. Still, to France's credit, it has been willing to tinker with the system to bring it closer and closer to the ideal it had in mind.

Why has the United States found it so difficult to do something similar? Curiously, while we relish and rely on innovation in the private sector, powerful interests have made it difficult to pull off creative solutions in the public sphere. Indeed, in many ways the current healthcare battle is merely a rerun of the show that's been playing for decades—in 1945,

when Harry Truman first proposed national health insurance (he failed); in 1965, when Lyndon Johnson signed Medicare and Medicaid into existence (it passed, but over the vehement objections of many doctors); and in 1993, when the Clintons took a crack at revamping the system.

That said, it's not just politics that's stopping us from having the kind of national health insurance the French have; it's also philosophy. While France and the United States were founded on many of the same ideals—liberty, equality—"the French have a different view of government," says Paul Dutton, PhD, a history professor at Northern Arizona University, who's written extensively on the two countries. While the French see government as the main protector of their rights, Americans want to be protected from government. Our anti-statist feelings exist even though we have plenty of state-run features in our lives. As one South Carolina resident barked at his congressman during a town hall meeting, "Keep your government hands off my Medicare!"

That's why some in France doubt we'll ever have the kind of solidarity-based health-care system they have.

"The American spirit is individual liberty, innovation," said Dr. Milliez, who spent 2 years working at Columbia University in New York City. "That's the dynamic of the nation. It relies on individual capacity to innovate and doesn't care too much about those who are lying on the road."

Ouch.

So just how good is the care provided by French doctors and hospitals to those poor souls lying on the road in France? While all the doctors I spoke with there expressed admiration for the medical research we do in the United States and for ultra-prestigious facilities like the Mayo Clinic, they all believe the care a patient receives in France is just as good, if not better.

Jean de Kervasdoué, the health economist, delivered a blunt assessment: "I always say I'd rather be sick in France than in America."

To Americans, the great paradoxical question of French health care is this:

How can the French offer high-quality care to everyone in the country, from cradle to grave, and still spend less per person—by more than a third—than we do? The French say it's really no mystery: They spend less because no one is trying to become rich delivering health care to the French people.

To our American ears, it sounds strange to forswear the profit motive, because our assumption is that private enterprise and the free market are more efficient than anything run by the government. (And with a Department of Defense famous for its $640 toilet seats, this is an understandable assumption.) Yet with health care, that seems not to be the case.

On the day I met with the Hôtel-Dieu's François Cremiéux—you remember, the roadie from Abba—he had just returned from a trip to the United States, where he'd met with some administrators at Boston Medical Center. Like a lot of people in French health care, he was baffled by the way we sometimes spend our health-care dollars. He told me that Boston Medical Center, for instance, has invested in nuclear-medicine equipment—despite the fact that two other hospitals in Boston, Beth Israel and Mass General, already have similar equipment.

"In France we'd have one machine and agreements among the hospitals to share it," he said. The waste, he argued, is in not just the cost of the redundant equipment but also the ripple effects it sets off. "The consequence is that in Boston, three hospitals are fighting for the nuclear medicine doctors, so the prices are going higher," he said. "That's nonsense. The citizen is paying because three doctors are being paid more than they should."

This sort of duplication of services, which happens all the time in the United States as hospitals and health systems pursue the most profitable parts of the market, is just one way our market-based health-care industry ends up being more expensive than France's public-private partnership. Take bureaucracy, for example. While the French have one set of rates and one centralized system for processing paperwork, each U.S. health insurer strikes its own deals with health systems, and each company has different ways of processing payments and reimbursements. The result: American hospitals and doctors employ teams of people to deal with all the red tape. Indeed, 7 cents out of every dollar we spend on health care goes toward keeping up with the paperwork. That's four times what the French spend. (One note of progress for us: The 2009 economic stimulus bill included $19 billion to help move toward electronic records; this will lessen, though by no means solve, the paperwork problem.)

Then there's the cost of competing for patients. While the French lay out next to nothing for marketing, American hospitals, health insurers, and drug companies spend more than $30 billion a year on advertising and promotion. They're essentially using a big chunk of our health-care dollars to encourage us to come back and spend more of our health-care dollars. Then again, from a bottom-line perspective, you can't argue with success: In 2009, even as unemployment topped 10 percent and more than 15 million Americans searched for work, the five largest U.S. health insurance firms

pulled in $12.2 billion in profits—a 56 percent increase over 2008.

Perhaps the most disconcerting part of our market-driven system is the way it skews the very type of care we receive. Over the past several decades, study after study has shown that the best, most efficient way to deal with major killers like cancer and heart disease is through a combination of prevention, lifestyle changes, and early screening. Alas, our health-care system does basically the exact opposite, funneling most of the money toward pricey drugs and procedures that people need only when they're already sick.

Now, this isn't because the people running the system are evil; it's because that's what the market dictates. There isn't much of a profit in selling prevention and lifestyle changes, but there's a really good one in selling pharmaceuticals, high-tech medical procedures, and high-deductible insurance policies—along with all the booze, fast food, and recliners that produce health problems in the first place.

The great irony, of course, is that there appears to be an inverse relationship between the amount of money a country spends on medical care and the health of its citizens. Since 1990, the United States not only has shelled out more for health care than any country in the world, but it also has the fastest spending-growth rate. In that same time, we've actually shown the third smallest increase in life expectancy.

That's why the French are so skeptical of market control of health care.

"We've seen that the market can't fully regulate the financial system," Cremiéux

DIY Health-Care Reform

We don't know when or how America will solve its health-care problems. The solution: Reform your own health care, with five simple ways to maximize care and minimize cost.

GO DIGITAL

Percentage of patients with a chronic condition who received duplicate tests over a 2-year period
USA: 20 PERCENT
FRANCE: 10 PERCENT

Percentage of doctors who routinely receive computerized reminders for patients' screening tests or guideline-based interventions
USA: 20 PERCENT
FRANCE: 27 PERCENT

Electronic records can eliminate drug conflicts and the unnecessary repetition of tests, says Stephen Neeleman, MD, the CEO of HealthEquity, a personal health-care financial services company. The software might even prompt your doctor to schedule screenings. Before you sign on with a physician, ask the staff if the office uses a system that lets you review your personal health-care record online.

NEGOTIATE

Out-of-pocket health-care spending per capita in 2006 (in U.S. dollars)
USA: $857
FRANCE: $232

Percentage of chronic-care patients with out-of-pocket medical expenses in 2010 that exceeded $1,000
USA: 41 PERCENT
FRANCE: 5 PERCENT

Before receiving treatment, request the procedure's CPT (current procedural terminology) code, the number insurers use to calculate provider reimbursements. Plug it into the American Medical Association database (https://catalog.ama-assn.org/Catalog/cpt/cpt_search.jsp), and then use the Medicare rate to bargain with your provider. Doctors often lose money with Medicare, so expect to pay a bit more, Dr. Neeleman says.

ACT PREEMPTIVELY

Percentage of adults who received all recommended screening tests and preventive care for their age and sex
USA: 50 PERCENT
FRANCE: N/A

Neglecting suggested screening tests could be a costly mistake, says Anne Dunlop, MD, director of preventive medicine at Emory University. "If you identify a disease early on, the consequences of both the disease and the treatment are far less severe," she says. Search recommended tests for your age on the U.S. Preventive Services Task Force Web site (ahrq.gov/clinic).

DIVIDE AND CONQUER

Percentage of adults with a chronic condition who did not receive a treatment because of cost in the past 2 years
USA: 38 PERCENT
FRANCE: 13 PERCENT

Ask your dentist to "straddle" costly procedures—half in December, half in January—to combine the yearly spending limits of two-plan years.

COORDINATE CARE

Percentage of adults who've seen the same doctor for 5 or more years
USA: 49 PERCENT
FRANCE: 75 PERCENT

Percentage of adults who saw four or more doctors in the past year who reported problems coordinating their medical tests/records
USA: 45 PERCENT
FRANCE: 27 PERCENT

Your primary-care doctor initiates preventive treatments and also coordinates specialty care, Dr. Dunlop says. And because he's familiar with you and your records, he can best counsel you on which procedures are appropriate and which are unnecessary. This reduces cost and the likelihood of treatment errors, the Commonwealth Fund reports.

said. "Americans have to understand that the market can't fully regulate the health system, either."

When I spoke with Dr. Milliez, he put it a little more smugly.

"Health is a common good," he said smugly. "It is not Pepsi-Cola."

The evening before I flew home, I was invited to meet with Jean de Kervasdoué. Among the French people, Kervasdoué is considered the Yoda of health care—a grandfatherly man who has a PhD from Cornell, who once ran the French hospital system, who has worked as a health-care consultant, and who now teaches, lectures, and writes about health economics.

I met him in his office deep inside the Conservatoire National des Arts et Métiers, yet another centuries-old building in Paris. When I arrived, he had two U.S. health-care reform plans on his desk—one Republican, one Democratic. I said, lightheartedly, that I bet he wasn't such a big fan of the Republican proposal, what with its reliance on market-driven solutions. His answer surprised me. "From what I've read, both of them are bad," he said.

Honestly. The French.

The problem, he said, is that while we keep focusing on the runaway costs of health care, cost isn't our only problem or even our main one. In Kervasdoué's view, our bigger issue is much more fundamental: It's our attitude about our health in general—the way we live.

Take, for example, the way we eat. "In France, people eat with somebody else. Always," Kervasdoué said. "And there is a lot of evidence that you eat less, and better, when you eat with somebody else.

When eating is a pleasure. And the French have a tradition of this. And we never eat between meals. When I go to your country, you have food all the time— doughnuts and coffee and fruits and more coffee."

You see the same sorts of differences between the French and the Americans, he continued, in many areas of life: in our attitudes about our jobs, in the number of days off we take, in our levels of stress, in our ideas about what it means to live well.

I looked at him. So was he saying America should adopt not only the French style of health care but also the French style of living? He laughed again; he was proposing an impossibility, and he knew it.

Then he told me about the Italians. In the late 1970s, Italy decided to revamp its national health system. In its eyes, the best system in the world was the British one, so Italy copied everything the British did. The problem? "They forgot they were not British," Kervasdoué said, chuckling.

"In England, you have waiting lists for care and nobody ever intervenes. But the Italians, they were always intervening, making calls and trying to cut the line. It didn't work."

His point is simple enough: A country's health system can succeed only if it's consistent with a country's character.

And that may be the ultimate triumph of French health care: It is, in both its values and its peculiarities, perfectly, almost maddeningly French. In fact, it's exactly what you'd expect from a society that is in late middle age, that has been around for more than 1,000 years and been through many struggles, that likes what it likes, and that now wants to slow down, enjoy its food and wine, and maybe not work so hard.

So here, for whatever it's worth, is what I think we can learn from the French—and what we should do about our health-care problems.

First, no matter what kinds of changes (if any) emerge out of our debate, we, like the French, ultimately need to find a solution that fits who we are as a country. Our political leaders have told us that only two alternatives exist when it comes to reform: Either the government is deeply involved in the system (Democrats), or the government lets the free market really take hold (Republicans). Alas, that seems to be not only a false set of choices but also a depressingly unimaginative one. The genius of America has always been its ability to look at things in a brand-new way, to see things that never were and find a way to make them real—whether it's connecting two coasts with railroad tracks, or knitting together a sprawling country with a highway system, or linking computers through wires and airwaves.

And so perhaps those past triumphs point the way forward when it comes to our health. None of those projects would have happened without some government involvement at the outset; and none could have made the impact they made without the imagination and hard work of private citizens. Couldn't a similar approach work in health care? Couldn't our government solicit outside-the-box ideas about taking care of our health, fund the 20 best ones for 5 years, and then let the venture capital guys and the masses take it from there?

I have seen enough fascinating (and possibly cockamamie) health-care notions out there—from open-source drug development to federal tax-return checkoffs that let people donate money to the uninsured—that I'd be shocked if there weren't, somewhere in this country, a Henry Ford of health and fitness, a Jonas Salk of insurance reform, a Steve Jobs of wellness, just poised to improve our lives with something really new.

Or maybe there will be many of them. The other thing we can learn from the French is that we should stop thinking of health-care reform as a one-and-done sort of thing. What France figured out decades ago, it seems, is that if you don't do it exactly right the first time—eh, you do not worry so much, you just keep trying, yes?

Ironically, that example just might provide the motto that keeps us motivated. The battle for a great health-care system: So important that not even the French surrendered.

Dr. FedEx

Would you like Express Saver shipping with that test? Medical tests can be delivered to your door. But does that make sense?

As doctors' fees rise, more people are turning to do-it-yourself medical tests. We asked experts to sort the helpful from the useless.

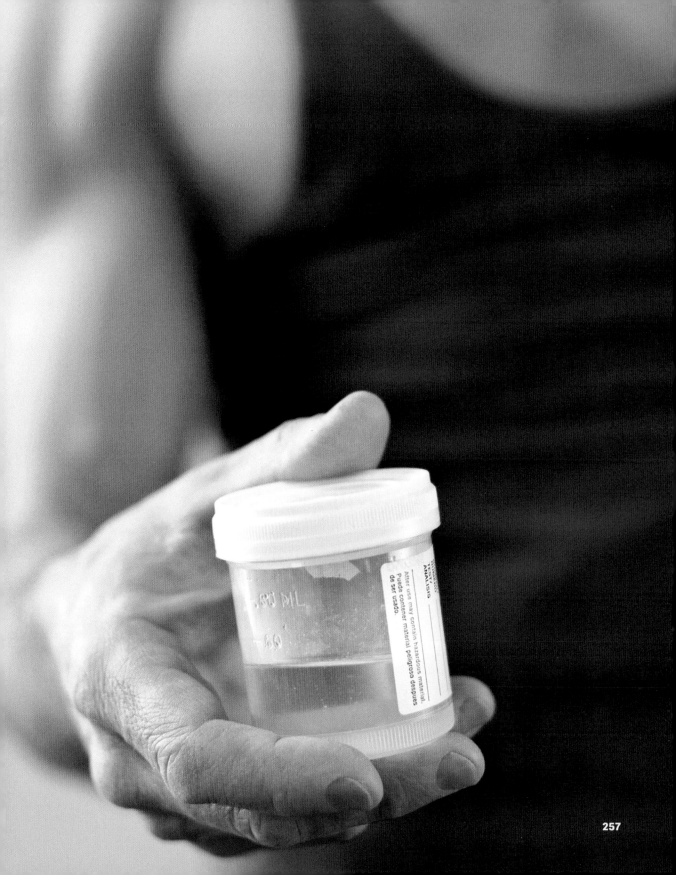

PSA Test

This finger-prick analysis—cost: $40—checks your blood for prostate-specific antigen, a protein that might signal prostate cancer. Dab your blood on a collection card, send it to a lab, and receive results in 5 days. Doctors say there's no need to take the test before age 40.

Does it work? Sometimes, but you'll need to follow up. If the PSA is lower than 1 nanogram per milliliter (ng/ml), take the test again in 5 years, says Judd W. Moul, MD, chief of urologic surgery at Duke University Medical Center. If it's over 1 ng/ml, test every year. And if it hits 2.5, see a urologist. A high PSA count doesn't always mean you have cancer, but you might need a prostate biopsy to prove that your prostate is healthy.

Not all mail-order tests are worth your time (or blood).

HIV-1 Test

The test, which costs $45, detects antibodies to HIV. Mail a blood sample to a lab to be scanned.

Does it work? Yes. Use the Home Access HIV-1 Test System ($45, homeaccess.com), which is the only FDA-approved test on the market.

"It's a viable, anonymous form of at-home HIV testing," says Richard MacKay, MD, an assistant professor of medicine and infectious diseases at Mount Sinai Hospital. But if you think you've contracted the virus within the past 3 to 6

weeks, see a physician. The at-home test might not be sensitive enough to detect the virus in its early stages, says Dr. MacKay.

Colon-Cancer Screening Test

A strip of collection paper changes color depending on the presence of blood in your stool. Fecal blood can signal colon polyps that could be cancerous. Cost? $40.

Does it work? Not really. It detects blood, not cancer.

"So at best, the test detects fewer than half of large advanced precancerous polyps, and it has little ability to detect common smaller precancerous polyps," says Patrick Pfau, MD, clinical services chief of gastroenterology and hepatology at the University of Wisconsin School of Medicine and Public Health. Ask your doctor for an endoscopic colonoscopy—that's the most accurate test, says Dr. Pfau.

Bring Backup

They call it an emergency room, but you'd never know it from the notoriously long wait times. In fact, a study in the *Archives of Internal Medicine* shows that the problem only worsened from 1997 to 2006). Your best bet: Bring a friend or a family member; they'll help keep you on the nurse's radar and can speak up if your condition changes.

Male Fertility Test

For $40, you produce a sperm sample, and a color-coded test gauges your fertility potential right then and there. A sperm concentration at or above 20 million per milliliter is good; below that level is bad.

Does it work? Not really. "This test is a crude measure of sperm count and may not be as accurate as tests available at a fertility clinic," says David Sandmire, MD, coauthor of *Medical Tests That Can Save Your Life*. And remember, low sperm count is only one possible cause for the inability to conceive. If you're worried about your fertility, see a specialist who can examine you more fully.

Home Cholesterol Test

The device scans a small amount of blood that you draw from your finger, and a built-in monitor shows your total cholesterol level. It costs $18.

Does it work? Not well enough. Steven Jones, MD, director of inpatient cardiology at Johns Hopkins School of Medicine, says the devices are not as reliable as hospital tests—and anyway, total cholesterol is an inaccurate gauge of a healthy heart. You're better off with a test that breaks down HDL, LDL, and triglyceride levels.

Express Lane to Better Health?

Chains like Walmart, Target, and CVS are adding health clinics for the treatment of minor wounds, infections, and flu, and for various tests and shots. Sounds odd, but a recent *Annals of Internal Medicine* report says that the care the clinics provide is similar to what you'd receive in a physician's office and slightly better than you'd get in the ER—and cheaper than both.

Great, right? Maybe. The *American Academy of Family Physicians* and the American Medical Association say the clinics are useful for minor issues, but the study's scope (one state) and focus (common health issues) was too narrow to draw big conclusions. Bottom line, they say: You're better off developing a relationship with your doctor, who can spot larger problems a clinic may not.

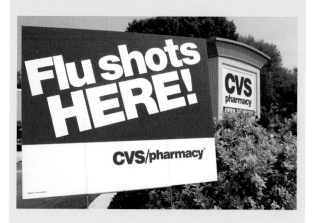

HARD TRUTH

60 Percentage of colon cancer cases that might have been caught earlier with screening

Too Much of a Good Thing?

Vegetables? Go crazy. Sex? Have at it. But pace yourself with these other health boosters.

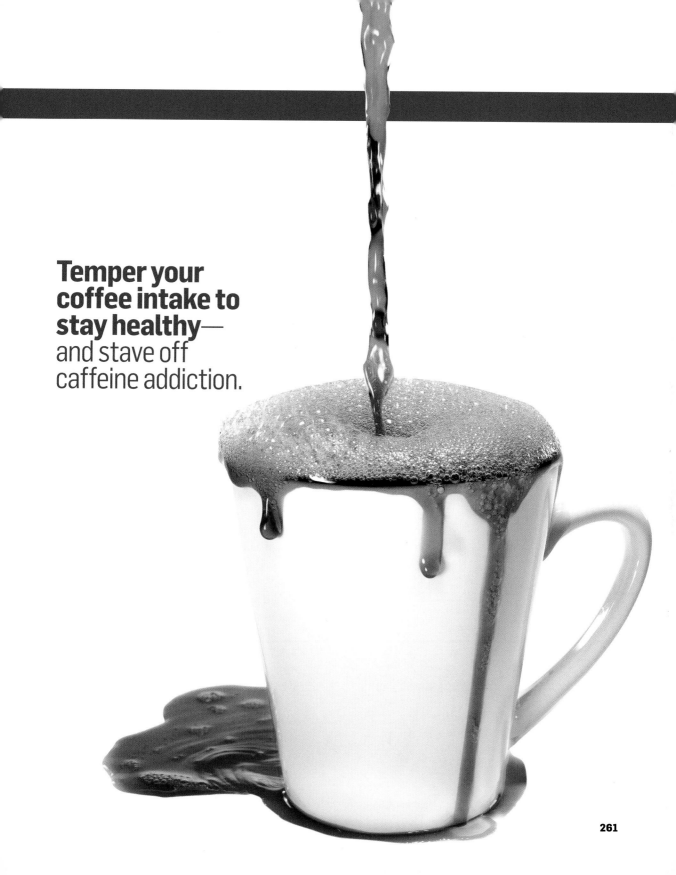

Temper your coffee intake to stay healthy—
and stave off caffeine addiction.

A life lived at full throttle can't be sustained. Eventually we start calling it a night and asking for the doggie bag after a couple of rounds. We begin feeling more sorry for than envious of Charlie Sheen. But what about overindulging in the stuff that seems so good for us? Sleep, for instance. Or coffee. Or antioxidants. If those things are inherently good—even lifesaving—can't we just gorge ourselves on them? After all, who ever heard of someone going on an antioxidant bender?

Nobody: That's the problem. So we combed the research and consulted experts across a range of specialties. In our process of elimination, we were thrilled to hear that it's difficult to OD on sex or masturbation. Ditto fruits and vegetables. But the dark sides of other health-enhancing moves surprised us. Toxicologists have an expression for this principle: "The dose makes the poison." That's never been truer than with these five "good" things.

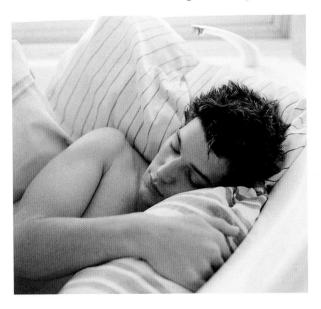

GOOD/BAD THING #1

Sleep

If a deficit of nightly sleep can make you gain weight and lose mental sharpness as well as increase your risk of cardiovascular disease, then scoring tons of shut-eye must be just what the doctor ordered, no? No. In a 2010 study in the journal *Sleep*, men who logged 9 or more hours a night were 43 percent more likely to have heart disease than 7-hour sleepers—regardless of their age, BMI, physical activity, alcohol use, and preexisting diseases.

But you may be among the minority of people who naturally need a lot of sleep—which is okay, as long as you feel refreshed the next day.

"If you're still sleepy, something may be affecting sleep quality, such as sleep apnea or restless leg syndrome," says Clete Kushida, MD, PhD, medical director of Stanford Sleep Medicine Center. "These conditions fragment sleep, so they can actually make you sleep longer."

If you suspect one of these is a factor, your physician can refer you to a sleep center for evaluation.

Wake up easier. If you're just sleeping too much, set your TV timer to wake you up—the light and noise combo is more rousing than an alarm clock, says Christopher Winter, MD, a *Men's Health* advisor and medical director of the Martha Jefferson Hospital Sleep Medicine Center in Charlottesville, Virginia.

"Light tells your brain to stop making the sleep hormone melatonin," he says. "This is better than leaving the curtain open—flickering TV light is more bothersome to your brain than steady light."

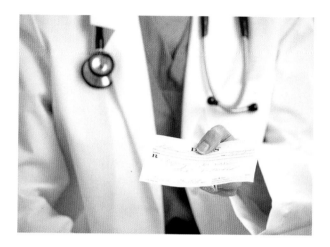

GOOD/BAD THING #2

Antibiotics

Use the right tools for the job. We wish doctors would internalize this message better. Many insist on banging in nails with screwdrivers by prescribing antibiotics—which fight bacterial infections—for viral ailments.

"When a doctor doesn't want to be wrong because there's a slight chance a patient has a bacterial infection, or if a patient insists, then antibiotics are more likely to be prescribed," says Lauri Hicks, DO, medical director of the Centers for Disease Control and Prevention's "Get Smart: Know When Antibiotics Work" campaign.

Upper-respiratory infections are classic examples. They account for 75 percent of all antibiotics prescribed by general practitioners, yet their cause is viral about 90 percent of the time. What's the harm? Antibiotic overuse can spawn resistance in fast-evolving bacteria, such as NDM-1 and the skin infection MRSA. Also, antibiotics can kill off beneficial bacteria in your body.

Battle better. Ask your doctor if your condition could resolve itself without a prescription, or whether a first-line antibiotic, such as amoxicillin or penicillin, would be more appropriate than a broad-spectrum antibiotic, like azythromycin.

"There's a perception that newer antibiotics are more effective, and that's not always the case," says Dr. Hicks. "Good old penicillin is still an important initial therapy, and it leaves options for further treatment."

GOOD/BAD THING #3

Coffee

Your daily java provides long-lasting health advantages. Recent research suggests a link between coffee consumption and lowered risks of Alzheimer's disease, liver cancer, and prostate cancer.

But beware the telltale buzz of caffeine addiction, which can set in if you slurp more than 300 milligrams of the stuff each day. (A 12-ounce Starbucks standard brew has 260.) As your body adjusts to regular caffeine exposure, your fatigue-regulating adenosine system—which is hijacked by caffeine—becomes more sensitive, and you'll feel sluggish in your noncaffeinated moments, according to a 2010 British study. The buzz that addicts feel is merely the emergence from fatigue-causing withdrawal symptoms.

Spread out your fix. Pace your daily intake.

"Better to spread it throughout the day to prevent overdose," says James D. Lane, PhD, the director of Duke University Medical Center's psychophysiology laboratory. "It's the high peak of caffeine in your blood that causes problems." If you normally drink 12 ounces with breakfast, limit yourself to half that in the morning and have the other half at lunchtime.

GOOD/BAD THING #4
Ibuprofen

When knees and muscles ache, wounded warriors in a hurry to heal dose up on "vitamin I"—ibuprofen. And if the recommended 400 milligrams of magic relief

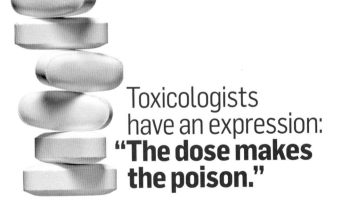

Toxicologists have an expression: **"The dose makes the poison."**

from pain and swelling don't quite do it, well, pop two more. In fact, why not head off workout pain by gulping several ibuprofen tablets before going running or playing hoops? So goes the logic that leads men to pop them like Tic Tacs.

Ibuprofen leads a broad pack of painkillers known as nonsteroidal anti-inflammatory drugs, or NSAIDs. These drugs decrease production of prostraglandins, which can act as pain and inflammation messengers. When used habitually or preventively, though, they deter those hormones from doing another vital job: generating tissue-building collagen.

Injured bone, ligament, and muscle can't heal as quickly or grow at the same rate, says Stuart T. Warden, PhD, an assistant professor in Indiana University's Department of Physical Therapy. "Taking ibuprofen before a workout won't reduce soreness and can actually decrease the effectiveness of exercise," he says. NSAIDs also inhibit cyclooxygenase, which is an enzyme thought to be involved in the protection of the heart and stomach linings; this effect can lead to an increased risk of heart attack in susceptible people, as well as nausea, diarrhea, and intestinal bleeding.

Ease the pain. Stop the prophylactic pill popping and head for the pool after your workout.

"The best treatment for muscle soreness is gentle exercise, like hydrotherapy—so walking or running in a pool for 20 minutes is one option," Warden says. The movement alleviates the fluid buildup that causes pain.

Antioxidants

Free radicals: They're as scary as they sound. These cell-damaging molecules are thought to contribute to arthritis, diabetes, stroke, cancer, and heart disease. Your potential lifesavers? Antioxidants. Those in beta-carotene and in vitamins C and E attack and neutralize the roaming free radicals. But antioxidant supplements are a different story—they might actually sideline your body's antioxidant defenses. In a German study, young men who exercised for 4 weeks saw an improvement in their sensitivity to insulin—a known exercise benefit that helps prevent type 2 diabetes—while those who exercised for 4 weeks while supplementing with vitamins C and E saw no boost.

Let nature do its thing. Score your antioxidant infusion from a balanced diet; you'll hedge your bets in favor of any still-unknown benefits, and avoid megadosing.

"It may be there is something in whole-food 'packaging' that makes the nutrients better absorbed or used than they would be in supplements," says Katherine Zeratsky, RD, LD, of the Mayo Clinic.

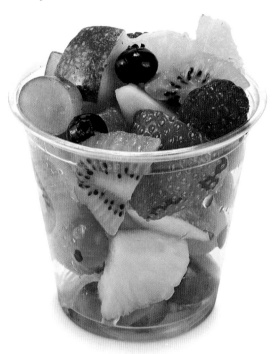

Drop That Scale! And That BP Cuff ...

Be careful that you aren't testing and measuring yourself into an obsession.

We're big fans of at-home health monitoring; the easier it is to measure your weight, body fat, blood pressure, and other vitals, the better. But there's a catch.

"With such easy access to technology, some people tend to monitor their health more closely than they ought to," says Elias Aboujaoude, MD, director of the Obsessive-Compulsive Disorder Clinic at Stanford University School of Medicine. When you find yourself unable to go to work or out on a date without weighing yourself first, it's time to step back and reevaluate your behavior, he says. Remind yourself that if your BMI or blood pressure hasn't dramatically changed in the past couple of days, it probably won't in the next few. Unless your doctor recommends otherwise, stick to weekly monitoring. Try unplugging the device or removing its batteries after each use, or place a note with the date of your next scheduled reading on your scale or BP monitor, Dr. Aboujaoude suggests. The idea is to place obstacles between you and the behavior you're trying to stop. If you still can't tear yourself away, stash the devices in the basement or someplace without easy access.

The Healing Power in Your iPod

Writer Bill Stieg reports: Music is an invisible force that can help lift your spirit, build your body, and improve your mind. Are you listening?

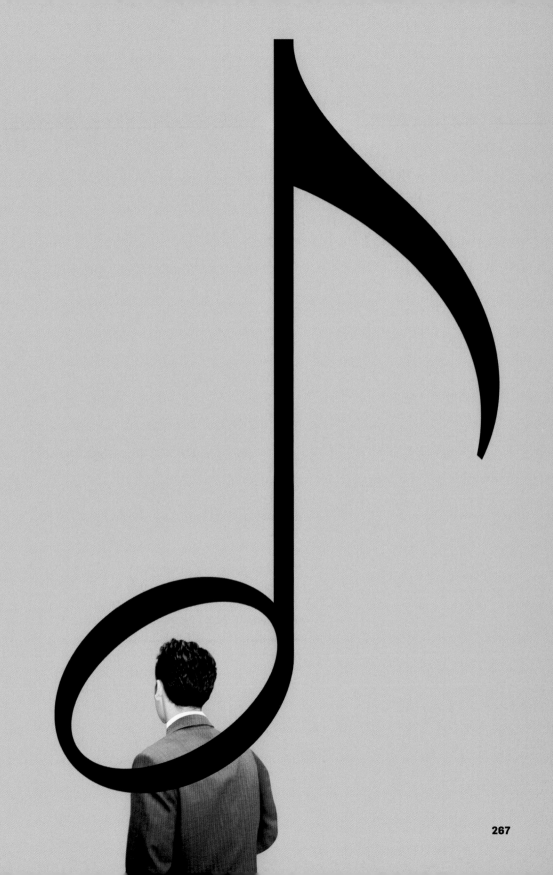

The opening chords make the hair on my arms stand up. A spotlighted Roy Bittan is at the piano, playing the quiet intro to "Racing in the Street," as Bruce Springsteen waits in the shadows. I first heard them perform this song 31 years ago, so nostalgia is a factor, no doubt. But 8 minutes later, by the time Bittan is crashing through the glorious chords of the song's extended coda, I've been transported, dazzled, exhilarated. There are quivers down my backbone.

This is a familiar sensation, one I indulge in to the tune of hundreds of dollars a year in concert tickets—from aging-boomer arena shows to ear-catching new bands in clubs. I go in knowing I'll howl like a fool at a Neil Young guitar solo, well up like a wuss as Carole King harmonizes with James Taylor—and love every minute.

Such is the power of music over me. And even though the volume usually isn't turned up to 11, music has a hold on nearly all of us—insidious, ubiquitous, and irresistible. Companies know this and have been messing with your vulnerable synapses for decades through shopping soundtracks and commercial jingles. But you too can tap into music's power (minus the amplifiers and overpriced tickets) if you want to work more efficiently, train harder, think quicker, and maybe even live longer.

Just Listen

It's 6:45 on a weekday morning, and I'm at the piano with a cup of coffee, plunking through the four simple chords of Hank Williams's "Weary Blues from Waitin'," a tune meant for guitar, which I don't play. When the cracked-voice country yodel on the last line of the chorus ("Oh sweet ma-a-ma, please come home") emerges from my amateur throat, it sounds lame. But it feels so good.

Today's immersion in music began 45 minutes earlier with "Black Coffee in Bed" by Squeeze and a carpet jingle ("800-588-2300, Empire Today") on MSNBC's *Morning Joe*. Then I heard snippets of Costello and Petty. Humming in the shower. The *Today* theme. At the piano, some Hank, and Radiohead's equally simple "Creep," complete with f-bombs. Driving to work, there were more songs on the radio and from CDs, and a jingle from a gas-pump screen. As I walk across the parking lot to the office, I helplessly hum the last song I heard.

This isn't my fault. I was—we all were—born this way.

"We're musical beings," says Teresa Lesiuk, PhD, an assistant professor of music therapy at the University of Miami. "It's like we're hardwired for music. We're ready to take it in, we're ready to interact with it."

Moreover, the experts I spoke with—

neurologists, musicologists, guitarists— all agree that man is probably exposed to music more frequently now than at any time in history.

"It's beginning to be looked at as a resource," Lesiuk says. "How can this help people?"

To start with, it helps me wake up. This morning, Joe Scarborough was nattering about the president when I heard the organ intro and thumping drums of Squeeze—a "bumper" for an impending commercial. I like this song. I opened my eyes. My brain was beginning to stir. Daniel Levitin, PhD, an associate professor of psychology at McGill University and the author of *This Is Your Brain on Music*, tells me I'm off to a good start. (He wasn't in my bedroom; we talked by phone.) Music with a beat, he says, leads to a brain process called spreading activation. "That's a fancy name for when a bunch of

neurons start firing at a certain rate, say in response to music, and other neurons that have nothing to do with music start firing in sympathy." Indeed, a Japanese study found that people who listened to music after a nap were less sleepy than those who didn't tune in.

I never realized it, but this shot of aural caffeine is amplified whenever I sit down at the piano in the morning.

"Playing an instrument activates disparate parts of your brain," says Levitin. "It's waking up the decision-making center, the motor center, the sensory center that feels the touch of the instrument on your fingertips, the auditory center, and the visual center, to the extent that you're reading music or watching your fingers."

Of course, the idea of playing music before breakfast might seem absurd to most sane people. But even a short session

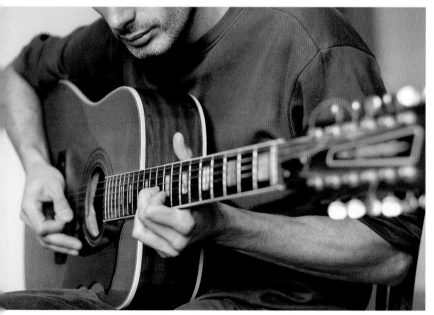

Human beings are easily hooked, experts say. **Our brains seem hardwired to respond to music.**

of Guitar Hero can serve the same purpose. My quick hit of piano noodling makes me feel ready for anything—or at least my drive to work.

We're probably **exposed to music more now** than at any time in history.

Can You Hear Me Now?

For the first part of my 45-minute commute, I listen to talk radio or news. But eventually I must have music; silence simply won't do. In fact, Australian research suggests that silence isn't ideal for driving. It lets you think about things other than driving.

My mix, using the radio and CD changer, is mostly indie and classic rock with the occasional nostalgic wild card, like marching band or Broadway or folk. And that's what matters for driving, a range of research shows: Within reason, music that makes you feel good is best for alertness, reaction time, and maintaining a safe speed.

Again, the key is "within reason," because research has also shown that the faster the music, the faster and less safely you'll drive. For example, a study from Israel discovered that a lot more speeding, red-light running, and accidents took place as the tempo of music increased. Similarly, a study from Memorial University of Newfoundland found that drivers listening to hard rock crashed more often on a simulated course than those listening

to industrial noise did. I know this from experience. I have avoided ZZ Top on freeways ever since "La Grange" led to a speeding ticket.

That said, it's still best to listen to something while you're behind the wheel. Levitin says the daydreaming reverie of driving causes many of us to sleep at the wheel, in a way. "If you choose the right music when you're driving, it can stimulate you enough to hold your interest and keep you conscious, aware, and awake," he says.

The problem, he adds, is that "if the music is too interesting or too absorbing, it draws you too deeply in and away from the road." Moderation seems to be the key—as with driving itself. Nothing too loud, too fast, or too distracting.

Once Americans arrive at the office, in the morning, they increasingly seal themselves off with earphones. A 2010 survey of workers who use computers (and don't interact with customers) found that 95 percent of them listen to music at least 30 minutes during the workday, usually through earphones, according to a 2010 survey by CIMI Corporation, a research firm in New Jersey.

Of course, for most of human history, music has been making physical labor—from rowing a Greek galley to mowing a half-acre lawn—more bearable. But can it help in the white-collar world?

Lesiuk, the University of Miami music therapist, has found that, generally speaking, if people listen to music of their choosing, they can decrease 9-to-5 fatigue, nervousness, and irritability while at the same time enhance their enthusiasm and relaxation. The net effect: They become better problem solvers.

Awaken the Musician Inside You

Piano lessons as a kid? Garage-band guitar in high school? Never played anything? Whatever your experience, technology makes it easier than ever to make music.

The instrument	The tech	The trick	The benefit
YOUR VOICE	*No need for public humiliation. Software (try karafun.com) lets you record yourself along with karaoke tracks (karaoke.com) or your own CDs.*	*Breathe better by relaxing your abs (you heard us!) and let your gut jut out so your diaphragm can do its work.*	*A lung and diaphragm workout. Plus, you may also boost your immune system, German studies show.*
PIANO	*Buy a teaching keyboard, like the Yamaha EZ-200 ($150, amazon.com). Keys light up so you can find the notes. Spare the fam—use headphones.*	*Simplify by just learning chords, and hum or sing the melody. Find chords on the Web or buy a "fake book" of melody, lyrics, and chords.*	*Less stress. In a study in Medical Science Monitor, keyboard players showed fewer immune-related genes in their blood, indicating lower stress.*
GUITAR	*You're not Ted Nugent yet. The software Amazing Slow Downer (roni music.com) lets you change the tempo of a song without altering the pitch.*	*Countless rock, folk, and country songs are based on just three chords. Learn G, C, and D, and hundreds of songs are within your reach.*	*Better language skills. Musicians' brain stems had more-robust linguistic encoding, a study found, which may explain their language-learning skills.*
DRUMS	*Go simple with the Remo medium Festival Djembe ($120, remo.com). Or pound Yamaha's DD45 portable electronic drums ($90, amazon.com).*	*Find a drum circle (drumcircles.net) for helpful support. At home, play along on an electronic pad with mid-tempo songs—and use headphones.*	*Upper-body training and less stress. Japanese researchers found that drumming breaks improved office workers' moods and lowered stress.*

Sources: John David De Haan, associate professor of voice, University of Minnesota; Pamela Pike, PhD, assistant professor of piano pedagogy, Louisiana State University; Joseph A. Baldassarre, DMA, professor emeritus of music, Boise State University; Jonathan Haas, director of the percussion studies program at NYU

Even a tiny dose of tunes can have an effect. One Italian study found that when people listened to up-tempo music, they experienced the biggest boost in bloodflow to their brains, compared with when they heard slower tunes or nothing at all. But Lesiuk believes there's probably a psychological component too. People can convince themselves that they won't work as well without a soundtrack. For instance, she's had IT workers decline to participate in her research because the experiment required that music be shut off for a period of time.

There are exceptions, and I'm one of them. While I'm sure I'm more efficient at physical efforts (like cleaning the garage) and visual tasks (like playing around in Photoshop) as music is playing, I can forget about reading or writing in the office. I can't concentrate. Lesiuk says hearing lyrics and reading words simultaneously probably divides my attention. She has also found that the more skilled someone is at a task, the better he or she does with music playing. If you're not skilled, music is just another stimulus that hurts your concentration.

Music diverts our attention during exercise, which lowers our level of perceived effort.

Not Following? Turn Down the Music

If any place seems to have sprouted more earbuds than the American office, it's the American gym. I used to be a purist, running roads and trails, and even the treadmill, without music. Now I'm less pure and more happy. An upbeat mix loaded into an old Nano makes my runs faster and more pleasant, no question.

This is not news. The link between rocking out and working out has been confirmed on treadmills and stationary bikes; cyclists use less oxygen while pedaling in time with tunes, and runners perceive less effort and have 15 percent greater endurance when matching tempo to stride.

One of the leading researchers in this field is Costas Karageorghis, PhD, of the sports psychology department at Brunel University in the United Kingdom. He helps organize a half marathon in London called Run to the Beat, during which live bands perform specially chosen songs along the route. Karageorghis says most athletes benefit from syncing their songs with their intended pace—starting with mid-tempo tunes, for instance, and then increasing the beat. If you know the music well, he says, you'll find it easier to push yourself during the most exhilarating passages, because athletes naturally increase effort at these moments.

It works on your strength too. Combining music and mental imagery helps muscular endurance. A Canadian study determined that lifters who played music while they pumped iron for 4 weeks completed 56 percent more repetitions of their 10-rep max. And if that doesn't convince you that the iPod is the best (legal) performance enhancer on the market, consider an Israeli study in which athletes who listened to upbeat music before a workout experienced a boost in peak power output, unlike when they warmed up in silence.

One way music helps us exercise is by diverting our attention, which lowers our level of perceived effort and makes "hard" seem more like "fun," Karageorghis says. Similarly, Australian researchers found that distracting free-throw shooters with upbeat music allowed them to perform without negative thoughts interfering, so they made more shots. I find that when I'm playing golf, I can block memories of bad shots by humming. (And I hum a lot on golf courses.)

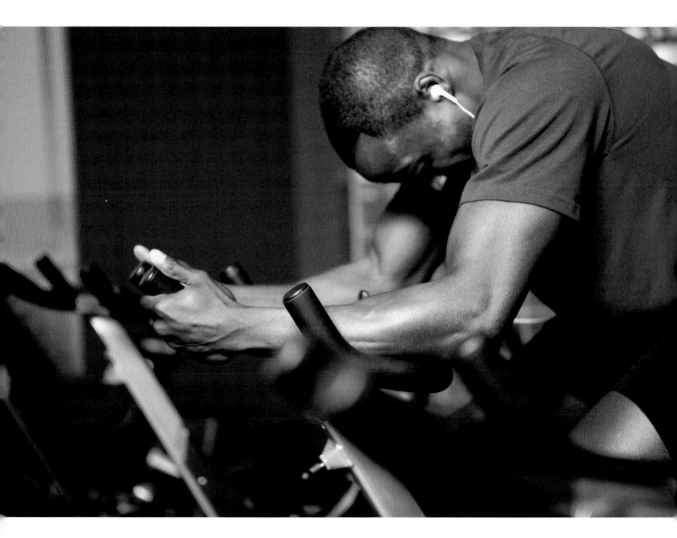

Crank Up the Muzak

There's one place in America where music is virtually unavoidable: the mall. Background music is a big, multinational business, with increasingly sophisticated research producing ever more targeted playlists. Muzak, the 78-year-old granddaddy of the field, sells its music services (for stores, offices, customers on hold) with promises to relax customers, encourage brand loyalty, improve employee productivity, and of course, boost sales.

An analysis of the data from 32 studies of background music in the *Journal of Business Research* finds clear implications for "return on investment" if music is piped into a business. The conclusions: Customers prefer music to silence, especially music they like. The slower and lower the volume, the longer they'll stay. This might not seem to explain the thumping soundtrack at Hollister, but in fact its young, female clientele loves it loud, the music fits the store's image, and "tempo has the greatest effect on arousal," the study review says. An excited girl is more likely to spend.

In a U.K. study, people would sign their name to support a charity regardless of the type of music playing, but if the music was uplifting, they'd volunteer to distribute leaflets too.

In another U.K. experiment, researchers compared bank environments that had easy-listening and classical music piped in with ones that had no music. The music actually made the banks seem more dynamic. The same researchers also conducted an experiment that compared bars with background music and those with no music or with music playing in the foreground. The background music, they found, made the bar seem more peaceful.

Listen Carefully

Noise of 85 decibels or louder can damage the hairs of your cochlea, a snail-shaped structure in your ears. Your iPod at full volume can hit 105 decibels. Worse, hearing loss tends to occur over time, unnoticed. "If you keep introducing noise trauma to the ear, you can cause permanent damage," says Theresa Shaw, a senior audiologist at New York University. Here's how to enjoy your music while saving your ears.

TURN IT DOWN.
"If the person next to you can hear what you're listening to on your iPod, it's too loud," Shaw says. One study showed that an iPod exceeds 85 decibels when it's set between 60 and 70 percent capacity.

SEAL YOURSELF OFF.
Ambient noise on planes and trains can top 100 decibels, tempting you to turn up your MP3 player. Use noise-canceling headphones like Audio-Technica's ATH-ANC7b ($200, shopaudiotechnica.com).

PLUG YOUR EARS.
Concerts can reach 115 decibels, but foam earplugs can cut that by 25 decibels. Try some Aearo ER20 plugs ($24, amazon.com: In a Brazilian study, musicians said they allowed them to clearly hear the music).

TAKE BREAKS.
Where loud music is playing, step outside for 15 minutes every 2 hours. The hairs on the cochleas can be overtaxed, causing a form of short-term hearing loss, and stepping away lets them recover.

DON'T BE DUMB.
Wear hearing-protection earmuffs when you mow the lawn or run any loud machinery. But don't slip your earbuds under the muffs to listen to music. You'll just negate their effectiveness, Shaw says.

One study even found that playing French or German music spurred shoppers to buy French or German wine.

Fair warning, then: Retailers are out to lull you into spending. Maybe it's best to listen to a podcast while you're at the mall.

An Rx for Music

I haven't been sick since the year 2000. It's weird. I'm also a (usually) happy guy. This can probably be attributed to genes, luck, and a wonderful family, but I can't help suspecting that—you guessed it— music is medicine too.

A review in the *American Journal of Public Health* calls music "the most accessible and most researched medium of art and healing." The review mentions the successful use of music to control pain in cancer patients as well as its role in improving their immune response, decreasing their anxiety, and reducing their psychological and physical symptoms. In one University of Wisconsin study, heart-attack patients who listened to relaxing music for 20 minutes showed slower heart and respiratory rates and less demand for oxygen—up to 1 hour after listening.

Then there's this research from the University of Maryland: Music that evokes joy can improve blood-vessel dilation by 26 percent. And scientists in Germany say that singing in a choir boosts immune function—and just listening to choral music lowers levels of the stress hormone cortisol.

I believe it. Around Thanksgiving I dig out a shoebox of Christmas CDs, and for the next 6 weeks our house sounds like an upscale department store. There's a CD of German carols and hymns by a boys' choir that move me beyond words, which is fitting because I can't understand a word they're singing.

One Canadian study I've read refers to the "chills phenomenon" of music: the physical indicators of emotional arousal, such as blood volume pulse and electrodermal activity. That Springsteen show did it for me and so does the choir: My dermis is electrified. The chills study validates this, charmingly: "Strongly felt emotions could be rewarding in themselves." I'll even sing along phonetically, recalling my days in junior-high choir, and can practically feel those blood vessels opening wide.

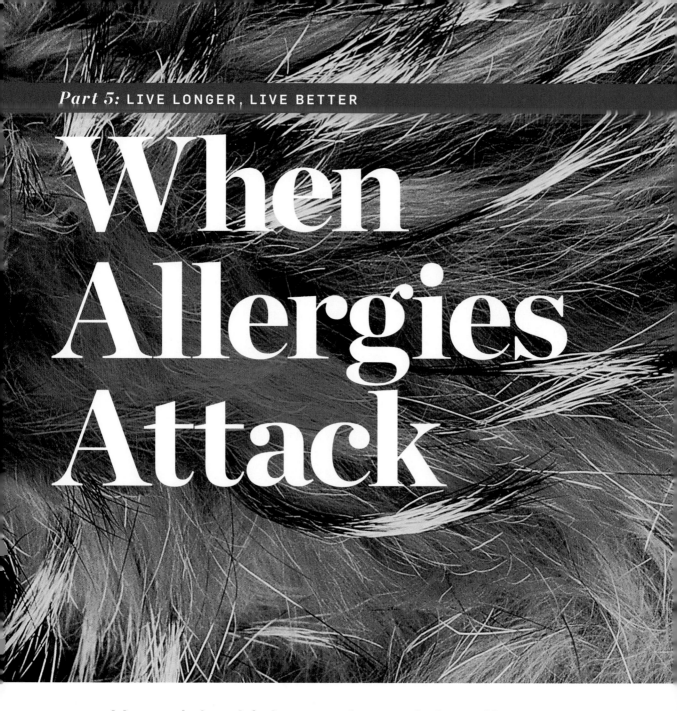

When Allergies Attack

You might think you cleared the allergy hurdle as a kid, but they can hit you at any time. Keep your defenses up with these tips.

Robert never had any allergies—nary a sniffle or a wheeze his entire life. Then he met his sister's new dog, a Lab named Finn. On a recent visit, Finn's copious dander ambushed the 39-year-old, causing sniffling, wheezing, runny eyes, scratchy throat, and relentless sneezing fits.

"I'd never had reactions to any animals," Robert said. "Now I won't come in the door without drugging myself up."

Allergists and immunologists are seeing more men like Robert, men who've been blindsided by new allergies.

"We used to think you couldn't develop allergies later in life," says immunologist Donata Vercelli, MD, a professor of cell biology and anatomy at the University of Arizona. "They usually arrived when you were young, and you typically outgrew them."

Adult-onset allergies might be part of a broader phenomenon. Scientists call it the hygiene hypothesis: The less you've been exposed to allergens in your life, the more likely you may be to develop allergies as an adult, according to a 2009 Australian review in *Allergy*. The theory is that when your system is out of practice, it becomes sloppy, Dr. Vercelli says. Instead of idly standing by, it launches all-out attacks against harmless dander and pollen, leaving you congested, itchy, and inflamed.

"Your immune system will work, not less effectively, but less appropriately," Dr. Vercelli says.

To hone your defenses, read on.

From the Air

The next time your boss blames your productivity dip on slacking, tell him it may be something in the air. Allergic rhinitis—a reaction that occurs inside the nasal passages and upper airways—costs employers millions in lost productivity and absenteeism each year. Often mistaken for bronchitis because both conditions cause coughing, it's actually triggered by pollen, pet dander, or dust mites.

When you're confronted with these invaders, a flood of chemicals—including histamine, bradykinin, and leukotrienes—dilates your mucous membranes, inflames your nose and throat, and causes your eyes to itch. Taking antihistamines such as Zyrtec, Claritin, or their generic forms can help prevent allergic rhinitis symptoms in most people—as long as they take the meds early in the day and not just when the symptoms appear. But these drugs target only one part of your reaction, histamine, says pulmonologist Paul Enright, MD, a professor of medicine at the University of Arizona. This may not be enough to clear you up.

YOUR STRATEGIES

When your throat starts to itch, raid the spice rack.

"Hot pepper, especially cayenne pepper, turns on mucus production," says James Dillard, MD, the *Men's Health* integrative-medicine advisor. "So if you have pollen sitting there, you may be able to rinse it out just by adding some pepper to your dish."

For persistent problems, ask your physician about allergen-specific immuno-therapy, which can shift your system to a nonallergic immune response. Currently, immunotherapy injections are the only FDA-approved treatment method for allergies. Some European countries recently approved an under-the-tongue tablet for grass-pollen sensitivity and are developing similar tablets to target allergies to dust mites and birch pollen. The FDA is investigating this treatment, and a 2008 study by the Naval Medical Center, in San Diego, found that allergists who've experimented with it viewed the treatment as safe and effective.

At home, turn down the thermostat. Warm indoor temperatures in winter can bring on a stuffy nose, irritated eyes, and wheezing, according to a recent U.S. government study. Make sure your house stays below 73°F, which is the temperature at which the symptoms began in study participants.

When it comes to pets, if you have an allergy and will be visiting a pet-friendly home, start using a nasal steroid spray 5 days beforehand, says George Pyrgos, MD, an allergy and immunology fellow at Johns Hopkins University. These products, including Nasonex and Flonase, help prevent inflammation.

From Your Food

Most likely you're not allergic to food. Only about 4 percent of adults are, and their reactions are generally limited to fish, shellfish, and nuts. But being among the other 96 percent doesn't mean you're entirely off the hook. Certain fish, when they're mishandled (inadequately refrigerated, for example) can release histamine, the same inflammatory chemical released by your immune system's mast cells.

"Some people eat fish and get a reaction that appears almost identical to a food allergic reaction," says Anju Peters, MD, an associate professor of allergy and immunology at Northwestern University.

Additionally, if your mouth itches every time you eat fruit, you may have oral allergy syndrome. That's because some types of pollen have proteins that are similar in structure to those of specific fruits. Such pairings include ragweed and melons, tree pollen and apples, and grass pollen and tomatoes.

"The similarities trick your immune system into thinking the trigger is one of these pollens when it's actually the fruit," says Dr. Pyrgos.

A Cold or Allergies?

Can't tell a cold from an allergy? You'll find out eventually: A cold lasts about a week; allergies can keep going for months. But at the start, know this.

EARLY SYMPTOMS: They may be identical at first, but allergies come with more itchiness and colds cause more coughing.

HOLD THE MEDICINE. Don't jump to take an antibiotic. It won't help either condition. Just treat the symptoms.

STAY VIGILANT. Monitor your symptoms. If nasal trouble doesn't improve or gets worse, you could have a sinus infection.

YOUR STRATEGIES

If you're uncertain about whether you're allergic to a specific food, consider requesting an allergen-detecting blood test called an ImmunoCAP. It's 95 to 98 percent accurate, according to a recent *Journal of Allergy and Clinical Immunology* study. In the case of oral allergy syndrome, Dr. Pyrgos recommends avoiding fruits, or eating them skinless, when your pollen sensitivity is high.

Through Your Skin

The winter complexion you probably attribute to cold, dry air could actually be atopic dermatitis, also known as eczema. It causes red, itchy skin and is triggered by unknown allergens. If you have it, you'll see tiny cracks in your skin. These fissures let in additional allergens and the natural bacteria on your skin (such as staph), giving them easy access to the immune cells waiting just below the surface. Or you might have contact dermatitis, in which one of nearly 3,000 triggers—such as nickel in a belt buckle or wristwatch—causes a similar reaction.

YOUR STRATEGIES

For eczema, apply a liberal layer of petroleum jelly to irritated areas after a shower to seal in moisture. Use only fragrance-free soaps, shampoos, and shaving products to avoid further irritation. For a persistent rash, apply hydrocortisone cream.

Because contact dermatitis symptoms don't show up for 24 to 72 hours, it might be difficult to pinpoint the cause. Identify the source with a doctor-administered

Allergic to Sex?

As if. But there are ways a little intimacy can cause the kind of reactions you weren't gunning for. Whether it's her lingering scent or a lingering itch from a latex condom, you can thwart these romantic gremlins.

COITUS INTER-OUCH. Some women develop allergies to proteins in their partners' semen, which can easily be misdiagnosed as vaginal itch. If she has other allergies, it may be worth being tested for it. Once diagnosed, you can use a condom, or she can try intravaginal immunotherapy. This treatment, a series of administered injections, desensitizes her to your semen.

NASAL NIGHTMARE. If her perfume makes you wheeze, you may have nonallergic rhinitis, says otolaryngologist Michael Benninger, MD, of the Cleveland Clinic. "True perfume allergies are rare, but the symptoms are the same—nasal obstruction and runny nose," he says. He suggests using an intranasal antihistamine, such as Astepro, 90 minutes before your date.

KISS OF DEATH. Never treat a good-night kiss lightly—especially if you have food allergies. Particles can linger in your date's saliva, which may mean itchy, swollen lips or even dangerous anaphylaxis, according to a Mount Sinai School of Medicine study. Offer her a piece of gum after dinner, and then wait an hour to make your move. This combo eliminates 99 percent of food residues.

BURNING RUBBERS. Latex allergies can be as unpleasant for women as they are for men. Either can break out in hives, have trouble breathing, or develop a rash, says Anju Peters, MD, an associate professor of allergy and immunology at Northwestern University. If she's allergic, use a polyurethane glove, such as Durex Avanti. It's as effective as latex, according to a recent Cochrane review.

TRUE (thin-layer rapid-use epicutaneous) test. Your doctor will stick a strip of allergens to your back for a few days to see if reactions develop.

If you have a nickel sensitivity, test your items with an Allertest Ni kit (allerderm.com, $20). If you want to keep using nickel products, coat them with the kit's Conceal Clear Coat or a layer of clear nail polish. Accidentally exposed? Smear on some hydrocortisone cream.

5 New Rules for a Healthy Heart

These key developments in cardio science will help your blood flow better than ever.

Are you doomed to heart disease? Given the fact that it's the most common killer of men, you'd be forgiven for thinking as much. But that's nonsense. Science has produced some nearly surefire strategies for not only treating a stricken ticker but also avoiding heart trouble in the first place.

And research is coming out almost daily that improves on what we already know. Our advice: Act on this wisdom. Sixty percent of young adults who did—by eating right, working out, keeping their BMIs in check, avoiding smoking, and going easy on the booze—kept their heart-disease risk low well into middle age, according to a new study from Northwestern University. Of people who ignored these basics, less than 5 percent stayed in the low-risk category.

"Your environment and the choices you make influence your risk more than genetics does," says study author Donald Lloyd-Jones, MD, chairman of North-western's preventive medicine department. "This is true even of the choices you made as far back as your youth and early adulthood."

We placed our finger on the pulse of heart research to find out which new approaches were most likely to improve your cardiovascular health. Follow our experts' advice and you'll be a lifelong member of the low-risk club, too.

Starting Point: Estimate Your Risk

In the past century, researchers have begun trying to predict heart-disease risk by manipulating key numbers. The Framingham Heart Model—an algorithm that factors in your age, blood pressure, cholesterol, and other figures—remains a widely used prediction tool.

"If you know your basic numbers, you can run an estimate yourself online and bring a printout to your doctor," says Michael Steinman, MD, an assistant professor of medicine at the University of California at San Francisco. "It's important to know at least your estimated risk."

NEW RULE: BROADEN THE EQUATION

Current research suggests that the Framingham Heart Model has some limitations: It doesn't consider family history, lifestyle, and body mass index. And according to a recent study published in *BMC Medicine*, roughly a third of heart trouble occurs in people labeled as low risk by common prediction models. So if you use the online tool, don't place a lot of stock in the results until you and your doctor have fully analyzed your family history and any bad habits you have, such as smoking or excessive drinking.

Furthermore, be careful about which Framingham model you use. There's a more complex equation-based version and a simpler points-based version. In a 2010 study, Dr. Steinman and his colleagues found that the points-based system was the less accurate one: It classified 17 percent of men into treatment categories that differed from ones they would have wound up in had the equation-based model been used.

"For some people on the borderline, this can make a difference in how aggressive their treatment will be," says Dr. Steinman. Find the equation-based version at MensHealth.com/heartmodel.

Starting Point: Train with Intervals

Swimming, running, biking: They're all terrific for your heart. And inserting periods of ultra-heavy heart pumping into your cardio routine (i.e., interval training, during which you reach 90-plus percent of your maximum heart rate) further boosts

What Your Heart's Trying to Tell You
Learn how to interpret the occasional telegram from your ticker, listed here from least to most severe.

LEAST SEVERE ← —————————————————→ MOST SEVERE

SHARP CHEST PAIN: Chest pain shouldn't be ignored, but it's not necessarily a heart attack. You may have pericarditis, an inflammation of the heart's outer membrane. "Pericarditis doesn't require urgent care," says Mehdi Razavi, MD, a cardiologist at the Texas Heart Institute. But see your doctor.

PRESSURE THAT WORSENS WITH EXERTION. This is probably angina, caused by a moderate arterial blockage, Dr. Razavi says. Beta-blockers can slow your heart rate and reduce your heart's oxygen needs to help prevent angina. An angioplasty may also be needed to treat the blockage.

LOWER JAW PAIN. This can be a less common sign of an infarction. "There have been horror stories of people going to the dentist when they were actually having heart attacks," Dr. Razavi says. While it may indeed be inflammation in your jaw joint, have an ER doctor check you out just to be safe.

SUDDEN, INTENSE PRESSURE. This may be a full-on heart attack. It differs from angina symptoms in that the pressure you feel is significantly more intense, Dr. Razavi says, and it may occur alongside a suite of other symptoms, such as sweating and nausea. Call 911.

your heart's efficiency over time.

"You're pushing the mitochondria in your cells to perform and adapt at a higher level," says Conrad Earnest, PhD, director of exercise biology at Pennington Biomedical Research Center in Baton Rouge, Louisiana. Intervals boost your heart's stroke volume as well as its efficiency, which is measured by peak oxygen uptake, or VO2 max. The impact is huge: After training with intervals, participants in a 2010 study in the *International Journal of Sports Medicine* saw an average improvement of 23 percent in stroke volume and a 17 percent increase in VO2 max. "Someone with a higher VO2 max tends to have a lower risk for metabolic and heart diseases," Earnest says.

NEW RULE: THROW YOUR WEIGHTS AROUND TOO

You can snare additional heart benefits by incorporating resistance training into your routine, says Earnest. According to a 2010 study in the *Journal of Strength and Conditioning Research*, weightlifting may improve bloodflow throughout your extremities, which eases your heart's workload. The study also found that your post-workout blood-pressure dip tends to last longer after weightlifting than after cardio exercise. Researchers speculate that the improved bloodflow could be the result of a boost in endothelial function, a measure of the health of your blood vessels. In the weight room, go for circuit training, during which you alternate between different muscle groups with minimal rest between them.

"There tends to be a larger circulatory response with circuit training," Earnest says. For the best exercises, head to MensHealth.com/circuittraining.

Starting Point: Cut Cholesterol with Fiber

Oatmeal, barley, and psyllium are rich sources of soluble fiber, which can help reduce your cholesterol. Barley and oatmeal contain betaglucans, soluble fibers that help lower your LDL cholesterol by preventing it from being absorbed into your bloodstream. Psyllium, found in cereals and fiber supplements, may slash your LDL by triggering an increase in your body's excretion of bile acid, the digestive fluid that cholesterol is converted into.

NEW RULE: ADD TOMATOES

Okay, maybe not to your oatmeal. But pour yourself a daily glass of tomato juice; it's rich in lycopene, a nutrient that might cut your body's production of LDL cholesterol. People who drank about a

Many patients on statins **might not need the drugs**.

glass and a half of tomato juice and ate 2 tablespoons of ketchup every day for 3 weeks reduced their LDL levels by an average of 8.5 percent, according to a study in the *British Journal of Nutrition*. Make sure you opt for low-salt varieties of ketchup and tomato juice, because sodium can raise blood pressure.

Starting Point: Watch Your Stress

That 60-hour-a-week job could send you to the ER. In a study in the journal *Stress*, researchers measured levels of the stress hormone cortisol in hair samples from 56 men who'd been hospitalized for heart attacks and from 56 men hospitalized for other reasons. For 3 months before the test, the heart-attack victims had cortisol levels that were a third higher than the control group's.

"It's a high-stress world," says John Ratey, MD, an associate clinical professor of psychiatry at Harvard medical school. "People are willing to take on more than ever."

If stress is making your head spin, walk up and down a short flight of stairs three times, he suggests. The exercise will release a calming concoction of chemicals in your brain, so you'll be more focused when you return to your desk.

NEW RULE: BANISH THE BLUES AS WELL

Stress can kill, but so can depression. After studying twins with genetic predispositions for depression and heart disease, researchers at Washington University in St. Louis concluded that depression—past or present—raises a man's risk of heart disease more than genetic or environmental factors do.

"The higher risk may come from the inflammation that certain mental health problems can cause," says *Men's Health* advisor Prediman K. Shah, MD, director of the division of cardiology at the Oppenheimer Atherosclerosis Research Center at Cedars-Sinai Medical Center.

Seek help for your head and you might help your heart: People who took SSRIs, a class of antidepressants, showed improved bloodflow as a result of slower platelet clumping, according to a 2010 study from Loyola University medical center.

Starting Point: Go for a Blood Test

Prescription statins are the gold standard for reducing cholesterol. For people at risk of heart disease, statins can lower the chance of having a heart attack by as much as 30 percent, according to the *British Medical Journal*. The trick is determining when you need to start popping the pills.

"For people with borderline cholesterol, the situation is murky," says Michael Blaha, MD, a cardiology fellow at Johns Hopkins University. Many doctors use a blood test that measures C-reactive protein (CRP), an inflammatory marker, to help make the final call. Your body makes more CRP when there's inflammation, which can be caused by the plaque buildup in your arteries. High cholesterol could be the culprit.

NEW RULE: ALSO CONSIDER A CT SCAN

The problem with the CRP test: Cholesterol may not be the only cause of inflammation, or even its main cause. Arthritis or a sinus infection, for example, can also inflame your insides, Dr. Blaha says. A 2010 study he coauthored shows that if you have borderline LDL and an elevated CRP, you should consider, well, another final call: a CT scan. This test can take the guesswork out of diagnosing atherosclerosis by allowing your doctor to see firsthand whether arterial buildup is a problem. The study concluded that many patients who'd been prescribed statins because of elevated CRPs might not have needed the drugs after all.

If your doctor's analysis does ultimately suggest that statins should be part of your treatment plan, he or she might give you 6 months to reduce your cholesterol before writing out a scrip. If that's the case, circle back to the cholesterol-reduction strategies mentioned earlier in this article, and work on bringing those levels down without an Rx. Hey, the clock's ticking . . .

The Magic Bullet for Prostate Cancer

The problem is, it's not magic.
And with a price tag of $200 million,
it's the most expensive medical device
in the history of the world.
Is it worth it?

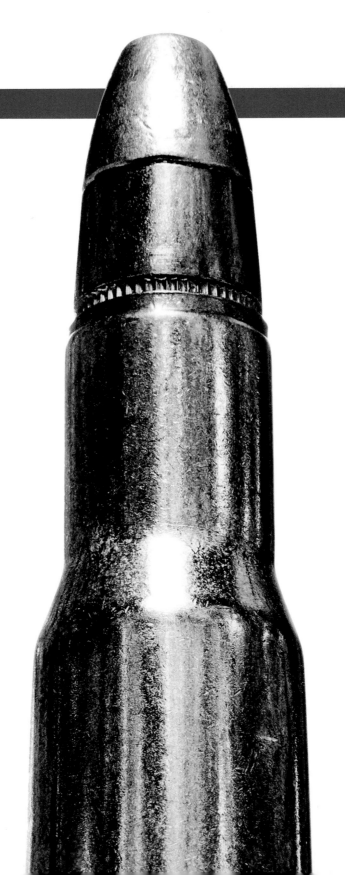

Oklahoma City was not John Bell's idea of a honeymoon spot. But somewhere between popping the question and setting a date came the difficult matter of his prostate.

Until the prostate problem, Bell was a fit 66-year-old who'd always boasted of remarkable health, provided he didn't count an unfortunate dart to the eye in his college days. But then a biopsy in September 2009 revealed a tumor in his prostate. His doctors—and there would be many before he was done—recommended surgery. Bell didn't like what he was hearing, though, about his prospects of impotence and incontinence. He was about to marry Sherry, a woman he had met 20 years earlier when her late husband and Bell were both dedicated Civil War reenactors. He wanted to be cured, no doubt, but for his honeymoon, he wanted his bayonet as fixed and as ready as any in Pickett's Charge.

Then his bride-to-be heard about something new: a treatment that zaps tumors with protons (subatomic particles that offered the promise of a cure with less collateral damage to healthy tissues). A little Internet sleuthing and consultation with a successful proton-beam patient convinced Bell.

"I was ready for something other than surgery," he says. Even better, a new proton center had just opened for business in Oklahoma City, right across the state line from his home near Dallas. The Bells were married in December 2009, and the following February he began treatment. The newlyweds spent 2 months at the nearby Town Village Retirement Community—radiation in the morning, sightseeing in the afternoon—and the groom returned home cancer-free—by all indications. Welcome to the atomic age for ailing prostates.

Once available at only two locations— one on each coast—proton-therapy centers are now the object of technolust, with many hospital administrators who don't have one wishing they did. When it opened for business in the summer of 2009, Oklahoma City's ProCure Proton Therapy Center, a concrete-and-glass edifice located just off the John Kilpatrick Turnpike, became the country's sixth proton-beam facility. Nine are now operating in the United States—two of them opened in the same week in October 2010—with at least four more on the way.

"I think people realize we have reached the limit on conventional radiation," says Sameer Keole, MD, medical director of the Oklahoma City center. "We haven't even scratched the surface of what we can do with protons."

There's one problem, though: It isn't certain that proton beams work better than conventional prostate-cancer treatments. And that bit of doubt has ignited one of the most contentious debates in modern prostate-cancer treatment. With construction costs that can exceed $200 million, a proton-beam generator could be the most expensive medical device ever made. In dramatic fashion, protons have raised a question we Americans find distasteful asking and even more distasteful answering: When is a lifesaving treatment worth its price?

But first things first: Is this therapy even an improvement?

"It's very good treatment," says Anthony Zietman, MD, of Massachusetts General Hospital in Boston, who is president of the American Society for Radiation Oncology. "It just doesn't appear to be superior treatment."

At least not for prostates, he says.

For tumors entrenched in exquisitely sensitive tissues, including the brain, eye, and spinal cord, and for most malignancies in children, doctors are enthusiastic about the potential of protons.

"I do not want to throw sand in the engine of proton-therapy development," Dr. Zietman says. "I think it's a game changer in radiotherapy. But the risk is it will discredit itself by concentrating on prostate cancer, where there's no obvious advantage, instead of concentrating on areas where a major advantage clearly exists."

One of those areas—childhood cancers—requires lengthy treatments, and insurance companies often cause hassles. A prostate patient spends 20 minutes in the machine, and the tab is usually picked up without hesitation by Medicare and most insurance companies.

"It's pretty clear that the economics of having a proton center depend heavily on using it to treat prostate cancer," says Sean Tunis, MD, director of the

Read This before Your Next PSA Test

The prostate-specific antigen (PSA) test is one step in diagnosing cancer, but it's far from foolproof. Only one in four men with moderately high PSA levels has prostate cancer, and some men with prostate cancer test normally.

"I like to think of PSA as 'Please Stay Alert,'" says Ash Tewari, MD, director of the LeFrak Center for Robotic Surgery at Weill Cornell Medical Center. Help your doctor make the most of your results by speaking up if any of these potentially PSA-altering conditions apply to you.

YOU TAKE MEDICATION CONTAINING FINASTE-RIDE. Propecia, the hair-loss drug, and Proscar, a drug used to treat prostate enlargement, can lower your PSA by half, Dr. Tewari says. Finasteride inhibits an enzyme that helps hormones act on your prostate, and without that enzyme, your prostate won't make as much PSA, whether you have cancer or not.

YOU'RE A PILL POPPER. Some common medications can lower your PSA if you've been taking them for 5 years or longer. A recent study in the *Journal of Clinical Oncology* found that men who took aspirin or ibuprofen, statins, or thiazide diuretics (blood pressure meds) had PSA levels 6 percent, 13 percent, and 26 percent lower, respectively, than men who didn't pop these pills.

YOU TAKE SUPPLEMENTS. One recent study in the journal *Prostate* showed that when men with high PSA readings took supplements containing curcumin and soy isoflavones, their levels dropped 45 percent. It's not clear whether some supplements alter just your PSA or your actual cancer risk. Make sure your doctor knows about any supplements you take, just in case.

YOU HAD A COLONOSCOPY. "Any manipulation in that area can affect PSA," Dr. Tewari says. The journal *International Urology and Nephrology* reported that nearly half of men had elevated PSA levels 24 hours after a colonoscopy; some had elevated levels a month later. For this reason, ask your doctor to test your PSA before a colonoscopy or digital rectal exam.

YOUR PROSTATE IS ENLARGED OR INFLAMED. Let your doctor know if you've experienced trauma in the area, if you have to pee more often, or if you experience a burning sensation when you pee. Those could be signs of benign prostatic hyperplasia (a noncancerous enlargement) or prostatitis (an inflammation or infection of the prostate). Both can raise your PSA.

Baltimore-based Center for Medical Technology Policy. Of the approximately 150 patients treated at ProCure's Oklahoma City facility in its first year of operation, 109 had prostate cancer. Even Dr. Keole concedes that the controversy comes down to money: "Prostate cases are easier to move through the insurance queue, and they make up roughly 50 percent of our cases. We're trying to lower that percentage, but many commercial payers are reluctant to cover lung cancer, and yes, even pediatric cases. They often drag their feet reviewing cases, creating 'denial by delay.' We sometimes have difficulty getting insurance coverage for even the most ideal non-prostate cases."

In an era when health care already consumes nearly 18 percent of the U.S. economy—and when medical bills are the

Protons vs. X-Rays: The Subatomic Smackdown

Proton-beam therapy and traditional x-ray radiation damage the DNA of cancerous prostate cells to kill them or stop their growth. But collateral damage from the beams determines if you come out of the treatment impotent, incontinent, or both.

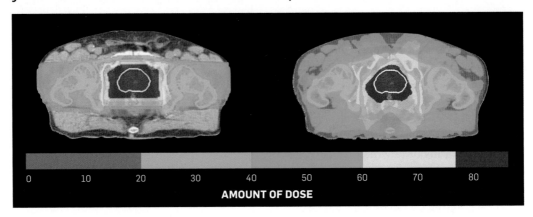

AMOUNT OF DOSE

PROTON-BEAM THERAPY

THE PROCESS: A cyclotron isolates protons from hydrogen atoms and accelerates them so that magnets can guide them to the tumor.

THE TARGET AREA: The mass and charge of protons make them deposit most of their dose at the tumor site; little radiation travels farther into other tissue, says Jason Efstathiou, MD, DPhil, a radiation oncologist at Massachusetts General Hospital.

STANDARD TARGETED RADIATION THERAPY

THE PROCESS: An accelerator smashes electrons into a tungsten target to form high-energy x-rays that are focused on and beamed to the cancer site.

THE TARGET AREA: The treatment delivers a lower dose of radiation over a larger area, but radiation from x-rays peaks shortly after entering the body and trails off slowly after hitting the tumor, so it might affect noncancerous tissues, Dr. Efstathiou says.

number one cause of personal bankruptcy, even though three out of four bankruptcy filers have health insurance—cost is indeed an issue. At the University of Pennsylvania's Roberts Proton Therapy Center, one of the world's largest, Medicare will reimburse $438 for a round of conventional radiation but will pay $1,282 for a proton blast. (Prostate-cancer treatment typically takes 44 sessions.) Private health insurers tend to follow Medicare's lead. Who picks up the difference? Mostly you—through the taxes you pay to fund Medicare, and through your health-insurance premiums.

Treatment is more expensive because protons are not easy to come by. The energy (and cancer-killing power) of traditional radiation comes when electrons are smashed into a metal plate, releasing their radioactive x-rays. The tumor-zapping energy of an electron can be harnessed by a device that fits easily into one treatment room. By contrast, the apparatus that beams the protons—which are stripped from hydrogen atoms and accelerated until they nearly reach the speed of light—weighs 220 tons. (That's heavier than three M1 tanks.) In its entirety, the machinery can take up more space than a football field.

Protons were suggested as an option for cancer treatment in the 1940s. Massachusetts General, where Dr. Zietman works, started collecting them from a Harvard cyclotron in the early 1960s. In the 1980s, James Slater, MD, a radiation oncologist at Loma Linda University medical center in California, was so convinced of their potential that he envisioned building a

Welcome to the **atomic age for ailing prostates**.

cancer-fighting accelerator.

"I did not like the side effects and the sickness we were producing with x-rays," says Dr. Slater, now 82 and still on the Loma Linda faculty. After an almost two-decade mission beginning in the 1970s, Dr. Slater and the medical center commissioned the Fermi National Accelerator Laboratory in Illinois to build a hospital-based proton accelerator, with part of the construction costs paid by the U.S. government. The first patient, a woman with melanoma on her eye, was treated in 1990.

What appealed to Dr. Slater, and what remains the main attraction of protons, is the idea that a stream of charged particles can be more easily controlled to match the irregular contours of a tumor. Both treatments—traditional x-rays and protons—disable a tumor's genetic structure, which has less capacity for self-repair than healthy tissues do. But x-rays barrel through the body, affecting all tissue in their path. One of Dr. Keole's defining professional moments was the day in medical school when he saw hair loss in a child who was being treated for a brain tumor—on the opposite side of her head. A proton beam delivers most of its radiation when it hits a tumor, and nearly stops cold.

"These patients really do make it through treatment much better," Dr. Keole says as he walks the halls of the Oklahoma center. At 39, he's one of

The machinery weighs 220 tons and takes up more space than a football field.

roughly 1 percent of radiation oncologists in the United States with experience in proton therapy.

Protons might have a theoretical edge, but so far there is little convincing proof to back up the claim that they do a better job of eliminating prostate cancer. This is not entirely surprising, given that a scientific comparison is lacking for all prostate-cancer treatments, Dr. Zietman says. Thanks to screening, the vast majority of the estimated 217,000 men diagnosed with the malignancy last year are in an early stage of the disease. Were it not for routine PSA testing, their tumors might have remained silent for a decade or two, or a lifetime. No one has compared the treatments—surgery, radiation, and their incarnations—in a scientifically rigorous way.

"Is surgery better than radiation? Who knows?" says Dr. Zietman, who calls prostate cancer "the bad boy of medicine" because of the scant data on which tumors are actually dangerous and which treatments work best.

"In this absence of knowledge, anything goes," he says. "Surgeons recommend their favorite surgery. Radiation oncologists recommend their favorite form of radiation." The least expensive option, which also happens to have the fewest side effects, is largely unused: active surveillance (also known as "watchful waiting"), in which a patient is closely monitored and receives treatment only when his cancer shows signs of growing.

To truly know whether proton therapy works best, large numbers of men would have to participate in a randomized trial, a study in which volunteers are randomly assigned to a treatment and followed for a decade or so to see who fares better. In a climate where Web-savvy men are already hooked on the promise of protons, such a study is proving difficult to launch. Dr. Zietman and Stephen Hahn, MD, Penn's chairman of radiation oncology, are trying. "Most men are coming to us convinced that protons are absolutely better," Dr. Hahn says. "The challenge is to discuss the available data, and why many of us feel as if we don't know whether it's better."

Another challenge of conducting a study: Even men who have unexpected side effects won't let go of the idea that protons are superior, says Dr. Zietman. They are so convinced they received the best treatment "they imagine the situation would have been even worse had they had another treatment," he says.

Oncologists have already learned a hard lesson about assumptions. In the 1980s, doctors began giving women with breast cancer colossal doses of chemotherapy to annihilate their tumors, and then replacing their bone marrow (which was also wiped out in the treatment) with a transplant. Preliminary study findings appeared so promising that scientists struggled to recruit trial volunteers who might not have received the treatment. But randomized trials finally revealed that women who received both chemo and a transplant didn't live any longer and suffered more adverse effects.

Prostate experts are in much the same position with proton therapy today, comparing the outcomes of proton treatment with the historical experience of standard radiation treatments. It's inexact science, but so far protons haven't outshone their competitors, either for treatment effectiveness or for side effects.

In September 2009, the U.S. Agency for Healthcare Research and Quality pronounced proton-beam treatment for cancer "promising but unproven." One of the largest proton studies, which appeared in March 2010 in the *Journal of the American Medical Association*, compared two groups of men who had received conformal, or targeted, doses of x-ray radiation followed by either a standard dose or a high dose of proton therapy. As part of the analysis, the researchers compared outcomes for these proton-beam patients with those for a group of men who had received only x-rays. They found the latter group's quality of life was similar to the proton group's. Dr. Zietman cites the increased precision of conventional x-rays as a reason the difference between the two has become so much harder to detect.

Dr. Keole points to recent study data, presented at the American Society for Radiation Oncology's 2010 meeting. In that study, 94 percent of men younger than 55 who'd had proton therapy at the University of Florida were sexually active 18 months later. (The study didn't provide a comparison for under-55 men who'd had surgery or x-ray treatments. Also, men under 55 may more easily recover their sexual mojo than older men can, so the study might have had some inherent bias.)

To say that nothing supports the use of protons, Dr. Keole says, "is simply false." Given the early data and the known physical properties of protons, he says, "I firmly believe they are superior to targeted x-ray treatments for prostate cancer."

It is that kind of endorsement that men like John Bell find when they start Googling. One of the biggest resources is protonbob.com, founded by Bob Marckini, a retired manufacturing executive from Massachusetts who flew to Loma Linda for treatment in 2000, and who has a missionary zeal in promoting protons through his website and self-published book *You Can Beat Prostate Cancer: And You Don't Need Surgery to Do It.* "You can't argue with the laws of physics," Marckini says.

Marckini was like most men with early prostate cancer: The threat of death was secondary to the threat of side effects. "There aren't too many things more important to a man than sexual function and bladder control," Marckini says. His own treatments were so exact that he hit the golf course every afternoon. "My friends were sending flowers and get-well cards, and I was feeling guilty."

Testimonials on Marckini's website often run along these lines: "I played golf and swam at the beach during my treatment," says one. The National Association for Proton Therapy assures patients that they can "play golf, tennis, swim, walk, run, work out in a gym, or go on a 'radiation vacation'"—which has

Sex and the Single Prostate

Every ejaculation can affect not only your sexual health but also your overall health, according to *Men's Health* advisor Judd W. Moul, MD, chief of urology at Duke University. Rule of thumb: More is better. So solicit the help of a loved one, or if necessary, give your gland a hand. What do you have to lose? Plenty.

EJACULATION REDUCES CANCER RISK. A study in the *Journal of the American Medical Association* showed that men who ejaculated 21 times a month or more were 33 percent less likely to develop prostate cancer.

"A man who is ejaculating regularly is probably clearing out the toxins that could be in his semen," Dr. Moul says. "And many urologists believe that infrequent ejaculations can lead to prostatitis, which might be a risk factor for prostate cancer." Consider a standing (heh) appointment for toxin clearing.

SEXERCISE HELPS IF YOU ARE DIAGNOSED WITH PROSTATE CANCER. Plenty of sexual exercise now could pay off in protective benefits later, in case you're among the 16 percent of men who will be diagnosed with prostate cancer.

"Sexual recovery after treatment tends to work best on young men who have good sexual function before the treatment," Dr. Moul says.

SEX CAN ELEVATE YOUR PSA SCORE. No, that isn't a good thing. But having sex within 2 days of your prostate-specific antigen (PSA) test could bump up your score without putting you at risk. The reason: When your prostate contracts during ejaculation, you release a small amount of PSA.

"For a normal guy coming in for a routine test, we don't make a point of telling him to abstain from sex before the test," Dr. Moul says, "but for men who are on the borderline or are coming in for a repeat test, we may ask them to abstain from ejaculation for 2 or 3 days."

actually become part of the appeal, in Dr. Zietman's view. That's because until recently, access to the treatment had been limited to men with the time and means to relocate, so patients felt as if they were joining a privileged club. "It's acquired a very high-end following," he says.

That sense of exclusivity will probably fade as more centers open for business. The cost might drop, too, which is a point that proton advocates make—as if a proton-beam generator were just another cellphone or flatscreen TV. But this rationale (i.e., we need more units to make the treatment affordable) bothers people like Elliott Fisher, MD, who, as director of the center for population health at the Dartmouth Institute for Health Policy and Clinical Practice, spends a lot of time contemplating the cost of health care.

"I believe in technological progress," he says. Nonetheless, "how many proton-beam accelerators do we need in a given city? How many in a given country? I want these decisions to be made thoughtfully."

Americans devote more of their paychecks to health care than workers in any other country worldwide, yet have a life expectancy that ranks 50th, just behind Portugal. Estimates vary widely, but studies suggest that a large portion of the steady rise in health-care costs can be attributed to new technologies.

"If we continue at this pace, health care will be unaffordable for our children," Dr. Fisher says.

Above all, says Bob Hill, the author of the self-published *Dead Men Don't Have Sex: A Guy's Guide to Surviving Prostate Cancer*, men shouldn't be so eager for protons that they ignore other options. Hill was diagnosed with prostate cancer 7 years ago, at age 47, and underwent surgery. Even if proton therapy didn't have lofty claims, men would be attracted to it because it represents the latest technology, he says. ("What do you think sells the newest plasma TV or GPS system?") He also says that a man who has a positive experience wants to convert others. "Once they go through this, guys almost become evangelists telling other guys this is the way to go. I had the same experience with laparoscopic surgery," he says. "The downside to that, for some guys, is that it makes them think they don't have any other options. Prostate cancer is typically a slow-growing cancer. I want men to take the time to make their own decisions."

For his part, John Bell remains happy with his choice of protons. He's had no side effects from the treatment. He sometimes has to enlist a little blue friend when he's ready for action, but he did before protons too. ("The way it goes" at his age, he laments.) He is unwavering in his belief that he received the best treatment. Maybe one day, researchers will know for certain whether he's right.

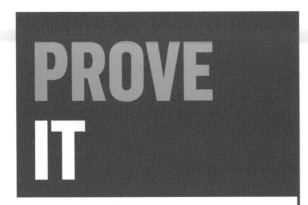

PROVE IT

BE SAFE AT HOME

Check the tags on your furniture: If it resists stains or flames or is made with pressed wood, it could contain chemicals that can mess with your hormones and may contribute to cancer.

Polybrominated diphenyl ethers (PBDEs)

Found in upholstered furniture treated with PBDE flame-retardant chemicals. Over time, PBDEs slowly disperse into surrounding air. Exposure to PBDE-laced dust may lower male hormone levels, a University of Michigan study showed.

Cut your risk: Control dust: Wipe surfaces weekly with a wet rag and use a vacuum with a HEPA filter.

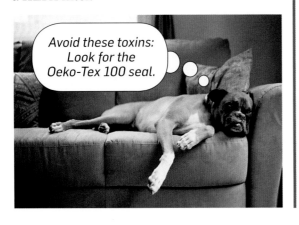

Avoid these toxins:
Look for the
Oeko-Tex 100 seal.

Porfluorinated chemicals (PFCs)

Found in upholstered furniture with stain-resistant coatings. Exposure might come when PFCs are emitted from your sofa into the air. A study in *Environmental Health Perspectives* linked high blood levels of some PFCs to high cholesterol.

Cut your risk: Dust and clean weekly, and opt out of professional stain-resistant coating treatments.

Formaldehyde

Found in furniture made of medium-density fiberboard or particleboard. Formaldehyde diffuses from inside your table to the surface. The International Agency for Research on Cancer lists formaldehyde as a carcinogen.

Cut your risk: Keep relative humidity at 40 to 50 percent in rooms with pressed-wood furniture.

Sources: Richard Corsi, PhD, a professor of environmental engineering at the University of Texas at Austin; and Tracey Woodruff, PhD, MPH, director of the University of California at San Francisco's Program on Reproductive Health and the Environment

GIVE FLU THE FINGERS

Hit the massage table now to stay out of the sick bed later. Massages may help you fend off the flu, according to a study in the *Journal of Alternative and Complementary Medicine.* People who received a 45-minute Swedish massage had an 18 percent spike in infection-fighting white blood cells.

"Deep massage may move white blood cells from a man's lymph nodes into his blood-stream," says study author Mark Rapaport, MD. Find a certified massage therapist at the American Massage Therapy Association site findamassagetherapist.org.

SIZE UP YOUR RISK

Sometimes the fight to stay healthy is a game of inches: A study from Norway found that tall men (6 feet or over) were twice as likely to form blood clots in their legs as guys shorter than 5 foot 8 inches. Tall, heavy men had an even higher risk.

Why the disadvantage? Tall men may have slower bloodflow in their femoral veins, which might increase the risk of blood clotting, says study author Knut Borch-Johnsen, MD, PhD. If you feel warmth, pain, tenderness, or swelling in one leg, see a doctor.

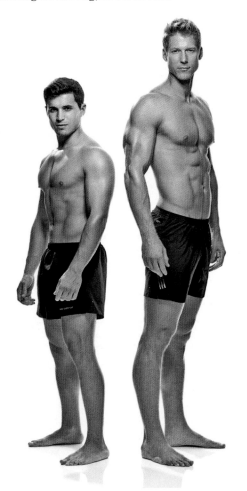

HARD TRUTH

22 Percentage decrease in your risk of developing a blood clot if you play sports at least once a week, according to *Journal of Thrombosis and Haemostasis*

BE FLUENT IN HEALTH

Se puede combatir el Alzheimer aprendiendo un segundo idioma. Translation: You can fight Alzheimer's disease by learning a second language. A study in the journal *Neurology* found that bilingual people fended off the disease 4 years longer than people who spoke just one tongue.

"Bilingual people may have enriched neural connections, better brain bloodflow, or both," says study author Fergus Craik, PhD. Buy a book or software to brush up on the language you took in school. Even that could be enough to boost your brain function, Craik says.

SWEAT OUT A COLD

Time to go viral with your workout. Regular cardio exercise can help ward off colds, say Appalachian State University researchers. In a 12-week study, people who exercised for at least 20 minutes a day 5 days a week caught fewer upper-respiratory infections than did their sedentary peers, and they also experienced milder symptoms when they were sick.

"During aerobic exercise, more natural killer cells and neutrophils—the army of the immune system—circulate in your body," says study author David C. Nieman, DrPH. Even 20 minutes of yard work or a brisk walk can give you an immunity boost.

PROVE IT

HEPA YOUR HEART

It's clear: Filtering the air in your home can cut your heart-disease risk, Canadian researchers report. In their study, people who used air purifiers with HEPA filters experienced a boost in blood-vessel function and a drop in inflammation. Airborne particles might cause lung irritation that impairs blood vessels throughout your body, says lead author Ryan Allen, PhD.

Before you buy a HEPA air purifier, check its clean air delivery rate for the square footage it filters.

TOWEL OFF

Hand dryers are full of hot air: Restroom air dryers can leave your hands covered with germs, according to a recent U.K. study. The reason: Air dryers won't budge residual germs that paper towels can slough off. Hot air the only option in the loo? You'll kill the most bugs by holding your hands steady under the dryer for at least 30 seconds.

BUY A FOG LIGHT

Do you have MZS (Morning Zombie Syndrome)? A timed dose of light can boost a.m. alertness, according to a study in the *Journal of Sleep Research*. When sleepers were exposed to gradually intensifying light in the half hour before waking, they felt more alert than those who were blasted with light when their alarms went off. Gradual light exposure might rev your sympathetic nervous system to help you wake up. Try a light-equipped alarm such as the Verilux Rise and Shine Natural Wake-Up Light Clock Radio ($100, bestbuy.com).

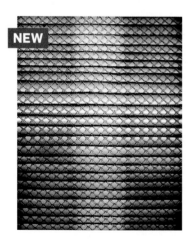

NEW

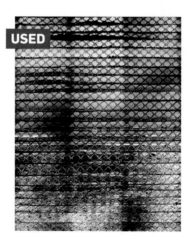

USED

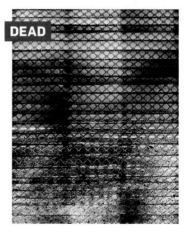

DEAD

LIMP TO THE BEDROOM

Talk about adding insult to injury: Popping OTC pain relievers for a few months could cause erectile dysfunction. In a Kaiser Permanente study, men who took nonsteroidal anti-inflammatories daily for 3 months were more likely to have ED. Chronic use might block chemicals that aid penile bloodflow, says author Steven J. Jacobsen, MD, PhD.

PROTECT YOUR DRUG SUPPLY

A lot can go wrong in the time it takes a pill to go from the manufacturer to your mouth: Heat, humidity, light, air, and other environmental factors can all degrade your drugs.

"Anything that affects the physical component of the drug can alter the way it's delivered and absorbed in your body," says Joyce Generali, MS, RPh, director of the Drug Information Center at the University of Kansas. Preserve the potency of your pills with these strategies.

Ask for your pills in their original bottle. The manufacturer's packaging seals out light, water, air, and germs better than the vials pharmacies provide, says Laura Bix, PhD, an associate professor of packaging at Michigan State University.

Store pill bottles in a cool, dark place. That's a cabinet or drawer—not in the kitchen or bathroom. Humidity can soften tablets, make gelcaps stick together, and alter the active ingredients in some medicines. It can even make multivitamins less effective, say scientists at Purdue University. When they subjected vitamin C to 86 percent humidity—the level in a kitchen where a pot of water is boiling—the vitamin began to degrade in 1 week. Vitamin C is a marker for how other vitamins would fare under similar conditions, say the study authors.

Take precautions if ordering online. If you order online, make sure the pharmacy uses temperature controls and requires that you sign for packages when they're delivered, Bix says.

Don't leave medicine in a parked car. The temperature inside can rise to about 40 degrees higher than outside temps.

When flying, don't pack pills in the luggage that you check. Temperatures in the cargo hold can fluctuate, Bix says.

Multiday pill organizers let in air and light. Try an airtight, watertight, opaque box like the Gasketed VitaCarry ($13, vitacarry.com).

Q: I occasionally smoked in the past. What can I do to reverse the damage to my lungs?

A: Your airbags need regular scrubbing and exercise. Even low levels of smoke exposure, including secondhand smoke, can lead to the formation of inflammation-causing and DNA-mutating free radicals.

But this damage may be reversible, says Irfan Rahman, PhD, an associate professor of environmental medicine at the University of Rochester Medical Center. "Eating foods high in antioxidants—such as the resveratrol found in red grapes, curcumin in turmeric, catechins in green tea, and sulforaphane in broccoli—can neutralize free radicals."

Rahman recommends making sure you eat at least one serving of antioxidant-rich produce at every meal.

Working out can deliver similar benefits. Exercise pushes your body's defense system into overdrive, increasing the activity of antioxidant enzymes in your lungs and decreasing free-radical production, reports a study in *Pulmonary Pharmacology and Therapeutics*. Your prescription for healthier lungs is cardio sessions of moderate to high intensity lasting 30 to 50 minutes. Do them at least 3 days a week, recommends study author Ricardo Pinho, PhD, a professor of physiology and biochemistry at Criciúma University in Brazil.

Q: How can I beat fatigue and sleep better?

A: Here's how Christopher Winter, MD, director of sleep medicine at the Martha Jefferson Hospital and a consultant to the San Francisco Giants, beats fatigue.

How to catch up on sleep: "For a small sleep debt, doze, but not for longer than 30 minutes; otherwise you can enter a deep-sleep phase and wake up groggy. If you're seriously sleep deprived, skip the nap and go to bed a couple of hours earlier than usual. Your waking time should stay constant."

How to fall asleep fast: "Our brains respond

HARD TRUTH

26 Percentage increase in your diabetes risk if you drink one or two sugary drinks a day versus less than one a month according to *Diabetes Care*

to bright light by inhibiting the production of melatonin, a chemical that makes us sleepy. I installed simple dimmer switches throughout my house, and I turn them down when it's getting late. Then, an hour before hitting the hay, I switch off the television and my smartphone."

How to catch z's on the road: "When I'm traveling, I request a hotel room that faces away from the sun and is located in the quietest part of the building. I always pack earplugs and a sleeping mask, and I bring duct tape to block out light under doors and around curtains so that the room is pitch-black."

Q: What actually happens to a man's brain when he has a concussion?

A: Think of your head as a big egg: The shell is your skull, the white is your cerebrospinal fluid, and the yolk is your brain. A violent impact causes the yolk to vibrate and sometimes even bash into the shell. If the force is strong enough, you'll end up with a concussion. And yet for all that trauma, there's often no evidence of injury because the damage is on the inside.

"It's known as the 'silent injury,'" says Mark Lovell, PhD, director of the University of Pittsburgh Medical Center's Sports Concussion Program. But don't assume that if you didn't black out, you're fine. Any knock to your head that results in vomiting, dilated pupils, or loss of smell or taste should be checked out by a neurologist. Same goes for headaches, dizziness, or memory loss that persists for longer than 5 days.

Here's the full bonk breakdown.

1. Impact: The most common causes of concussion are falls, motor vehicle accidents, impacts related to sports, and explosions. In each case, the trauma causes enough force—either linear (forward and back) or rotational (side to side)—to make your brain slosh around in its syrupy cushion of fluid and hit the skull wall.

2. Firestorm: Any serious brain trauma can damage your neurons, the cells that govern the flow of chemical messengers known as neurotransmitters. Worst case, those damaged neurons lose control of the neurotransmitters, allowing them to accelerate to as much as five times their normal speed. The resulting chemical firestorm can lead to memory loss, blurred vision, dizziness, headache, and nausea.

3. Hibernation: Mission control—your brain's cortex—detects the neurotransmitter imbalance and tries to fix the neurons by calling for a surge of healing glucose. At the same time, calcium neurotransmitters start constricting the blood vessels, delaying glucose from reaching the neurons. Your brain function slows until bloodflow returns to normal.

4. Recovery: It can take several weeks for your neurons to heal. But if you sustain another concussion during this period, you could suffer permanent damage and a lifetime of headaches—even, down the road, dementia. Your best bet: Rest and refrain from any activity with a high risk of a head bonk. Headaches? Take acetaminophen; do not use aspirin or ibuprofen, which may increase your risk of brain bleeding.

YOU ASKED

Q: I have a blood-pressure monitor in my office and noticed that my BP jumps all over the place. Is that normal?

A: Are you guzzling java and butting heads with your boss? Blood pressure fluctuates in healthy people, but those peaks and valleys can be accentuated by external factors such as caffeine and stress, says Steven E. Nissen, MD, chairman of the Cleveland Clinic's Department of Cardiovascular Medicine.

"A variation of up to 10 millimeters of mercury (mmHg) from your baseline BP is normal," says Dr. Nissen. See the BP Roller Coaster graph below to identify triggers. To determine your baseline, take a reading when you're relaxed—midmorning and mid-afternoon—at the same times each day, for 2 weeks, says Dr. Nissen; take two readings each session and discard the first one. If you still see variations greater than 10 mmHg, you could be experiencing labile hypertension—regular, excessive blood-pressure spikes—and should consult your physician, says Dr. Nissen. Your doc will probably advise diet changes, such as slashing your salt intake to 1,500 milligrams a day, and might discuss BP meds.

The BP roller coaster

For a physically active man in his late 20s with a baseline BP of 120/80.

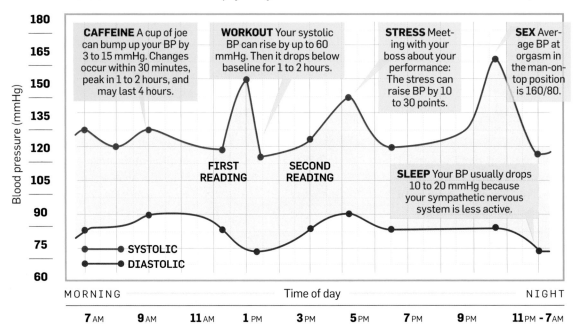

CAFFEINE A cup of joe can bump up your BP by 3 to 15 mmHg. Changes occur within 30 minutes, peak in 1 to 2 hours, and may last 4 hours.

WORKOUT Your systolic BP can rise by up to 60 mmHg. Then it drops below baseline for 1 to 2 hours.

STRESS Meeting with your boss about your performance: The stress can raise BP by 10 to 30 points.

SEX Average BP at orgasm in the man-on-top position is 160/80.

SLEEP Your BP usually drops 10 to 20 mmHg because your sympathetic nervous system is less active.

FIRST READING

SECOND READING

Blood pressure (mmHg)

SYSTOLIC
DIASTOLIC

MORNING — Time of day — NIGHT

7 AM 9 AM 11 AM 1 PM 3 PM 5 PM 7 PM 9 PM 11 PM – 7 AM

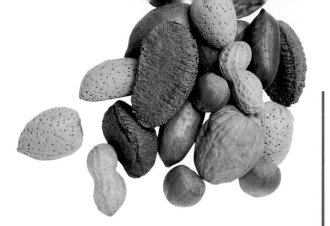

Q: Why are triglyceride levels so important, and what's the best way to lower my score?

A: These blood fats increase your risk of heart disease and stroke because they mess with your circulation in two critical ways.

"First, when your triglycerides are high, your body makes the harmful LDL cholesterol particles smaller, which means they can lodge in artery walls more easily," says Patrick McBride, MD, MPH, a cardiologist at the University of Wisconsin. Second, your body produces less HDL (good) cholesterol, its primary defense against the buildup of artery blockages from plaque.

Aim to keep your triglyceride count below 150 milligrams per deciliter (mg/dl), and have a lipid panel done every 5 years—or every year if you have high cholesterol, says Dr. McBride.

To lower yours, exercise at least 3 days a week for a minimum of 45 minutes a day. And tweak your diet: Eat more vegetables and whole grains and fewer refined carbs; choose monounsaturated fats (olive oil and canola oil, for example) over saturated fats; and limit alcohol to no more than two drinks daily. Crunching nuts can also help: People who ate 2½ ounces of nuts daily for 3 to 8 weeks reduced high triglyceride levels by as much as 10 percent, according to a study published in the *Archives of Internal Medicine*.

Q: I'm worried that my father may be heading toward diabetes, but he's not concerned. What are some risk factors?

A: Ask your dad some personal questions: Is his waist bigger than 40 inches? Does he exercise less than three times a week? If the answers are yes, he might be at risk of developing diabetes. And is he both urinating excessively and feeling constantly thirsty? If the answers to those last two questions are both yes, drag him straight to the doctor. He might already have diabetes.

If he resists, tell him this: The Centers for Disease Control and Prevention estimates that there are 5.7 million undiagnosed cases of diabetes in the United States, and having the disease doubles his chances of dying at any age compared with a person who's diabetes-free.

"Being overweight and inactive hinders the body's ability to use insulin, raising blood sugar," says Vivian Fonseca, MD, the American Diabetes Association's president for medicine and science. "One way your body sheds excess glucose is through urination."

Your dad will probably be given an A1C blood test, which can be used to diagnose diabetes without fasting. Encourage healthy lifestyle changes by offering to do them with him, says Dr. Fonseca. People who have prediabetes (fasting blood sugar between 100 and 126 milligrams per deciliter, or mg/dl) can reduce their risk of developing full-blown diabetes by 58 percent with moderate physical exercise 150 minutes a week and a 7 percent reduction in body weight, according to the Diabetes Prevention Program.

YOU ASKED

Q: Is there a natural Viagra?

A: There's no surefire boner builder that can match the little blue pill or its chemical cousins, Levitra and Cialis. These ED meds can take a man from flaccid to fully engorged in 30 to 60 minutes—while even the best natural supplements are hit-or-miss in terms of timing and duration.

Before you self-medicate with a natural supplement, know that ED can be the initial sign of a serious underlying condition, such as heart disease, says Larry Lipshultz, MD, a professor of urology at Baylor College of Medicine. That means you could be missing early and potentially lifesaving warning signs. But what if your erections are hard and you just want them harder?

Then you could consider a supplement. Of what's available, Korean red ginseng is the best, Dr. Lipshultz says: Most men respond well with few side effects. In one Brazilian study, two-thirds of the men who popped 1,000 milligrams of Korean red ginseng three times a day for 12 weeks reported having harder, longer-lasting erections than before the study. The downside: You'll have to take the stuff every day.

Q: I'm fine, but my erections aren't as hard as they used to be. What's up?

A: Your erection is a barometer of your overall health, so limp on over to your GP. "Everyone occasionally has softer erections due to stress, lack of sleep, increased alcohol consumption, and other factors," says Dr. Lipshultz. "But if the erections are consistently weak, it could be an early sign of heart disease, diabetes, or low testosterone."

Ask your doctor to test your endothelial function, cholesterol, and testosterone levels. If the problem is simply that your testosterone is a little low, you can take the following three steps to give it (and your erections) a lift.

Step 1: When you train with weights, make sure you lift slowly, taking 6 seconds per rep (3 up, 3 down). Slow lifting increases your body's T production more than faster lifting does, according to a recent Japanese study.

Step 2: Recommit to a solid 8 hours of sleep

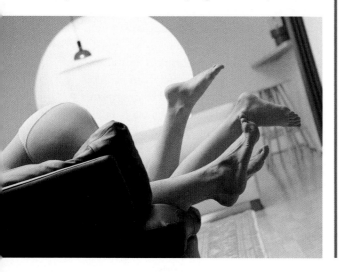

every night; a shut-eye shortage can disrupt testosterone production.

Step 3: Eat a diet high in monounsaturated fats, such as those found in almonds and olive oil; these fats are the building blocks of the he-man hormone.

Now if after all of those efforts, your testosterone levels have actually dipped lower—below 300 nanograms per deciliter (ng/dl)—talk to your doctor about testosterone replacement therapy.

Q: **I'm chained to a desk all day and have recurring back pain. How can I banish it?**

A: Stand up for yourself, man!
"Sitting weakens your glutes and abs and causes tightness of the hip flexors, all of which can contribute to chronic back pain," says Michelle Gittler, MD, medical director of the back program at Schwab Rehabilitation Hospital in Chicago.

Standing can decrease your chances of dying of cardiovascular disease by 42 percent, a Canadian study found. Plus, some researchers believe that standing not only requires you to use more energy but also may activate a fat-burning gene in your legs.

Your mission: Build a workstation that allows you to sit as well as stand—the ideal ratio is 45 minutes standing to 15 sitting. The simplest solution is to find two lightweight but sturdy supports you can place on your desk to elevate the keyboard and monitor. We like either a pair of large wooden bins, one upside down and one vertical, like the Feathergrain Wood Bins ($25, containerstore.com), or the Allsop Metal Art Monitor Stand for your keyboard ($23, amazon.com) and an oak Safco Vertical Desktop Sorter for your monitor ($85, amazon.com).

"Your arms should be bent 90 degrees as you type, and your eyes should be level with the top of your monitor," says Bill Hartman, PT, CSCS, co-owner of Indianapolis Fitness and Sports Training. Start by standing for 20 minutes every hour and add time as your fitness improves. If your office doesn't allow stand-up desks, try these spine-saving moves at MensHealth.com/mhlists/work_stretches/index.php.

Q: **All the cold remedies in the drugstore just relieve symptoms. Is there anything that actually battles the virus?**

A: In this fight, your immune system is on its own.
"There's no antiviral treatment for a cold," says Birgit Winther, MD, an associate professor of otolaryngology at the University of Virginia.

But there is some good news: An over-the-counter drug might help disable your enemy. A recent study in the *American Journal of Rhinology and Allergy* found that people who used a decongestant nasal spray containing oxymetazoline (such as Afrin) three times a day had lower levels of the rhinovirus in their mucus. By wiping out some of the virus, you might be able to slow its spread through your body, says Dr. Winther, who coauthored the study. Just make sure you wait to use the spray until the second and third days of your cold, when rhinovirus levels are at their peak concentration in your mucus. Plus, spraying for longer than 3 days can cause swollen blood vessels, leading to more congestion.

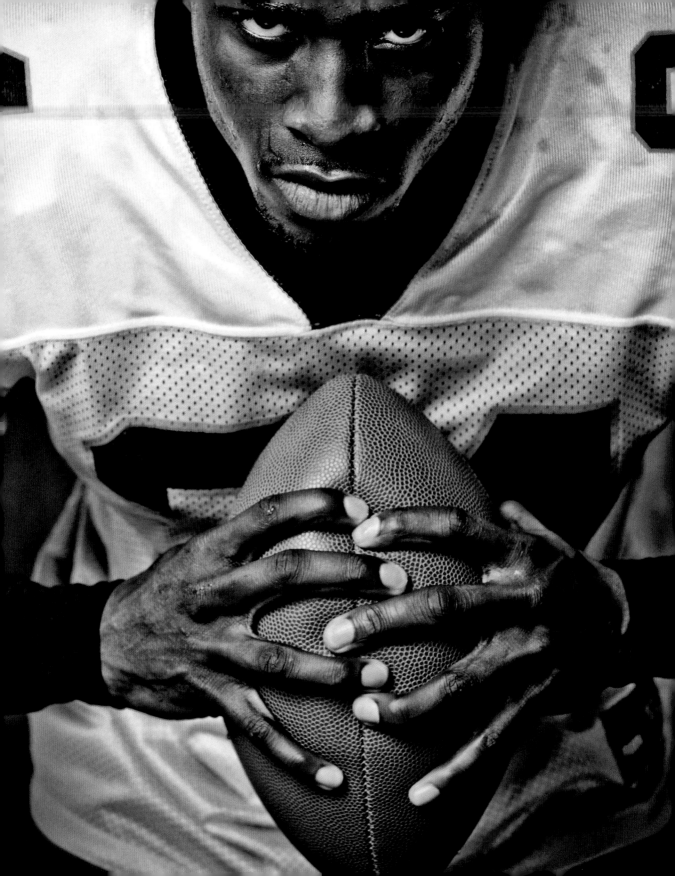

Improve Your Game

Your Records— Smashed

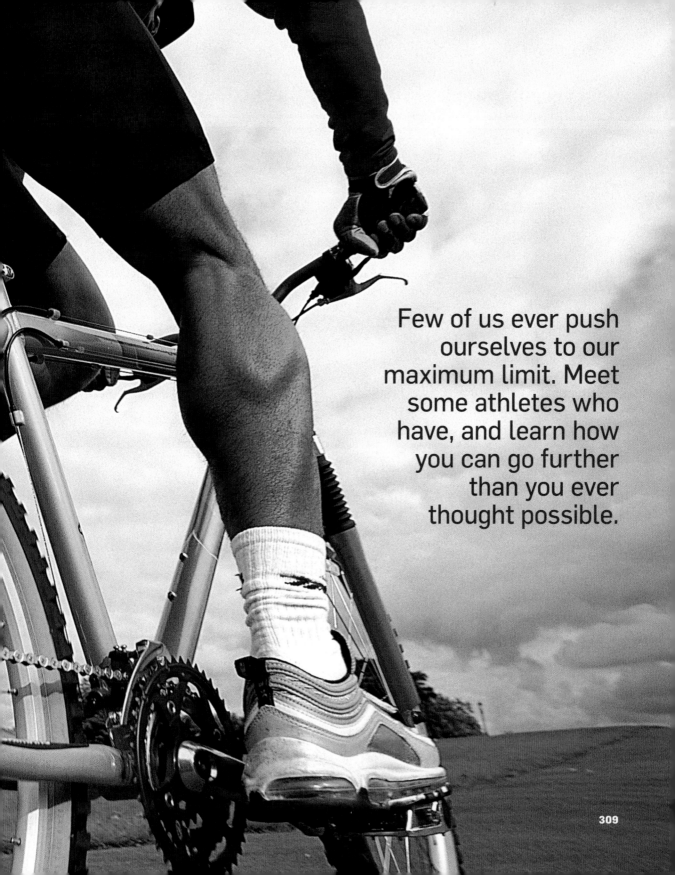

Few of us ever push ourselves to our maximum limit. Meet some athletes who have, and learn how you can go further than you ever thought possible.

Feeling stuck? Frustrated? Blocked?
Here are the keys to opening up your future.

Chris McCormack has won more than 200 triathlons. If he starts a race, he, by his own reckoning, has a 75 percent chance of winning it. Only a handful of humans have taken less than 8 hours to complete an Ironman, with its 2.4-mile swim, 112-mile bike ride, and 26.2-mile run. But McCormack has done it four times, on two different courses.

So when you ask him about when he came closest to his max performance, the furthest he could push himself in a race, you'd think he'd mention one of those wins. He doesn't. Instead, he talks about the 2006 Ironman World Championship in

Hawaii, a race in which he finished second.

"It was the absolute maximum I could possibly take my body," he says. "Your body allows you to go there only once or twice in your life."

To understand how and why he arrived at that point, it helps to know some context. The first time McCormack competed in Hawaii, in 2002, he said to a reporter, "I'm here to win." That comment had everyone rooting against him. He was leading for a while, but then cramped up and quit with 20 miles of the run to go. He walked the last few miles in 2003, dropped out again in

Max Profile #1
A.J. Roberts, 27, powerlifter

WHO HE IS: A native Brit, A.J. Roberts came to the United States as a 175-pound teenage exchange student. His plan was to play basketball. He'd been a national-level player in England and wanted to sharpen his game against American talent. He also played football and was on the track team.

"I just happened to end up in a really small town," he says. "They encouraged me to play football. Football culture is weightlifting culture." By the time he graduated, he weighed 200 pounds and held school records in all the major lifts.

WHAT HE DID: A paperwork snafu made Roberts ineligible to try out for college football, so he gravitated to powerlifting and

began training seriously in 2004. His training partner was Brent Mikesell, a high school math and phys.ed. teacher who had set a world record with a 1,075-pound squat. Although Roberts's personal record in the squat was less than half that, he knew he'd learn from his partner.

"There was never the thought that his regimen wouldn't work for me," Roberts says. "I just expected to keep adding weight."

MAX MOMENT: In March 2011, Roberts set an all-time record in the 308-pound weight class with a 2,825 total. He achieved this with personal records in the squat (1,140), bench press (870), and deadlift (815).

HOW HE IMPROVES: "Everybody I talk to is more successful than me," Roberts says. Although he has a world-record total, he works out with guys at Westside Barbell who have better individual lifts.

HOW YOU CAN IMPROVE: Roberts, who is also a coach, stresses the importance of using your full range of motion in training—and not sacrificing form for strength, which can happen in the competitive atmosphere of a gym. Most important, he says, is to find someone stronger than you are.

"Strength is strength," he says. "Anyone can increase it. If I were just a regular guy in the gym, I'd find the strongest person there and work with him."

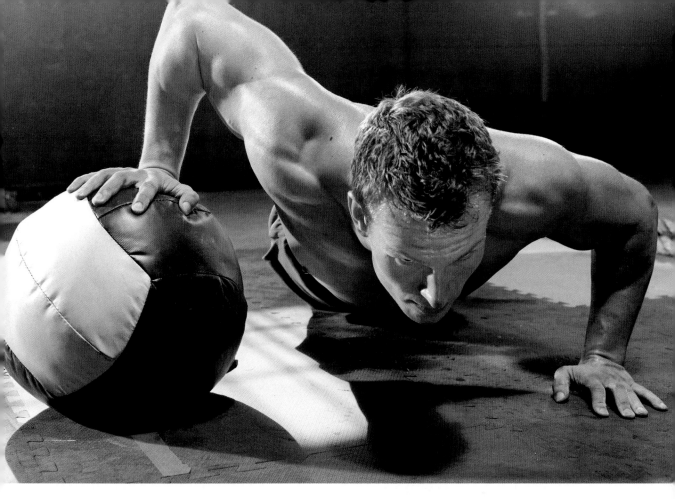

2004, and finished sixth in 2005.

Then came 2006, when McCormack went all-out, ran a technically perfect race . . . and still finished 71 seconds behind the winner.

You'd think he would've been as devastated emotionally as he was physically—and after the race he was a wreck, taking 2 liters of fluid through an IV in the medical tent. Instead, here's how McCormack describes the moment: "There's

Max Rule #1

Program hoppers tend to fail, so pick a training regimen and stick with it to achieve maximum performance.

nothing more satisfying."

Contrast that with the experience of powerlifter A.J. Roberts. On the best day of his career, Roberts gave what might have been less than his absolute best performance. He'll never know.

Powerlifting is a brutal pursuit. Travel and gear are expensive, nobody makes any money, and anybody who's good at it is in pain much of the time. A personal-record effort in the squat might burst so many capillaries in a guy's eyeballs that he'd look like he was coming off a 12-day bender. There's only one good reason to compete: to pull and push heavy things that no sane person would try to move without a forklift.

That's what Roberts was doing at a powerlifting meet on March 6, 2011. He did it so well that he didn't miss a single lift the entire day. In powerlifting you have three tries in each of, usually, three contested lifts—squat, bench press, and deadlift—and he completed all nine attempts. By the end of the day, he had set personal records in each lift, and the sum of those lifts was a world record for the 308-pound weight class. The only guy in the sport to reach a higher total outweighed Roberts by more than 50 pounds.

"I left the meet happy for one day," Roberts says. "It was a surreal feeling to go through the day hitting numbers and thinking, I wonder what I could do if I really pushed it? Maybe I limited myself."

That's the paradox of max effort, however you define it and however you pursue it: Your best possible performance isn't necessarily the one that brings home the trophy. And bringing home the trophy doesn't necessarily mean you did the best you could have done.

The Agony of Victory

Let's step away from these champions for a moment and talk about someone who matters more: you. Chances are, you aren't a champion in anything more prestigious than the office fantasy football league.

Max Rule #2

Know your kryptonite. Understanding your weaknesses positions you to conquer them.

Have you ever gone to your max? That is, have you trained for something specific, like strength or endurance, and reached what you thought was your body's limit? If you work out for purely aesthetic reasons, have you ever been in the best possible shape you could achieve? You can expand the question to team sports: Have you practiced and trained to the point where you thought you maxed out your ability in that sport, and played it at the highest level you could?

It's not really a simple question, is it? First, you have to distinguish between a personal record and a max performance. You can go out today and set a PR in anything, as long as it's something you've never done before. If it's something you have done, you can find a way to do it slightly harder, better, or faster. Finish one more rep, run one more block, pick up the pace on that final lap, and you have a PR.

A max performance is something else. It can come only from dedicated training toward a specific goal.

What Is a Max?

There's one school of thought, popularized by South African sports scientist Timothy Noakes, MD, DSc, that maintains it's impossible to reach your body's absolute limit.

"Your body won't allow you to push beyond a certain level," says Thomas W. Rowland, MD, author of *The Athlete's Clock,* a book that explores all aspects of peak performance. "You shut down."

Dr. Rowland uses the example of a treadmill stress test to make his point. If you've never taken one, it goes something like this: A technician hooks up electrodes to your chest and tells you to start walking on the treadmill. The slope becomes steeper and the pace faster in 3-minute increments. At some point you have to start running. And then you run until one of three things happens: He stops the test because he's detected a problem with your heart; he ends the test when you hit a target heart rate; or you give up.

In the "you give up" scenario, imagine that your doctor offers you $2 million to keep going for another minute. "You'd do it," Dr. Rowland says. "You could go beyond what your brain has told you to do."

You still wouldn't run so hard that you'd hurt yourself, but you would find a way to earn that $2 million. You can call this the Yoda theory of peak performance: "Always in motion is your maximum."

University of Texas at Austin exercise scientist Edward Coyle, PhD, agrees, but only if we're talking about untrained individuals. The higher the level of training and experience an athlete has, the closer he or she can push toward that limit. "A lot of times with athletes, you can see that they're doing all they can just to stay upright," Coyle says. "I don't think even a million dollars would make a difference."

Amby Burfoot's winning performance of 2:22:17 in the 1968 Boston Marathon seems to support Coyle's position. Burfoot was a 21-year-old all-American in cross-country at Wesleyan University, where he was a senior.

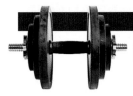

Max Profile #2
Nate Miyaki, 33, bodybuilder

WHO HE IS: Growing up in Northern California, Nate Miyaki remembers being a "pretty good" athlete.

"But I never looked the part," he says, thanks to what he calls "skinny-fat genetics." He had a slight frame with an aversion to muscle and a propensity to hold fat. Because he was too small for his favorite sport, football, he began training in capoeira, an acrobatic martial art that originated in Brazil.

WHAT HE DID: After college at the University of California at Berkeley, Miyaki's acrobatic skills won him a job as a pro wrestler.

"My character was the Kamikaze Kid," he says, an allusion to the Asian half of his Japanese-Irish ancestry. "I would do crazy flips off the ropes."

Although pro wrestling is staged, "the impact is real," Miyaki says, and his body couldn't take the pounding from guys twice his size. So, improbably, he gravitated to bodybuilding.

"As I dieted down and started training, I thought, 'Why not take it a step further? Have I ever taken anything 100 percent, all the way?'"

MAX MOMENT: Miyaki competes in natural bodybuilding, a far cry from the pro version. At 155 pounds and with a body-fat percentage in the low single digits, he won his weight class in the first show he entered, in 2004. After taking a 5-year hiatus from competition, he showed up even leaner and lighter for his first contest in 2009, which he also won.

HOW HE IMPROVES: His programs always match his goals. When the goal is a better-looking physique, he stays away from heavy and explosive lifts and focuses on slower, more controlled movements that keep muscles under tension longer.

HOW YOU CAN IMPROVE: Miyaki finds flexing on stage boring. But he needs a goal, and recommends that his clients have one as well.

"It's too hard to say out of thin air, 'I'm going to push myself to the limit.' What's going to make you stick to that plan?" You don't need to compete in public; Miyaki started with a friendly bet to see who could be in the best shape by summer's end.

"In the middle of the race I did a little surge, and only one guy went with me," recalls Burfoot, a longtime *Runner's World* editor and columnist. He knew he couldn't outsprint that guy at the end of the race.

"My only hope was to completely destroy myself on the hills. He was still with me at the top. He cramped up on the downhill, and I staggered to the end. I had put it all out there at 21 miles. I staggered in a little bit ahead of him and everyone else."

So was that Burfoot's max, his best possible performance? Actually, it wasn't. That came 8 months later, at a marathon in Japan. Burfoot ran it in 2:14:29, within a second of the American record at the time. But he finished sixth. "Winning the

Max Rule #2

Be patient: Only when you're struggling to improve by 1 or 2 percent a year are you near a max.

Boston Marathon was a huge accomplishment," Burfoot says, "but I participate in a sport ruled by the watch." And the watch says the race in Japan was his max. The one he didn't win. Read on to discover how to achieve yours.

How to Reach Your Max

Now that we know what a max is, let's ask two crucial questions: How do you reach

Max Profile #3
Brian Sell, 34, marathoner

WHO HE IS: Brian Sell was never considered a world-class talent in high school or college. But he never stopped improving.

"It was a linear progression," he says. "I had bad races, but pretty much every year I improved."

WHAT HE DID: After college in Pennsylvania, Sell entered a marathon-training program in Michigan.

"I put real life on hold for a year," Sell says. "If I didn't accomplish big things, I'd quit and go back to school." He ran his first marathon in 2:19:58, which qualified him in 2004 for an all-expenses-paid trip to the U.S. Olympic trials. There he took the lead at 7 miles and still led after 22. But his inexperience nearly killed him.

"I panicked and blew right past [the water stations]," he recalls. "I don't remember the last 2 miles. I sort of remember crossing the finish line and falling over and waking up 10 or 15 minutes later with an IV in my arm." He finished 12th. Only the top three go to the Olympics.

HOW HE IMPROVED: That experience motivated Sell to train harder so he could make the 2008 team. In the weeks leading up to a race, he would run an astounding 165 miles a week.

"I felt I had to," he says. "I didn't have great high school PRs like the guys I was facing in the trials. I figured I had to work harder to be on the same level as them."

MAX MOMENT: The payoff for all that training came in late 2007, when Sell ran 2:11:40 at the U.S. Olympic trials, putting him on the team for the 2008 Games and completing one of the most improbable rises in American marathon history.

HOW HE KNEW IT WAS TIME TO MOVE ON: Sell finished a disappointing 22nd in Beijing, and after running in the New York City Marathon in 2009, he knew he'd lost his edge. Married with two children, he enrolled in grad school at Penn State.

"I see metaphors for running everywhere," he says. "There are guys who go out in a marathon and burn out in the first few miles. Slow and steady wins the race. That applies in life too."

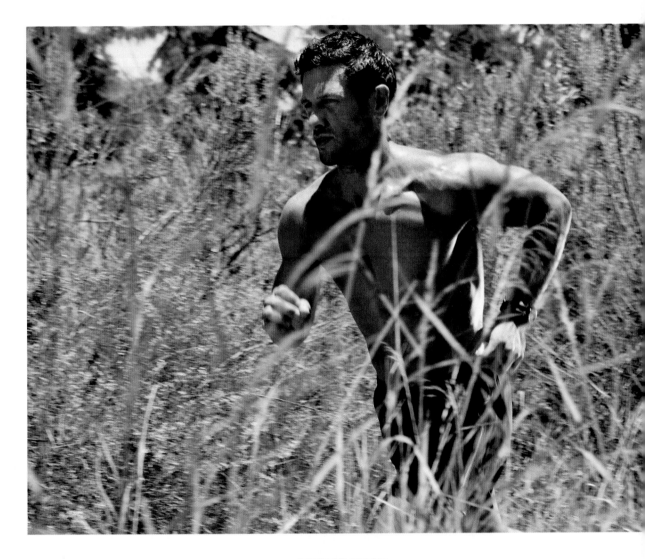

true peak performance? And how do you know when you've arrived there?

The authors, athletes, and academics we interviewed have different areas of expertise, but they all described similar paths to an all-out effort. No matter what area you want to focus on as you work toward your max—strength, endurance, or appearance—your process will include the following elements.

PREPARATION

It has to be something you're passionate about. You'll pay a price for a true max. Even if you are never injured, and even if your training expenses fit easily into your budget, an all-out pursuit of a fitness goal is more than a hobby. It eats into all of your work time, family time, and leisure time.

"Sport is selfish," McCormack says.

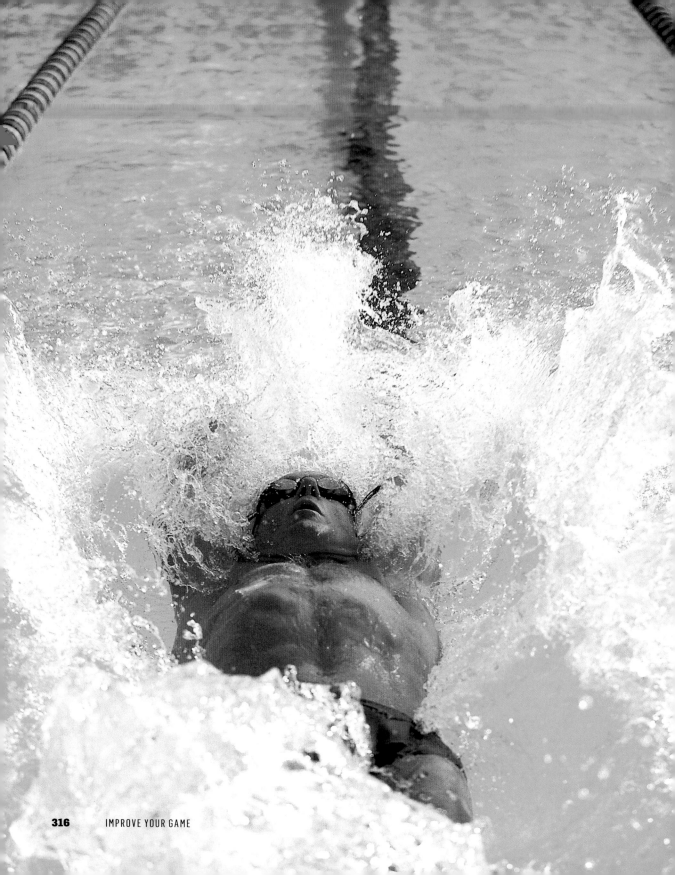

"Whether you're running or powerlifting, you're self-obsessed."

You'll bore friends and coworkers with stories about workouts and races, and you might even put a strain on your relationships at home. If a max isn't worth that price, you aren't likely to achieve it.

Plan to pursue it for years, not weeks or months. "You can show big improvements in the first year or two," Coyle says. "You can improve by 10 to 20 percent." Coaches call those "newbie gains." Only when you're struggling to improve by 1 or 2 percent a year are you anywhere near a max.

TRAINING

Work with people who know more than you do. The best athletes in solitary sports such as running and powerlifting often have mentors who won championships or set records. Burfoot's high school track coach, John J. Kelley, was a Boston Marathon champion and two-time Olympian. Burfoot's teammate and roommate was world-record-holding runner Bill Rodgers, and the two of them competed against another dominant marathoner of their time, Frank Shorter.

For most of us, training with a champion is not realistic. Even if there's one nearby, a pro might not have the time or interest to work with someone at our level. But you can almost certainly find a local gym that specializes in whatever you're pursuing, or a running, cycling, or swimming club you can join. If even these options are impractical, there's always an online community or coaching program you can join.

Your knowledge and skill led you to where you are today. You need something else in order to go beyond your current level—another base of knowledge or point of view. You don't know what you don't know about reaching your goals until you spend time around people who've already achieved them.

Find the right program and then stick with it. McCormack describes athletes who jump from program to program and trainer to trainer as "scattered people." "They don't have enough of a foundation," he says. "You should make a decision and go with it."

Program hoppers are doomed to fail, Roberts says. "They see results because it's a new program. When it fails, they jump to the next program. They never achieve the results they should."

How do you know which program or

Mad for Max

Here's the pursuit, in numbers.

Average height gain of 100-meter sprinters between 1900 and 2002: 6.4 inches

Improvement in world-record performance, 1900 to 2007:

100-meter dash	8.1 percent
Marathon	21.5 percent
Shot put	48.8 percent

Average decline in weightlifting performance between ages 35–40 and 45–50: 13 percent

Name of the first sports drink, introduced in 1924: Corpse Reviver

Powerlift most often performed by elite lifters in training: Clean

Guinness record for most consecutive days of marathon runs, set by Akinori Kusuda of Japan in 2009: 52 days

Record time for swimming the English Channel, set by Petar Stoychev of Bulgaria in 2007: 6:57:50

gym or coach is right for you? Look for consistent results from the people who use the program. Roberts trains at Westside Barbell in Columbus, Ohio, under the guidance of Louie Simmons, a powerlifting champion who has trained generations of winners.

"It's not like Westside is the only gym in the world that cranks out top lifters," says Roberts. But its results are consistent. Lifters who train there stick with the program and succeed with it.

Understand your weaknesses. Bodybuilder and personal trainer Nate Miyaki offers this advice: "Know your kryp-

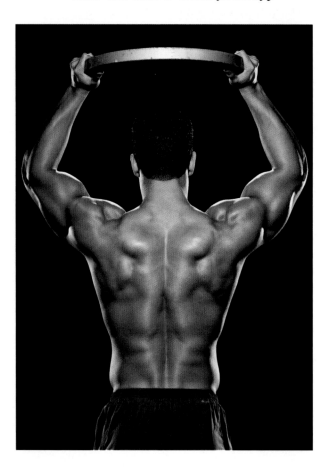

tonite." It might be something external, like a particular exercise that hurts your shoulder or a training method that leaves you with creaky knees. Or it could be a temptation, something that breaks down your willpower rather than your muscles or joints.

"You have to know the things that will pull you away from your goal," Miyaki says. "If you don't have the willpower to go out to dinner and skip dessert, you probably shouldn't go out to dinner. The farther away you are from your kryptonite, the less power it has. You stop craving it."

Focus your workouts. If you saw a triathlete, a bodybuilder, and a powerlifter working out in the same gym, their exercises and techniques would be as different as their bodies. But those are merely tactics. Their strategies might be identical.

McCormack says in his book, *I'm Here to Win* (yes, that ill-advised boast), that each of his workouts starts with the most important work of the day, followed by supplemental training that he might skip if he needs the extra time to recover.

Competitive lifters also build workouts around daily goals. A powerlifter might train four times a week, using two workouts to improve his bench press and the other two for squats and deadlifts. The most important exercise comes first, following a warmup. The other stuff matters, but you always want your best effort to go toward the lifts you'll eventually max out on.

Physique-focused gym rats tend to have the least structured training. They rely on instincts and experience to modulate the volume and intensity of a workout, but they still enter the gym with the goal of working specific muscle groups to whatever level of exhaustion they can tolerate that day.

PERFORMANCE

Pick your moment. If you're looking for a max effort in strength, and you can pick your own starting time, go for mid- to late afternoon. That's when your body creates the perfect circumstances to excel. Your core temperature is highest, bloodflow to your muscles surges, and your nerves fire faster. Your testosterone level may also be more responsive and rise with exercise.

For endurance, though, air temperature may be more important than your body's readiness.

"It's going to be different for every individual," Dr. Rowland says. "Some people run better in the heat, some in the cold."

All of this is moot if you're in a race or some other competition. Endurance events typically start in the morning, when all the competitors are fighting their bodies' circadian schedules.

Grade yourself on a curve. Performance is always circumstantial. Your max effort might not look like a max on the scorecard. An all-out effort in crappy weather might be the high point of your career, no matter where you finish or how long it took. If you're in a competition, there's always the chance someone else will hit his max on your best day, pushing you out of the winner's circle. Sometimes an official blows a call. Only you know

what went into your performance, and what you took out of it.

Wait before evaluating. A true max is evident only in retrospect. The longer you pursue something, the more opportunities you'll have for an all-out effort. What you once thought was your max might turn out to be something else—a great effort, possibly a personal record, but not your best. The reverse is also true: What you thought was just a PR may turn out, in retrospect, to have been your true max. You won't really know until you start to go backward.

And this brings us back to Chris McCormack and his performance in the 2006 Ironman World Championship in Hawaii—the one he remembers as the hardest he's ever pushed himself, even though he finished second. He grew up watching triathlons on television and says he never understood how the athletes could drive themselves to the point of collapse. Now he knows.

"Sport in its purest form is to test yourself," McCormack says. "The win might be the greatest moment. But as a competitor looking for that max performance, I was nowhere near it the year I won the race."

That's right. He went back the next year and won. He won again in 2010. And he still remembers 2006 as the one that pushed him to his max.

So what is a true max?

It's not always a win. But it sure as hell makes you a winner.

The Perfectly Balanced Body

Strength, power, and endurance will take you only so far without good balance. Writer and trainer Andrew Heffernan, CSCS, explains how athletes always stay on their feet—and how you can, too.

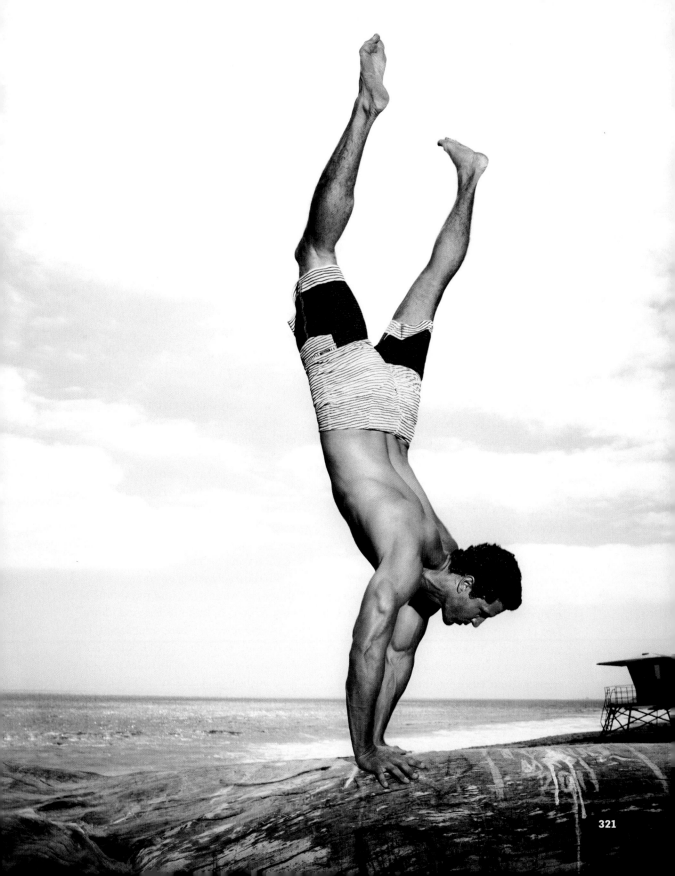

I've split my head open on a bunny slope. Tripped in martial arts class. Wiped out bicycling on bone-dry pavement. And I'm a good athlete—honest.

For years, I shrugged off this mystery of balance. I assumed it was innate—some guys had it, some didn't. Turns out I was wrong. You can train for balance like you do for strength, power, and endurance. It's just that I'd never bothered.

I realized how bad my balance was when I took my 7-year-old daughter roller-skating. Ten minutes in, she said, "Daddy, can you let go of my hand? You're kind of pulling me off balance." She didn't fall once in the next hour. But without a little girl to steady me, I ate hardwood a half dozen times.

At 41, I'm a black belt, a triathlete, and a trainer. But the huge textbook I studied to earn my trainer certification, *Essentials of Strength Training and Conditioning,* includes one paragraph on the subject of balance. And I was just now beginning to learn how my fitness had suffered because of it.

So I set out to learn more—and do more. Improving your balance, I found, can help you lift more weight, have more productive workouts, and play any sport with more power and agility while staying free of injury. An unbalanced body is a weaker body. To achieve more of what you want from your workouts, you need to exercise your equilibrium.

The Science of Balance

The first step to fixing a problem is quantifying just how bad it is. Physical therapist Bill Hartman, PT, CSCS,

coauthor of *Muscle Imbalances Revealed* and co-owner of Indianapolis Fitness and Sports Training, recommends this simple test: Stand on one foot and lift the opposite knee to hip height. Hold that position for 10 seconds and repeat on your opposite foot. Then try the same test with your eyes closed. If you fall or if your elevated knee drops, Hartman says, your balance is off. This means you're more vulnerable to fall-related injuries, such as ankle sprains, than your better-balanced brethren are.

I was okay on my right foot. Standing on my left, though, eyes closed, I lasted all of 5 seconds.

Oops.

Balance, I soon learned, is complicated. Therapists sometimes refer to it as "reflexive stabilization" because it happens unconsciously, virtually every second of every day, thanks to a synthesis of information from at least three sources.

"Balance depends on input from your inner ear, your eyes, and numerous sensors in your skin, muscles, and joints," says chiropractor Craig Liebenson, DC, founder of L.A. Sports and Spine, a rehabilitation center that includes pro athletes in a variety of sports among its clients.

Though the inner-ear mechanism can sometimes go out of whack and cause problems such as chronic vertigo, Liebenson says the inner ear is rarely the source of average-guy balance troubles like mine. Ditto for eyesight, which has to be seriously impaired to affect a person's sense of balance.

That leaves the clue finders in your muscles, connective tissue, and joints, collectively known as proprioceptors. They manage the moment-to-moment awareness of the relative positions of the different parts of your body. That process, called proprioception, varies widely from person to person. Fortunately for me, it's highly trainable. But what, exactly, do I need to train?

A Stable Foundation

Balance is context-specific. You might have it in one situation and lose it in another, as you know if you've ever watched Hall of Fame basketball player Charles Barkley swing a golf club. So even if you ace Hartman's sobriety test, there's no guarantee you'll be able to apply that skill the next time you go in for a layup.

So physical therapist Gray Cook, CSCS,

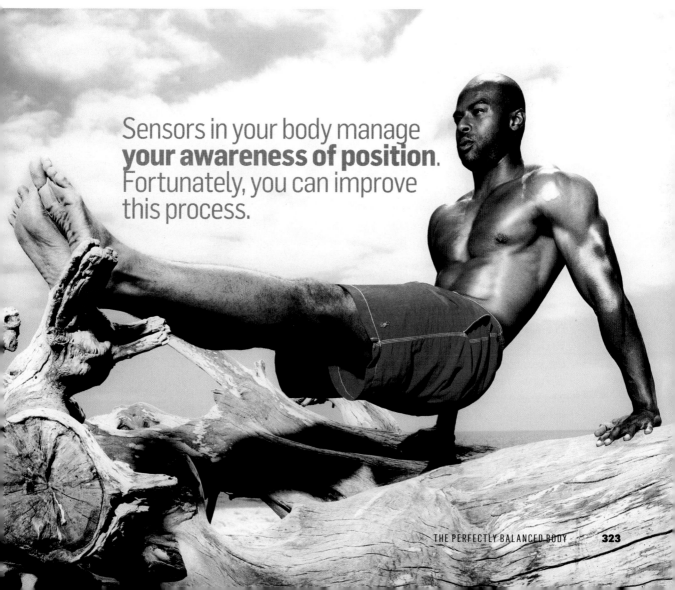

Sensors in your body manage **your awareness of position**. Fortunately, you can improve this process.

created the Functional Movement Screen, a multistep test of what he calls "movement competency." The FMS analyzes reflexive stability in basic movement patterns such as stepping, lunging, twisting, and squatting—the building blocks of everything we do in and out of the gym. Modern life has dulled our instinctual ability to perform these patterns.

"The active population of 120 years ago probably had greater levels of movement competency. Their exercise was more natural and less highly specialized," says Cook. "This afforded them natural symmetry and balanced movement."

Now, he says, we sit way too much, and when we do exercise, it's with repetitive movements, such as treadmill running, cycling, and lifting routines that emphasize beach muscles.

"When most people talk about fitness, they mean physical capacity—how much weight they can curl, how fast they can run," Cook says. "But numerical information about strength and speed tells you nothing about the quality of your movement."

Quality counts, as researchers discovered when they used Cook's FMS to test pro football players during the preseason. Players with lower scores were more than 10 times as likely to suffer injuries during the season as those with higher scores. (To test yourself, turn to "How Balanced Are You?," on page 328, and try the at-home version.) Remember, the low-scoring players were still professional athletes—probably faster, stronger, and better conditioned than anyone reading this book. But Cook's test shows that impressive fitness is often built on a shaky foundation.

I'm a prime example. Back in high school, when I was hell bent on becoming strong, I'd lift as much weight as I could, as often as I could. I bench-pressed before I mastered the pushup, and squatted with weight before I could squat correctly without it. And I never really stopped.

I'm not saying strength and speed don't matter," Cook says. But a body that doesn't move well is always at risk no matter how strong and fast it might be. "It's like driving with a flat tire," Cook says. "You can tinker with the engine all you want, with sets and reps of all your favorite exercises. But until you inflate that tire, you're never going to drive any faster."

Improving your balance, though, does

The Unnatural: Baseball's Lefty-Righty

"Even the most balanced person in the world isn't symmetrical," says Eric Cressey, MS, CSCS, cofounder of Cressey Performance.

"Think about it: The heart is on one side of the body. One lung has three lobes while the other has two. The liver is on the right. We're innately asymmetrical."

Cressey should know. He trains elite amateur and pro baseball players, who are among the most unbalanced athletes in the world. They throw with one hand, catch with the other, and run the bases by sprinting counterclockwise. He specializes in training pitchers, the most asymmetrical players in a uniquely asymmetrical sport.

Over the years, Cressey has noticed that among the ballplayers he trains are an unusual number who are ambidextrous, including many pitchers who throw with one hand and write with the other.

Lefty hitters enjoy the advantage of being a step closer to first base, but they often struggle against southpaw pitchers, who are highly valued. Off the diamond, though, lefties must function in a world designed mostly for right-handers.

more than keep you in the game. A recent study at Indiana State University showed that high scores on certain movement competency tests, while not predictive of athletic ability, correlated with better performance on tests of power, agility, and strength. A 2011 study published in *Sports Medicine* suggested that balance training improves markers of pure athleticism—the vertical jump and shuttle run, for example. The same study showed that elite golfers and soccer players had better balance than less-proficient players. So it might be your balance that's keeping you from breaking 90 or completing that pass with the game on the line.

A Balanced Approach

You don't have to abandon the gym and take up the unicycle to sharpen your movement skills. In fact, research suggests that the ideal approach to balance training is, well, a balanced one. The experts I interviewed agree that balance training works best as an adjunct to and not a replacement for the fitness training you already do (or should be doing).

There's no reason you can't train for balance, strength, and performance simultaneously. Start with these tweaks to your routine.

KEEP YOUR FEET ON THE GROUND

A few years back, if you'd told a trainer you wanted to improve your balance, he'd stick you on a Swiss ball and have you do circus tricks.

"You're certainly training your balance when you stand on an unstable surface," says Eric Cressey, MS, CSCS, cofounder of

Improve your balance by including **asymmetrical exercises** in your workouts. They'll **help keep you stable** in awkward situations and reinforce your core.

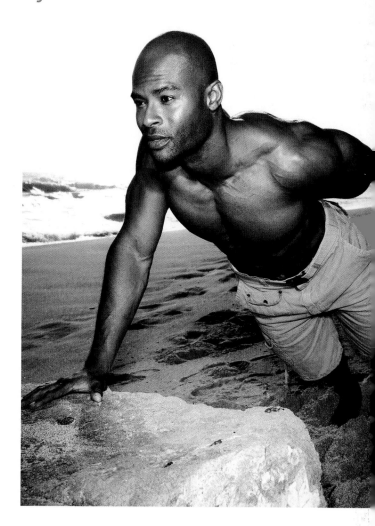

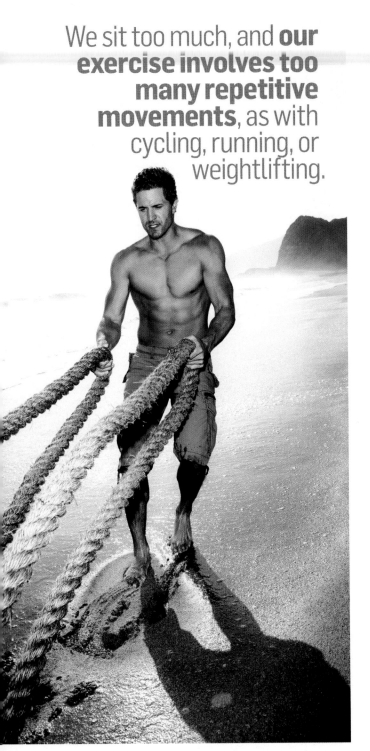

We sit too much, and **our exercise involves too many repetitive movements**, as with cycling, running, or weightlifting.

Cressey Performance in Hudson, Massachusetts. "But is there carryover to athletics? Will standing on a Swiss ball help Adrian Peterson stay upright with a 300-pound lineman trying to drag him down? I'd say that's a stretch."

Cressey's own study, published in the *Journal of Strength and Conditioning Research* in 2007, showed that soccer players who did a lower-body exercise with both feet on the floor saw greater improvements in power, speed, and jumping ability than those who did the same exercise on an unstable surface. These stable exercises, says Cressey, can enhance your balance proficiency.

TRAIN ONE SIDE AT A TIME

Life isn't symmetrical. If all you ever do in the gym are two-arm, two-leg moves like barbell squats, deadlifts, presses, and rows, you may find yourself ill-prepared when called on to lift an unbalanced load—like that couch your girlfriend needs you to help lift up her front steps.

Asymmetrical exercises—including single-arm presses and rows, and deadlifts and lunges holding a weight in one hand—can help prepare your body for the challenges that would otherwise knock you off balance. And unlike unstable-surface training, these moves allow you to use serious weights: You can build size and strength while improving balance. As a bonus, they give your core muscles a terrific workout.

BE A GENERALIST

An elite athlete has to specialize in one activity. But specialization is the enemy of the weekend jock.

"Doing any activity too much or too long eventually throws off the balance between opposing muscle groups," Cook says.

So even if you're the best bench-presser in the gym, spend at least as much time on exercises for the other half of your body, and from time to time let the bench gather some dust. If you live in a place where you can run or swim or ride year-round, take a few months off from weightlifting each year to give your overworked muscles time to recover and your underutilized muscles a chance to catch up.

STAY SKILLFUL

Exercise shouldn't always be a numbers game. Round out your lifting or running with activities that help you develop new skills or reinforce the ones you already have. I'm a big fan of martial arts and a system called the Feldenkrais Method, which improves your movement efficiency. Friends rave about yoga, tai chi, and Pilates. All are great ways to keep your brain and body engaged in learning new ways to move and to control movement. You also can't go wrong with less-structured activities, such as climbing, paddling, jumping rope, or working a speed bag. These can all improve balance, timing, reflexes, and athleticism as they build fitness.

"The best fitness program isn't overly rigid," says Frank Forencich, founder of Seattle-based Exuberant Animal. "It's not tied to any particular place or time schedule."

Another alternative: On a nice day, simply take your normal workout outside.

A trail run beats the snot out of an hour on a treadmill.

"A rich sensory environment with uneven terrain and unpredictable obstacles is ideal for improving your balance," Forencich says.

AVOID THE CHAIR

Sitting is bad for us, yet we keep doing it. Virtually every major workplace or lifestyle shift in the past 20 years has involved more sitting and less of everything else. But unless the apocalypse comes and forces us to forage for our survival, it's hard to see us spending less time staring at computer and TV screens. So what's a deskbound guy to do?

Take microbreaks. "It takes 20 minutes for your ligaments to deform," Liebenson says. He suggests standing up at least three times an hour. Stretch, extend your spine, breathe deeply, and focus on a distant object for 30 to 60 seconds. "The best chair is the one you leave often," he says.

After a few weeks of following the experts' advice, I could sense a big difference. I stood taller, I sat up straighter, and my workouts seemed more productive. I was still better on my right foot than my left, but I passed the closed-eye balance test with ease.

The real test, though, came on my return trip to Moonlight Rollerway with my daughter. She lapped me repeatedly for the better part of an hour. But this time, both of us stayed on our feet. Maybe it's just a small step in the big scheme of things, but for this 41-year-old former klutz, it was an epic leap forward—and a well-balanced landing.

How Balanced Are You?

The following five tests, from Gray Cook's *Athletic Body in Balance*, are simple but very challenging.

"Perfect" is the only passing grade. Anything less means you have work to do. If you feel any pain, stop and have it checked out.

HERE ARE THE RULES: Give yourself three tries on each exercise. Repeat the entire test every few months to see how your workout is helping. If you're not improving, you need to switch up your routine.

HERE ARE THE TOOLS: You'll need some masking tape, a 4-foot-long broomstick or dowel, and a standard doorway. You might also want to keep a serving of humble pie at the ready.

DEEP SQUAT

Grab the stick overhand with your hands slightly beyond shoulder-width apart. Stand inside the doorway and turn sideways to face the frame. Set your feet shoulder-width apart with your toes 12 inches from the door frame. Lift the stick overhead and lock your arms. (If you're too tall to do this, you'll have to straighten your arms as you squat.) Keep your feet flat as you slowly squat as low as possible. Reverse the movement and return to the starting position.

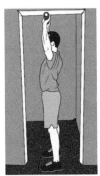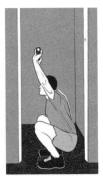

YOU PASS IF:

- Your hips are below your knees at the bottom of the squat.
- Your feet remain flat.
- Your toes are pointed straight ahead.
- Your knees remain in line with your feet.
- Neither the stick nor any part of your body touches the door frame at any point.

IF YOU FAIL:

- Spend more time stretching your ankles, hips, and shoulders, and add overhead squats with a light barbell to your workout routine.

HURDLE STEP

Run a strip of masking tape across the doorway at a height just below your kneecap. Stand with your feet together, facing the "hurdle," toes directly beneath the tape. Place the stick across your shoulders as you would for a barbell squat. This is the starting position. Step over the tape with your right foot. Tap your right heel lightly on the floor on the opposite side of the tape. Step back over the tape. Repeat this move with your left foot.

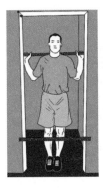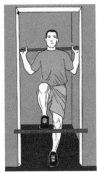

YOU PASS IF:

- You don't touch the tape going forward and back with either foot.
- Your hips, knees, and ankles keep their original alignment—nothing twists or bends in or out.
- The stick remains parallel to the floor.

IF YOU FAIL:

- Work on core stability with planks and side planks, and improve your hip mobility with walking lunges.

INLINE LUNGE

Cut a strip of masking tape the length of your lower leg. Lay the length of the strip through the doorway, centered between the jambs. Stand with the toes of one foot on the back end of the tape, and the heel of the other foot on the front end. Place the stick across your shoulders. Keeping your torso upright and front foot on the floor, slowly lower your back knee to the tape. Reverse to the starting position. Switch feet and repeat.

YOU PASS IF:

- Your upper body remains perpendicular to the floor, with minimal movement.
- Your feet stay on the ends of the tape.
- Your back knee touches the tape behind your front heel.
- The stick remains parallel to the floor without touching the door frame.

IF YOU FAIL:

- Use more balance-challenging lower-body exercises in your workouts, including lunges, single-leg deadlifts, and stepups.

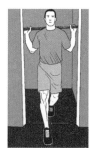

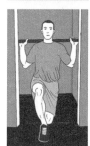

STRAIGHT-LEG RAISE

Lie on your back inside and perpendicular to the doorway, with the midpoint of your thigh even with the frame. Extend your arms straight out to your sides, palms up. Start with both legs straight, heels together, and ankles flexed 90 degrees. Raise your left leg as high as you can, keeping your right leg flat on the floor and both legs straight. Repeat with your right leg.

YOU PASS IF:

- The raised leg remains straight throughout the test.
- The ankle bone on the raised leg clears the door jamb.
- Your head and arms remain on the floor in their original position.
- The leg on the floor remains straight and still, with the toes pointing up.

IF YOU FAIL:

- Work on stretching your hamstrings without rounding your lower back, as in the downward-facing dog yoga stretch and the stiff-leg deadlift.

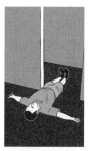

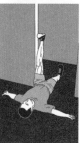

SEATED ROTATION

Sit cross-legged on the floor inside the doorway, with one foot on each jamb. Hold the stick across the front of your shoulders so it touches your collarbone. Keeping your back straight, rotate your shoulders as far as you can to each side.

YOU PASS IF:

- You touch the stick to the door frame on each side.
- The dowel remains level and in contact with your collarbone.
- Your spine remains upright—no forward or backward lean.

IF YOU FAIL:

- Focus on upper-body rotational movements, including single-arm cable rows and dumbbell rows.

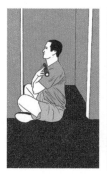

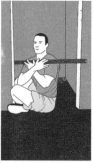

A Man in His Prime

David Beckham is about to change the way you think about your "best" years.

A long time ago, someone somewhere said something horrible about men . . . and it stuck. It's the nasty schoolyard rumor that won't go away, like when you heard that your best friend's brother had head lice in the fourth grade. It wasn't true. But the kid never lived it down. An equally destructive whopper about men was dumped out there decades ago, and we're still plagued by it:

Men peak at age 18.

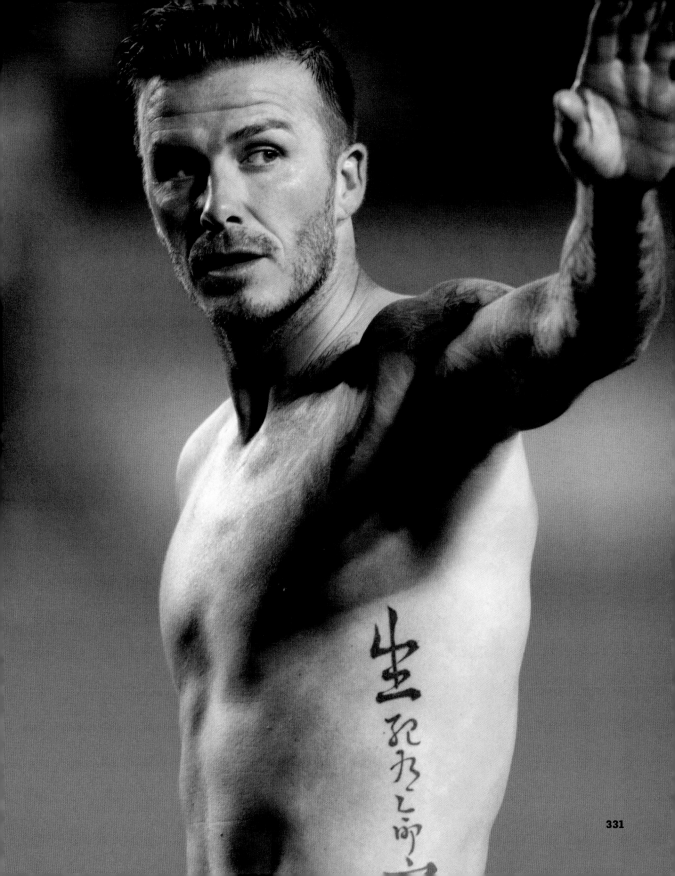

Maybe you can show in a lab that the reproductive potential of the average 18-year-old male is peaking (eight times a day, baby!). You can write newspaper stories about his time in the 100-meter against Central Catholic, or his passer rating, or his four gold medals in the district swimming finals. You can give him a high school diploma. Hell, you can also send that guy off to war and into a voting booth (not necessarily in that order).

And according to popular lore, that's the story of a man—the best he'll ever be.

We should know better. It's time to revise that number. In fact, let's double it.

Age 37. That's a more realistic prime— a time of achievement, family, and friendship, with equal parts reflection on the past and anticipation for the future. It's an accurate time to measure a man's self-worth. Our case study: David Beckham.

You've heard of him. You don't even have to be a soccer fan. He's probably the most famous athlete on earth. He married one of the most famous women on the planet. He has money. He has four kids (all sired after age 18, by the way). He's accomplished everything a man in his profession can accomplish, and he's done it at the highest level.

And the idiots out there say he's over the hill. Past his prime. A "Yesterday Man," according to the U.K.'s *Mirror*. A "self-serving" jock who should "step down for the good of his national team," an ESPN columnist wrote. Everyone seems to agree that Beckham is not as fast as he once was, but an athlete, like any man, shouldn't be measured by just one standard. We might try—with rulers, with hood ornaments, with trophy cases and trophy wives—but it's never a complete picture.

When you start counting up the real benchmarks of success, the ones that actually mean something, you see just how many there are. And how the ones that receive the most attention are, in fact, the least valuable.

Let's take a look at the worthy metrics, with Beckham as our guide. The best part? No matter which side of 37 you're on, if you're excelling in these areas, you're in your prime. If you're not excelling? There's plenty here to think about, and it's never too late to start.

Metric #1

You accept change. Dynamic men waste little time—at any age—sitting on bar stools talking about how great they were at 18. Dynamic men evolve. Case in point: Beckham, who's still playing soccer at age 37. People see an aging athlete change his game, and say, "He's done." That's not true. The guys who struggle are the ones who refuse to adapt to their age and march onto the field expecting the same results as before. Beckham has remade his game to take advantage of what he can still do better than most. He plays deep in central midfield, watching and waiting to intercept the ball and then passing it with his legendary accuracy.

"You have to change," he says. "I'm still running 12 miles a game. [But] I've definitely become more aware on the field. I know what my limits are, what I can achieve, and which passes I can play. I have adapted to my age."

The result? The L.A. Galaxy won the

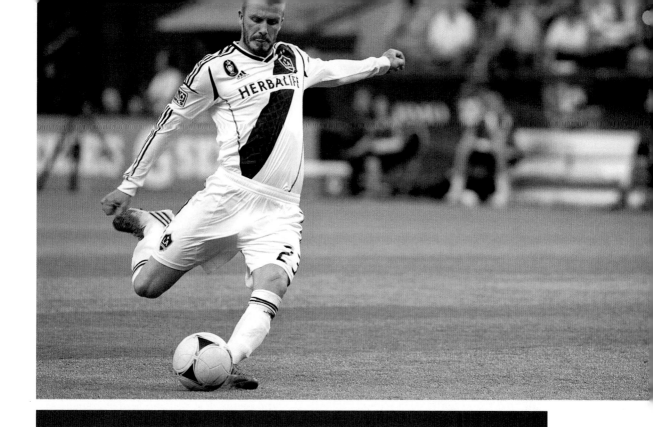

Don't Play Your Age
Beckham turned 37 last year.

"Most players are gone at this point," says Ben Yauss, strength and conditioning coach of the L.A. Galaxy, where Beckham returns next season. "But by adjusting his fitness regimen to his age, we keep him at the top of his game. Follow Beckham's lead to stay on top of yours.

PRIME YOUR MUSCLES. Beckham is known for being the first to arrive at practice.

"He's usually ready to work an hour before practice starts," Yauss says. But it's not to impress his coaches. Twenty years on the field has taught Beckham that exercising cold is a fast track to the disabled list. "Warming up ensures that his joints and muscles are ready for action," says Yauss, who has Beckham prime his body with dynamic movements like the kneeling hip flexor stretch, hip raise, and reverse lunge—all of which improve active flexibility and excite the central nervous system.

ADD SOME RESISTANCE. Like most men in their 30s, Beckham faces a gradual decline in performance. To curb those losses, he supplements his regular gym workouts with resistance-band and resisted-movement exercises.

"Adding them to sprints, kicks, and lateral movements helps build explosive power," Yauss says. One of Beckham's moves for glute strength: the band lateral shuffle. To try it, loop a resistance band around both legs just above your knees and stand with your feet shoulder-width apart. Next, take 10 wide steps to your left and then 10 wide steps to your right. That's 1 set; do 3.

ROLL IT OUT. To help his body bounce back after 90 minutes on the pitch—or after especially tough training—Beckham focuses on soft-tissue work.

"Five to 10 minutes of massage or foam rolling makes sure he's not stiff or sore the next day," Yauss says.

Such gentle manipulation boosts bloodflow to tired muscles, speeding recovery. It's also an essential part of his mid-30s mantra: Exercise in balance. "It's not just lifting or running or stretching or flexibility work—it's a combination of all of them," says Yauss. "By taking a holistic approach to fitness, David is able to stay healthy all season long and dribble circles around guys 15 years his junior."

MLS Cup in 2011, earning Beckham a club championship in a third country, after England and Spain.

Metric #2

You shed vanity. Yes, Beckham is a notorious popinjay. But the vanity we refer to isn't about looking good; it's about needing adulation to maintain self-worth. For Beckham it's simple: He respects his fans but he's not addicted to their cheers. He lives a real life beyond work.

"I've got friends at the different teams I've played for, but family is the most important thing to me. That will always be the case. I've got my wife. I've got my four kids. I've got parents, grandparents still, and three really good friends. It's all you need. I'd rather have three really good friends than 20 good friends."

Metric #3

You bring out the best in yourself. Do you know your worst trait? The smart guys leverage theirs into something useful.

"I am a very stubborn person," Beckham says, so he uses it as fuel. "I think it's helped me over my career. I'm sure it has hindered me at times as well, but not too many times. I know that if I set my mind to something, even if people are saying I can't do it, I will achieve it."

Metric #4

You approach fatherhood like a man. Any guy can knock up a woman. But even with the biggest surprise pregnancy, you still have, oh, 9 months to think about what kind of father you want to be. Too few men do this. Beckham, though, has a parenting ethos.

"It would be easy for our kids to sit back and not work for anything," he says, "but they're not like that. They're as competitive as Victoria and me. We're very lucky with our boys: They want to win. They want to work at something. They know their values. That's the way we've brought them up so far, and that's the way we'll continue to bring them up."

Metric #5

You manage your self-destructive tendencies. Men find all manner of ways to implode. Some choose classics like booze and drugs. But you can also overspend or cheat your employer. What's your poison? Beckham, despite all available vices, has managed to keep his self-discipline.

"Sportsmen have changed over the past 10 to 15 years. When I came into the Manchester United squad, you still heard about players going out for a few beers after a game. That doesn't happen very much now. The real professional players look after themselves a lot better than they did 10 years ago, and that's obviously how you see the likes of Ryan Giggs or myself still playing at the top level."

Metric #6

You thrive in crisis. In March 2010, Beckham tore his Achilles tendon, ruining his chance of playing in the 2010 World Cup. It could've been a career-ending injury. In the past 4 years, a lot of men have faced their own potential career killers, through firings and layoffs. How do you react when something bad happens?

Here's how Beckham responded: "There was only 1 day when I doubted that I'd get back to playing. It was 2 days after the operation, when my bandages came off and I saw the scar. It was very different from what I'd seen a few days before, and it scared me. I think that's the only time I've really felt that I wouldn't play football again. I was emotional. . . . I've played this sport for quite a few years. To think that I wouldn't be doing it anymore upset me. But it lasted only for the day. My kids walked into the room, and that took my mind off it. From then I was determined, absolutely determined, to get back. The surgeon told me I'd be back playing in 9 months." He smiles. "I was back in just under 6."

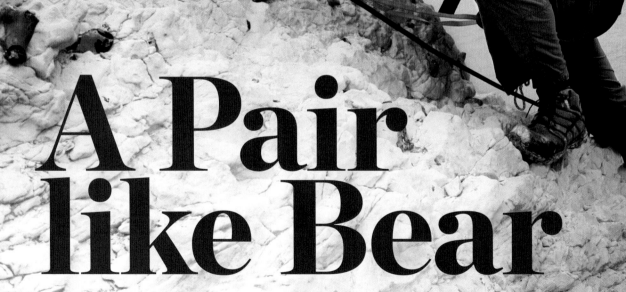

A Pair
like Bear

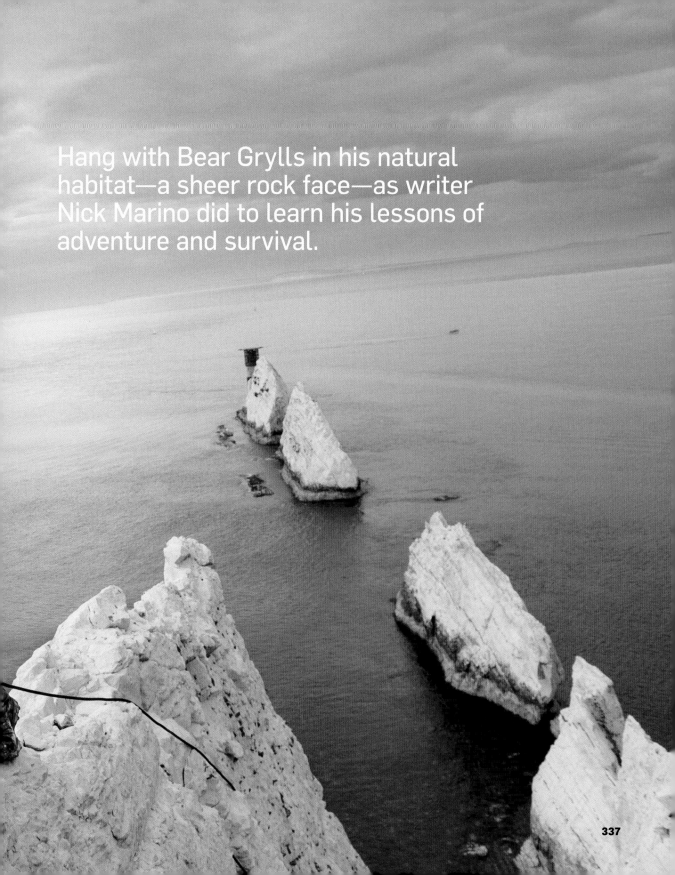

Hang with Bear Grylls in his natural habitat—a sheer rock face—as writer Nick Marino did to learn his lessons of adventure and survival.

Two hundred feet up, with the waters of the English Channel lapping below, Bear Grylls wants to know how I am with heights. We're strapped into harnesses and standing on a chalk cliff at the Isle of Wight's westernmost tip. In 5 minutes we'll rappel down the cliff—part of a formation, called the Needles, that juts out like shark teeth—and now he asks? I allow that heights might possibly rattle my nerves.

"Fear is normal," he says, surely not for the first time. "It's a tool that sharpens us for what we need to do."

The idea is that I'll descend first, with Grylls following. It's only fitting that a journalist with zero climbing experience would show the *Man vs. Wild* star (who has twice summited Everest—once on foot and once in a paraglider) how it's done. We'll venture in succession onto a ridge that's perhaps 6 inches across, and from there lower ourselves with ropes to a small ledge halfway down the cliff. There we'll pause to conduct an interview, and through this process the *Men's Health* reader will learn how he can live more adventurously. Grylls advises me to shuffle onto the ridge, hook my rope into a crack in the cliff, and then rappel.

"Just don't look down," he says. And then it's go time.

The tricky thing about chalk is that it crumbles—you don't need climbing experience to know this—and, true to form, a chunk of cliff breaks apart beneath me once I'm about 10 feet out onto the ridge. Pebbles tumble down. And so, it seems, will I.

"Don't worry," Grylls calls out, seeming more concerned about the rock than about

me. "It's only an ancient national monument."

Grylls can joke because he knows I'm safe. He trusts our rigging. I might feel as if I'm one false move away from a death dive, but feelings don't necessarily match reality. The truth is that even if I let go, I'd simply dangle in my harness. Eventually this sinks in. I ease myself backward and down, backward and down, backward and then . . . down to the ledge.

Grylls follows, strolling backward with little apparent effort. He lands on the ledge and fishes into his backpack for a stainless-steel thermos engraved with his name—a gift from his patrol sergeant back in the British special forces, where he served 4 years before breaking his back in a skydiving accident. He twists off the thermos cap.

"I was always brought up to have a cup of tea at halfway up a rock face."

Edward Michael Bear Grylls has explored the outdoors ever since he was a child here on the island.

"We did a load of boating and sailing and kayaking and climbing and horse riding around here," he tells me. "It wasn't a complicated life. It was a great life." But it was only after the accident

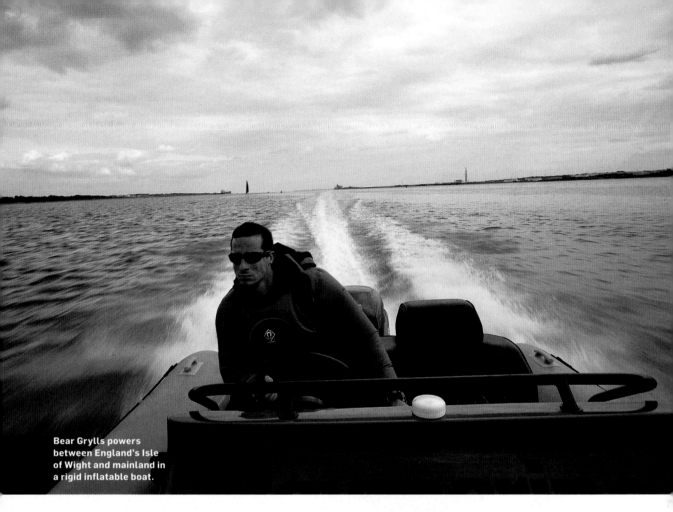

Bear Grylls powers between England's Isle of Wight and mainland in a rigid inflatable boat.

that he became a celebrated adventurer.

That sense of adventure comes from his father, a Royal Marines commando who later became a wine importer and a member of Parliament.

"My dad's not around any longer," Grylls says, "but I'm a dad to three young kids, and there's always a special bond when you climb and you have to trust each other with your lives."

In the age of overprotective parenting, it's bracing to hear Grylls describe paragliding with his 2-year-old son, Huckleberry (as in Finn), and kayaking with 8-year-old Jesse. The middle Grylls child, Marmaduke, is named after the World

Your Adventure Checklist

This simple gear could save your life.

Zip-top bags: You'll need these to waterproof your gear.

"They could save your life," Grylls says. "You know, people go out with a cellphone, put it on top of the rocks; then it rains, and the phone's dead." Throw your wallet in there too.

Extra socks and gloves: Socks get wet. Gloves are dropped.

"Somebody loses a glove in a cold environment," Grylls says, "and they can die because they'll suffer a frostbitten hand and can't use the hand. I've had a lot more riding on a spare pair of gloves than you might imagine."

Tarp: Rain or shine, "the priority is always protection from the weather. So if you're in the desert, you need something for shade."

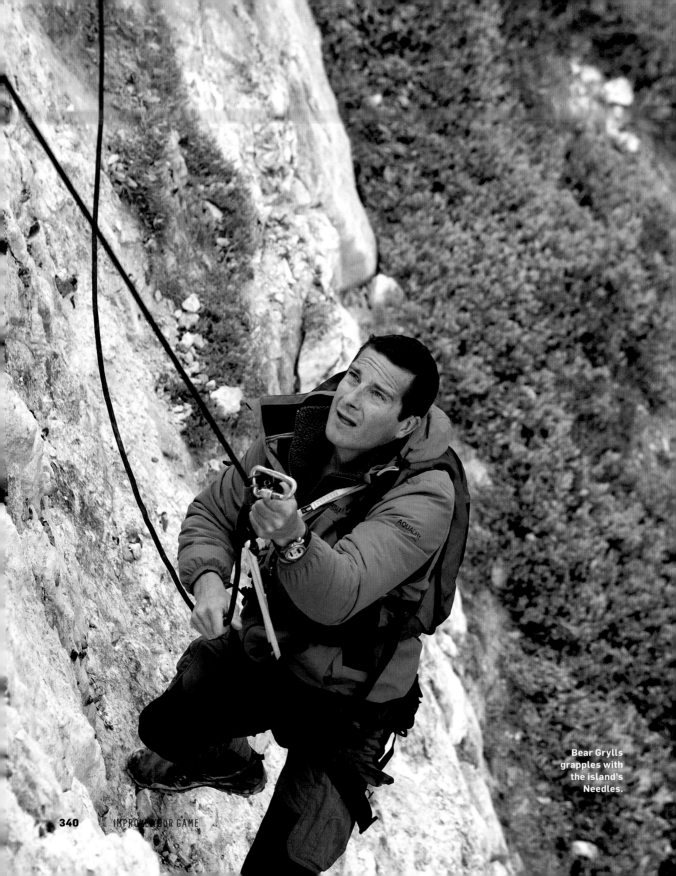

Bear Grylls grapples with the island's Needles.

War II flying ace Marmaduke Pattle. Grylls is a man who treats bravery as a sacred heirloom handed down from father to son.

"The problem is, they now watch my TV show, so they love it a bit too much. I am now actually trying to scale it back with them. Their teachers have said to me, 'That's all well and good having Jesse give me a detailed description of how to rappel out of a helicopter, but his mathematics are suffering.'"

Man vs. Wild, now in its sixth season, drops Grylls into dangerous and remote terrain—jungles, deserts, volcanoes, glaciers—and then follows him as he battles the elements. His two most notorious survival tactics involved guzzling his own

Ratchet Up Your Nerve
To summon your courage, follow this playbook.

ANTICIPATE HAZARDS, AND PLAN AROUND THEM.

You don't need the heart of a lion to face danger like Bear. You do, however, need to resourcefully strategize for safety.

"Being brave isn't the absence of fear," Grylls says. "Being brave is having that fear but finding a way through it."

DETACH FROM YOUR ANXIETIES.

Objectively examine your situation. Then harness your fear, which Grylls says exists "to fire up your sensors and give you the edge to make sure you hear well, see well, act strongly, and perform well in a big moment."

TRUST YOUR GUT.

Grylls says he has a reliable inner voice, and a rather insistent voice of doubt.

"The doubting voice is not the one to listen to. The doubting voice is just that little boy going, 'Have you double-checked everything? Are you sure?' But yes, it's fine. The inner voice is the one that says, 'You're okay to do this,' 'This is the right girl to marry,' or 'This is okay to climb this rock face.' And life's journey is to distinguish between the two voices."

MAKE RISK A HABIT.

Once you've conquered a few dangerous situations, you know you can handle the next one. Previous experience teaches you when to take a calculated risk and when it's time to pull back. It also helps you avoid panic.

"When it overwhelms you—and we've all been there—it controls you; people freeze. I've seen it a lot with people on mountains, and it's often the people you don't expect."

TALK TO YOURSELF.

In difficult moments, Grylls allows himself to pause.

"I just go, 'Okay, I'll stop for a second. I'm just going to breathe and look at it. I'll check my safety—I have confidence in that—and then I'm going to remind myself that I'm way more likely to be hit by a bus. I don't have a problem here.' And then I get on with it."

urine and crawling inside a camel carcass for shelter. Grylls, 38, freely acknowledges that he'd like to move on from the show. But it's become such a juggernaut—1.2 billion viewers in 180 countries, the promo materials boast—that it's hard to just shut down. Plus, he has product lines to maintain: his clothes, his books, his knives. The dude even has his own deodorant.

"When I'm in *Man vs. Wild* mode, it's not pleasure," Grylls says. "Every sensor is firing and I'm on reserve power all the time and I'm digging deep—and that's the magic of it as well, and that's raw and it's great. But pleasure for me is good friends coming, picking some adventure—whether it's a weekend thing or a day thing or a weeklong thing—and then planning it and building it and researching it and training for it."

And this, he believes, is something every man can do. Maybe even something every man *should* do. Adventure builds character and camaraderie. Adventure breaks us out of our daily routines. Adventure reminds us we're alive.

Grylls stashes the tea, and we prepare to climb back up. By the time I reach the top, both hands are bleeding and my adrenaline is surging, as Grylls knew it would be.

"You feel a complete buzz when you reach the top of that," he tells me before we ascend, "because you did it. And I feel exactly the same, and that's the magic and attraction of adventure."

Three Adventure Sports to Try Now
Make one of Bear's favorites your next challenge.

ROCK CLIMBING:

"Go with a friend, take a class, find a wall in your city, and learn some skills," Grylls says. "And then push yourself a bit. Research some cool routes nearby, go out and try some easy ones, take someone who's done it before, and just grow. Adventure should be 80 percent 'I think this is manageable,' but it's good to have that last 20 percent where you're right outside your comfort zone. Still safe, but outside your comfort zone."

PARAGLIDING:

"I took my kids paragliding yesterday," Grylls says. "Huckleberry is 2. I strapped him in—it was an adult harness. I wrapped it around him a few times, and we jumped off this hill. It wasn't like a vertical hill or anything. It was a gentle hill, and I ran down, just holding the bottom of his feet, and he was going, 'I'm flying! I'm flying!' My 8-year-old loves it and doesn't want me to hold him, and he takes off on his own, goes up 20 feet and comes down." Grylls says he taught himself the sport. But that's not advisable. "Take a class."

KAYAKING:

"You can do it with your kids, you can do it on your own. You can start off just on a lake. You can learn how to kayak well, how to roll it, and then take it to a river. But again, be careful, research the river, and get some help and some guiding, because rivers are things I've learned to really respect. And I always give myself a 20 percent margin of error."

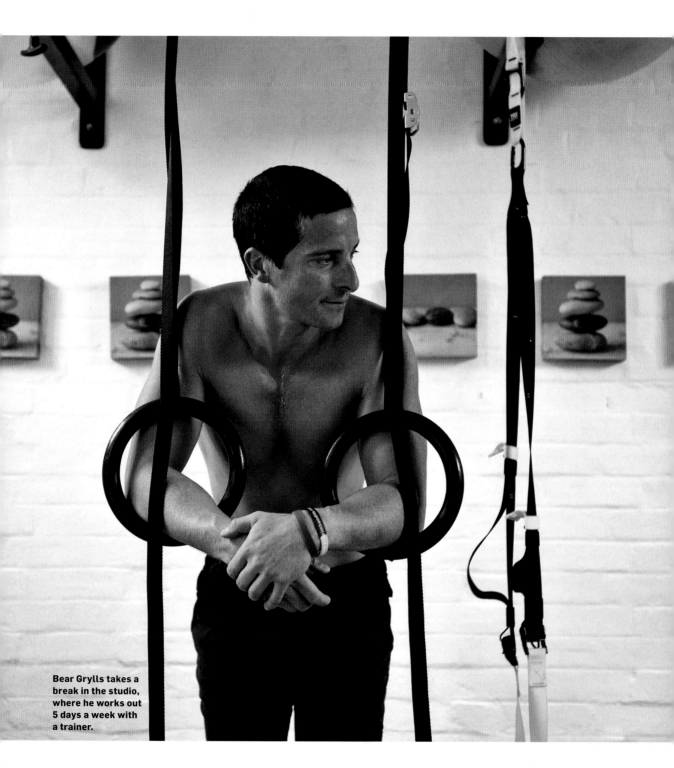

Bear Grylls takes a break in the studio, where he works out 5 days a week with a trainer.

Flying Higher

When will they play? NBA sensation Blake Griffin couldn't wait for an answer.

Blake Griffin says it's just a small cut.

On the second floor of a modern home overlooking L.A.'s Manhattan Beach, the 23-year-old Clippers power forward props his bandaged right foot on a brown ottoman and reclines into the matching sectional. Behind the conjoined living room and kitchen space, a bank of large windows displays the sequined blue ocean.

It's all very nice to look at, the spoils of budding NBA stardom. The high-profile tenant looks somehow familiar and unfamiliar at the same time. You never see this dude relaxing—it's like his 4WD suddenly developed a new gear: park. Why? Three days earlier Griffin was out in that sequined water when he felt a sharp pain in his foot. Then, blood. Griffin doesn't know what did the piercing, but it produced a seven-stitch wound that knocked him on his ass for a week.

"I've been sitting around, bored out of my mind," he says.

It's just a little break in his skin that led to a short break in his routine. But for Blake Griffin, any sort of rest is unusual. The man's world is defined by hustle.

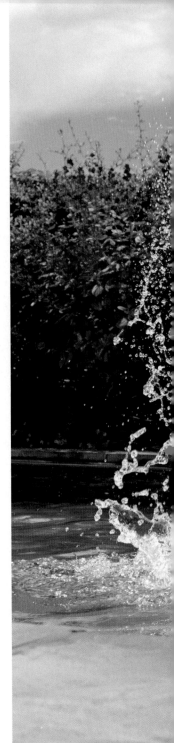

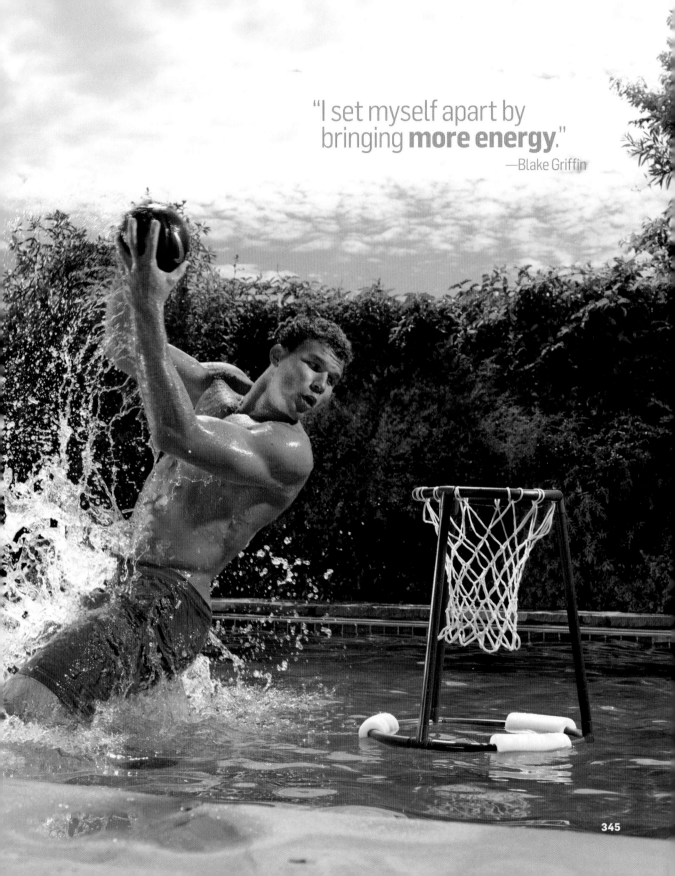

"I set myself apart by bringing **more energy**."
—Blake Griffin

When Griffin made his NBA debut season, he registered 20 points and 14 rebounds in his very first game. Within weeks he had established himself as a force in the post and a revelation above it, his dunks making him a stock character on *SportsCenter*. When the All-Star break arrived, Griffin became the first rookie to make the team since Yao Ming in 2003. Then he won the Slam Dunk Contest by jumping over a car. For the season he averaged 22.5 points and 12.1 boards, reinvigorated the NBA's most pathetic franchise, and was unanimously voted Rookie of the Year. His impact was so pro-

found that former Warriors coach Keith Smart told the *San Francisco Chronicle*, "I don't think we've ever seen a guy whose energy level is that high." Griffin aims to keep it that way.

"Energy is something you can control," he says. "In everything you do, you're going to face people more talented than you. I set myself apart by bringing more energy than they do."

This isn't always as simple as it sounds. As the number-one pick in the 2009 NBA draft, Griffin was expected to immediately inject life into the moribund Clippers. Then he tweaked his knee in the team's final preseason game. Trainers thought rehab would suffice, but the hinge healed improperly, so Griffin needed surgery. That meant 3 more months of the same tedious rehab he had just completed. It's one thing to summon boundless energy while garnering six national Player of the Year awards during his sophomore campaign at the University of Oklahoma. It's another to stoke that fire when the crowd consists of a physical therapist.

During those months of rehab, he built booster rockets into his vertical leap, which is now a staggering 38 inches. The naysayers questioned whether he'd ever fully recover, so he emerged more motivated than ever. The stage was set for his breakout. He hit his high mark, right on cue, but then found that even his explosive highlights weren't enough.

"I constantly heard that all I do is dunk," Griffin says. "And I can understand it. There aren't *SportsCenter* clips of me shooting 15-footers."

No ambitious person wants to be one-dimensional; the greats in every arena

Why I Moonlight

By Blake Griffin

As many of us have learned during the NBA lockout, you can't do the same thing for 8 months straight—in our case, our workout routines. You have to pace yourself and take breaks. For anybody, the key to working hard is variety. There are so many different ways to keep life fresh and stay motivated. Find something you enjoy: When it comes to exercise, if you like being outdoors, try running, hiking, or mountain climbing.

Since working out is actually my job, I try to find something else that I enjoy doing and make sure I carve out the time to do it. For me, that "something else" is learning about the world of comedy. Though I'm not an actor by any means, I have fun in that environment. That's why I did an internship at Funny or Die and worked on *Sports Show with Norm Macdonald*. But I always make sure that when I'm doing something on the side, it never stops me from working out. I put my training first. That way I know I'm prepared, because that's what's most important to me. It's just that once I'm done, I'd rather spend my free time doing an activity I enjoy, as opposed to just relaxing—during the off-season, at least. During the season, it's a big deal for me to even go out to eat at a restaurant.

have complete games. So Griffin went into this off-season committed to developing his shooting.

Every morning, and again a few nights a week, Griffin works on his shots: off the dribble, facing up—game-situation fare. He says the performance that gave him the most pride was a January 17, 2011, tilt against the Pacers. He scored 47 points but had only one dunk.

"Most of my baskets came from mid-range jumpers," he says. "I was the finesse player people said I couldn't be. I'm excited to show how I've added to that part of my game."

The contract dispute between NBA team owners and the Players Association at the start of the 2011–12 season once again put Griffin on the shelf. While waiting for the squabble to end, Griffin supplemented his shooting drills with an hour of yoga 3 days a week, heading off to the gym afterward for a workout. In a standard off-season week, he does an hour of strength and conditioning work 3 to 5 days a week.

Griffin's relentless work ethic came from his dad, who coached him throughout high school.

"My dad pushed me harder than any other coach would have," he says. "He stressed that when you're on the court, it's time to do work. That really rubbed off on me."

Then Griffin sliced his foot open. Yes, it was just a minor injury, more of an annoyance than a serious setback, but it served as yet another reminder that there will be times when he can't play. Eventually he'll be ushered off the court for good.

"A lot of older guys have told me how quickly it goes by," he says, "and that suddenly I'll be in panic mode, trying to figure out what to do next. I figure it's never too early to start planning ahead."

To that end, Griffin spent a portion of his lockout-plagued summer channeling his extra energy into something positive—an unpaid internship (not that he needed the money) working on videos at the humor Web site Funny or Die.

"I wanted to see that side of comedy," Griffin says. "After my workouts, I'd spend the day at the Web site offices. I'd like to get involved with TV in some capacity when I'm done playing. Next summer I may even write my own videos."

Griffin has also done improvised interviews for MySpace and a segment on *Sports Show with Norm Macdonald*. (Producers should start calling Griffin's agent . . . now.)

Griffin worries that people might see his extracurriculars as distractions, but like any career-minded worker, he believes in using his current gig as a foundation for future options. It's called foresight. After all, injuries happen. So do labor disputes. Having a backup plan is just one more hustle play.

How to Play Everything Better

With a few simple secrets, you can win
at pretty much anything in life.

**Runner-up, sister kisser, loser . . . no one will ever put
you and those descriptions in the same sentence again.
Here's how to play the game—and win!**

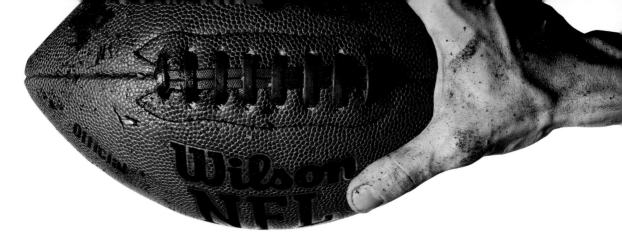

BOOM THE BALL HIGH AND DEEP

Former Dallas Cowboys All-Pro kicker Shayne Graham helps you put the foot in football.

Take your position. Deep, accurate punts require controlled form. Grip the ball with your dominant hand as if you were giving a handshake, nestling it between your thumb and fingers (A). Extend your arm forward as far as you can and hold the ball horizontally, with the nose pointing slightly to your left (or to your right if you're left-handed). Keep the laces up (B).

Make contact. Starting with your kicking foot, take two steps forward to build momentum, and then swing your foot out to meet your hand (C). Make contact with the ball as late as you can so you're almost kicking it straight out of your fingers. If you drop the ball too early, you're more likely to have a wayward punt. If you kick smoothly, the ball will fly farther than if you simply blast the ball.

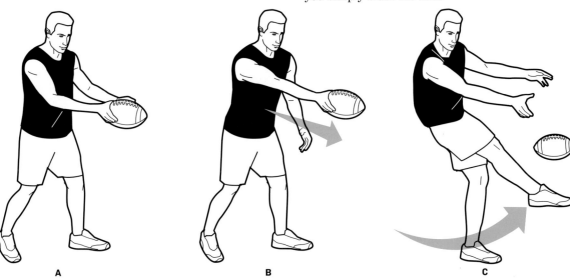

A   B   C

BUILD A BACKYARD ICE RINK

Leverage ice-cold temps to construct a private skating rink on your property. (Penalty box not included.)

Gather your supplies. Estimated cost: $350.

> Mason's string (at least 160')
> 20: 24" rebar
> 10: 16' Douglas fir 2x6s
> 6: 1' 2x6s
> 2 lb 2" deck screws
> 2 lb 3" deck screws
> 1: 40'x100' spool 4mm plastic liner

Scope your turf. On a flat area, measure a 32'x48" rectangle with string and pound a piece of rebar about 18" into the ground at each corner. Clear away any rocks or sticks.

Bracket the rink. Run the fir 2x6s along the inside of the string, joining them with the 1' 2x6s and 2" deck screws.

Secure the corners. At each corner, connect the boards with 3" deck screws—driven in at angles—to form a rectangle. Pound rebar outside each corner so that all the corners are braced by two pieces of rebar. Also, place two pieces of rebar at the joints along the length and width of the rink's frame.

Lay out a liner. Plastic liner will compress your grass without killing it. Cover the box with plastic and push down at the edges to form a reservoir. Now trim the outside so the plastic overlaps your rink brace by a foot around the perimeter. Staple the plastic to the outside of the frame.

Fill 'er up. Fill your rink with 1" to 1½" of water. Let it freeze overnight and add a second layer the next day. Let that sit for two nights. Filling it in stages will ensure optimal results. Test to make sure the ice is solid before skating.

Smooth the ice. Keep the Zamboni in the garage. If the ice is uneven, spray water on it and allow it to freeze. New ice!

Source: Jason Cameron, licensed contractor and host of DIY Network's *Man Caves* and *Desperate Landscapes*

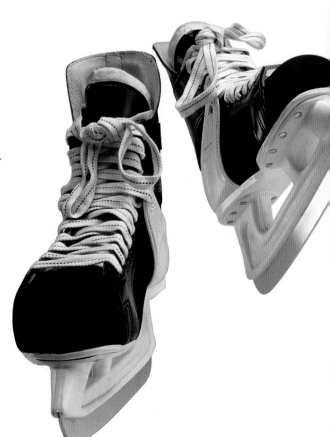

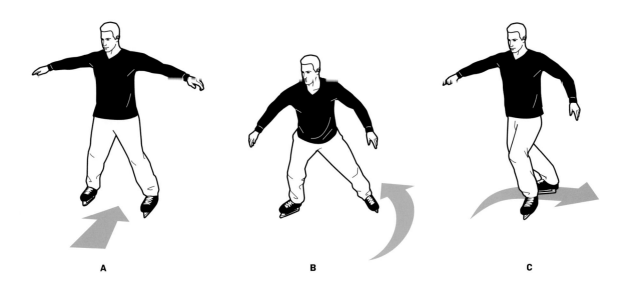

A   **B**   **C**

SKATE BACKWARD

Play better D during pickup hockey—or just impress your girl on a winter date.

Step 1: Stand strong. Come to a stop. With your feet shoulder-width apart, hold your arms out for balance (A). Bend your knees, which will help your hips provide push-off power.

Step 2: Build momentum. Alternating your feet, start making slow, smooth cuts backward into the ice and slightly out to the side, turning your skates no more than 15 to 20 degrees from the path you want to travel. Squeeze your thighs together to bring your skates inward.

Step 3: Stop—or turn. To slow and stop, put pressure on the inside edge of either blade and slowly drag it against the ice perpendicular to the direction you're moving (B). To turn around, bend your knees and rotate your shoulders against your hips. Then snap around by reversing that motion as you straighten your knees (C).

Source: Ryan Bradley, 2011 men's U.S. figure skating champion

BUILD A FROZEN FORTRESS

Give your kids the advantage in a neighborhood snowball war.

Check your powder. Snow crumbles easily when it's fresh, so wait out the storm. If you can't wait, bring out a watering can of cold water. Sprinkle the water over the snow you're using until the powder reaches a denser consistency.

Build your fort. Grab some bread pans, head outside, and start making bricks. Fill each tin with snow and pack tightly. Slam it upside down on the ground and lift the tin quickly upward to prevent sticking. Sprinkle cold water over the first few layers to make them icier and stron-

ger. As you build upward, use fluffier, less-dense bricks so they won't crush your walls. Make the walls about 4 feet high and leave the top open so your kid can launch an attack.

Bolster your defenses. During construction, insert cardboard toilet-paper tubes (for spotting enemies) between bricks. Pile a mound of snow into a corner and carve out a burrow about the size of a lunch box. Fill that with juice boxes, grapes, or a thermos of hot chocolate.

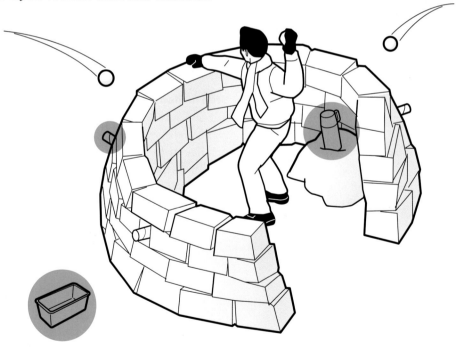

Sources: Joanne Seelig, family programs manager for the National Building Museum; and Andrew McMartin, executive director of the PINE Project

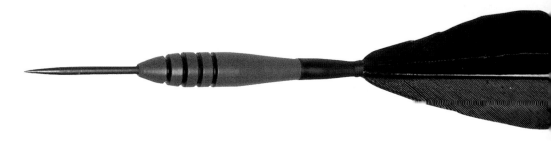

DOMINATE THE PUB DARTBOARD

Lesson one: Don't throw anything if you can't focus on your bull's-eye. Also . . .

Give the shoulder. Newbs usually face the dartboard, a stance that allows for errant throws. Instead, stand with the shoulder of your throwing arm facing the board. This locks your arm, ensuring darts fly true.

Plant your feet. If you lunge (or worse, jump) in an attempt to add oomph to your throw, you'll send your dart off course. Your throwing power should come from your biceps, elbow, and wrist. Keep your body rigid to create a good foundation.

Don't throw elbows. Your elbow should naturally move slightly upward or downward to adjust for the height of your target on the board.

Ease your grip. The tighter you clamp down on the dart, the harder it is to transition into a quick, smooth release.

Stay focused. Aim for an exact point on the board—not a section. The more focused your eyes are, the less space you subconsciously allow your arm to move and cause a miss.

Source: Gary Boyd, professional darter for the American Darters Association and winner of the 2011 ADA National Professional Men's Singles Championship

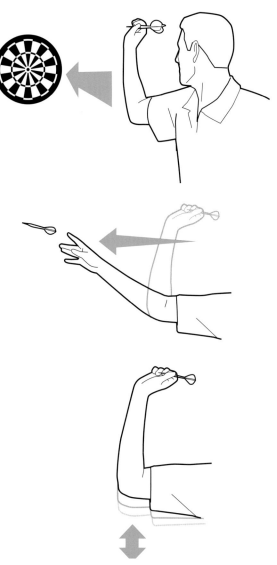

SAVE FACE ON THE CLIMBING WALL

Reaching the summit of Mount Bogus is no easy feat, but the payoffs are huge: a total-body workout, plus bragging rights.

Prep for your ascent. Walls require softer shoes than outdoor climbing does. Look for climbing shoes with slightly downturned toes, such as the Evolv Geshido ($140, evolvsports.com). Also use a chalk bag to keep your hands dry.

Bury your fear. Nervous about falling? Climb 10 feet up, and then ask your belayer to hold you tightly with the rope. Let go. You won't budge. Now climb!

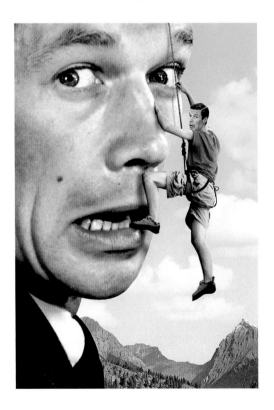

Lift with your legs. Center your weight on the holds using the most stable part of your shoes—the area around your big toe. Then push up with your legs. Use only your hands to stay upright and balanced.

Decode handholds. There are five basic holds in real-world climbing. The best walls replicate local conditions.

- Edges: You'll usually find these on granite and quartzite where rock has cracked or flaked off.
- Pockets: These are hollowed-out holds typically seen on limestone.
- Knobs: These protrude from all types of rock and are better stood on than grabbed.
- Slopers: These flat or curved surfaces, found on sandstone, generally slope downward. Create friction by making as much contact as you can with your fingers and palm.
- Pinches: Find these outcrops on limestone.

Slow down. Look for spots to take breaks, and focus on keeping your torso in a vertical plane above your feet, neither too close to the wall nor too far back.

Sources: Steph Davis, a top-rated professional rock climber; and Brooke Sandahl, vice president of Metolius Climbing

SET UP THE PERFECT HOME GYM

Convert your workout dungeon into a space you'll actually want to spend time in.

Fortify your floor. Carpet fibers can trap sweat odors. Opt for roll-out rubber flooring; this can protect your floor from dropped weights and make body-weight exercises, like pushups or planks, more comfortable.

Add some color. Use warm tones like red, yellow, or orange on the walls. In a 2011 study in *Perceptual and Motor Skills,* these colors were seen as stimulating, while cool hues were associated with restfulness.

Motivate! A wall mirror opens up the space and helps you check your form. For inspiration, hang a print of a historic sports moment from artletics.com, or order a canvas photo of your own at canvaspop.com.

Stop gym funk. Place a Smelleze Gym Deodorizer Pouch ($25, noodor.com) in a corner to stanch the stench. Improve the room's airflow with an oscillating fan. (A ceiling fan could interfere with jumping exercises.)

Achieve more muscle with less space. No room for a full-size gym? Use this instead.

- Cable weight station: JC Predator Bands ($50, ihpcombat.com) hook to a door or fixed object. You can add resistance by doubling or tripling them up.
- Full set of dumbbells: Lift with the Powerblock Sport 5.0 Adjustable

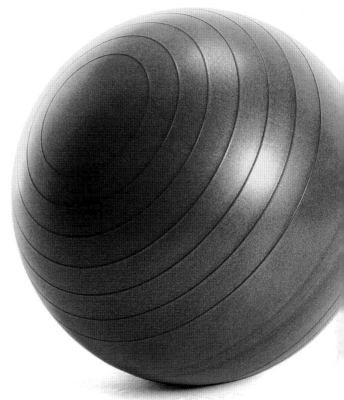

Dumbbell set ($300, powerblock.com). They quickly adjust between 5 and 50 pounds.

- Bench: Curls, presses—all are more challenging on a Swiss ball ($35 to $55, theragear.com) because your core stabilizes your body.

Sources: Gabe Valencia, CSCS, co-owner of Focus Integrated Fitness in New York City; and Trip Haenisch, a designer based in Los Angeles

WIN AT THE GO-KART TRACK

Make like Kyle Busch and leave your competitors chasing your tiny tire tracks.

A **Sit up straight.** Better posture in the kart leads to greater turning control. Sit upright with your arms slightly bent. This will help you apply even pressure to the steering wheel, decreasing your risk of a spinout.

B **Study the course.** The track should have a map showing the suggested "line"—the fastest path through each turn—and braking points. Braking points vary depending on your weight, so experiment on your first few laps. In some turns, you might be better off not braking at all—just lift off the gas instead.

C **Aim for speed, not position.** Most tracks score each race based on fastest laps, not relative positions. If that's the case, hang back so you have a clear track to produce the best time, or stick behind the fastest guy so you can follow his line and stay motivated to pass him.

D **Pass like a pro.** Stuck behind someone? In order to pass him, you'll need to carry more speed through the next turn than he does. Brake as little as possible, accelerate past him at the apex, and keep the hammer down all the way through the exit.

E **Master the turn.** Brake or lift your foot off the gas before the turn. Stay on the inside of your lane, accelerate as you exit, and allow the kart to drift to the outside. You'll cut seconds off your time.

Source: Kevin Williams, World Karting Association board member

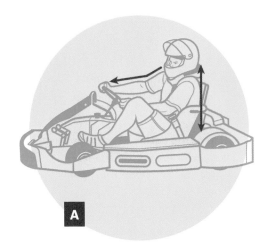

A

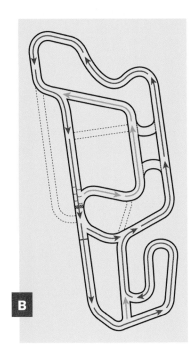

B

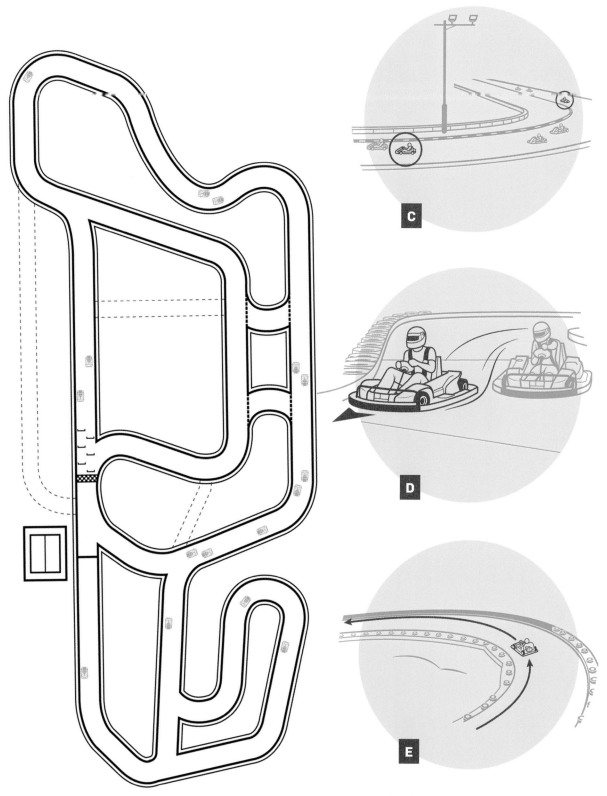

SPIN A BASKETBALL ON YOUR FINGER

Practice these steps for at least 6 minutes a day. Within a week you'll stop wobbling and start wowing, says Joseph Odhiambo, the world record holder for fingertip basketball spinning.

Do some prep. Deflate the ball slightly. This creates more surface area where your finger touches the ball, making it easier to control.

Set up your spin. Hold the ball (seams vertical) with your dominant hand on the far side and your other hand on the side facing you. Keep your elbows bent and tucked close to your body. The ball should be about 4 inches from your chin.

Let 'er rip. Snap both wrists to start the ball spinning; slower is better at first. The seams should pass by without wobbling. Quickly catch the ball with the pad of your index finger. Count to one. Then try again until you can last for a count of two, then three, and so on. Be sure to stop when you reach each count; this helps build confidence and control.

Keep it up. In 8 seconds, the ball will slow. Bend your finger slightly toward you and try to move the ball to your fingernail, keeping your elbow tucked to your body. This reduces friction between ball and finger, helping maintain spin. Now start lightly batting the ball with all four fingers of your free hand. Whistle "Sweet Georgia Brown."

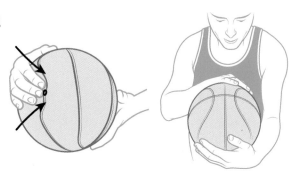

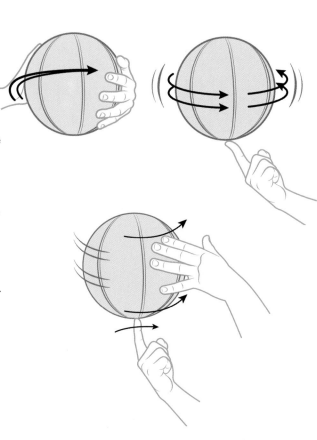

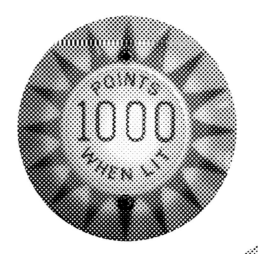

BE A PINBALL WIZARD

Stay on the table longer to blow away the high score, set by some dude called MetalManiac67.

Avoid the traps. Game designers often stick tempting targets with high point values near rubber posts that deflect your ball toward the drain lane. Aim for low-risk areas of the playfield. These are usually bumpers, drop targets, or sub-playfields—the confined areas your ball ricochets around in for a while before bouncing out again.

Control your shots. Don't kick the ball away every time it heads for your flipper or you'll never have control. You'll also increase your risk of errant shots. Instead, let the ball hit the flipper and bounce to the next flipper—then hold down the flipper button to "cradle" the ball. Release the flipper and aim your shot.

Score big. Modern machines use flashing lights and arrows to direct novice gamers through the playfield. Ignore them. Points accrue better in multiball mode, so do whatever you can to activate it. Once you're in multiball mode, don't go on a flipper frenzy. As in normal game play, controlling your shots is the key to high scores.

Source: Keith Elwin, Pinball World Championship winner 3 years running

PROVE
IT

WASH UP

According to *Medicine and Science in Sports and Exercise,* superbacteria MRSA can survive on artificial turf for 60 days when mucin (a component of snot and saliva) is present. Ugh.

RUN LIKE AN OLD LADY

In distance races, women and older folks maintain their pace better and finish stronger than men do, a University of Dayton study found.

"Men, particularly young men, tend to go out fast and blow through their carb stores," says study coauthor Paul Vanderburgh, EdD. Use training runs to get a feel for your planned pace—and stick to it in the race. Running with a pace group can help.

RUN, DON'T SWIM

By some health measures, runners lead swimmers, according to University of Texas at Austin research on recreational athletes.

Average Pulse Pressure

Runner: 47 millimeters of mercury (mmHg)
Swimmer: 54 mmHg

Pulse pressure can indicate arterial stiffness;

lower is better. Swimming puts demands on the nervous system that may trigger constriction, says study author Hirofumi Tanaka, PhD.

Resting Heart Rate

Runner: 50 beats per minute
Swimmer: 58 beats per minute

The heart of a runner (who is upright and fighting gravity) tends to pump out more blood volume than that of a prone swimmer. So a runner's heart doesn't have to beat as fast.

Body-Fat Percentage

Runner: 18%
Swimmer: 24%

Cold water may stimulate appetite; "this could prevent body-fat loss," says Tanaka. More body fat may also lead to higher blood pressure and LDL cholesterol in swimmers.

Blood-Vessel Dilation

Runner: 8.2%
Swimmer: 3.8%

Running helps relax the smooth muscles in artery walls so blood can flow more freely. Swimming doesn't have the same effect. Higher body fat may be to blame.

HARD TRUTH

19 Percentage of game time a basketball player is above 95 percent of his maximal heart rate zone according to the *Journal of Strength and Conditioning Research*

RUN HARDER

Short of breath? Run harder, but not as far. High-intensity, low-volume training helps your body use oxygen more efficiently, say researchers in Norway. Runners who worked at 82 to 92 percent of their heart-rate max for a third of their training time significantly improved speed and running economy in just 10 weeks—improvement that typically can take years. This kind of training adapts your heart and muscles to stress and helps your lungs take in more oxygen, says author Eystein Enoksen, PhD. So, on a 45-minute outing, run 15 minutes (spread out) in that higher heart-rate zone.

CYCLE HOT AND COLD

Your summer workouts will pay off in the fall. Adding low-intensity training to hot-weather workouts improves your performance in the cold, a recent study from the University of Oregon found. Cyclists who added low-intensity workouts in 100°F heat increased their power by 7 percent during a cold-weather event, while those who did the same workouts in cooler temps made smaller gains.

Study author Santiago Lorenzo, PhD, says heat acclimation raises plasma volume—the liquid part of the blood. This might increase delivery of blood and oxygen to your muscles, so you can exercise harder and sweat sooner for better thermoregulation. Layering tees may have a similar effect—but be careful not to overheat, he says.

GET FULL-COURT FIT

Point guards can cover lots of ground, a running test finds. Basketball players cover about 4½

miles a game on average, but they shouldn't train like distance runners, says Bruce Pearl, Tennessee University's head coach.

Take it outside. Each Monday in the preseason, the Tennessee Volunteers run sprints uphill to a Neyland Stadium gate. It's less pounding on the joints than running downhill or on level ground. Try it on a 50-yard hill with a slight incline.

Go soft. Bounding drills (skipping, single-leg jumps, broad jumps) can bolster your legs, but do them on a soft surface.

"We don't do a lot of preseason training on hardwood because the wear and tear can take out your knees," Pearl says.

Time your breaks. "Don't play to exhaustion—play to fatigue," says Pearl. "If you're hyperventilating, you'll have to sit out a whole lot longer." When you need a blow, wave in a sub, rest for a minute or two, and then jump back in, he says.

DISTANCES COVERED IN SHUTTLE-RUN TEST

Point guard: 2,724 meters

Power forward: 2,067 meters

Shooting guard: 1,907 meters

Center: 1,227 meters

Small forward: 2,031 meters

JUMP FOR YOUR BRAIN

Your weekly pickup game might do more than keep you in shape, a recent Korean study found. Brain scans of basketball players revealed that the striatum, an area thought to process and store muscle memory, was larger in athletes than in nonathletes. Other research has found that basketball players also tend to have larger cerebellums (seen in skilled musicians too).

PROVE IT

GET SMART, MEATHEAD

Carbs give you endurance, but protein might boost mental toughness. In a recent British study, cyclists who doubled their daily protein intake performed better in a time trial after intense training than cyclists who took in a normal amount. They also showed fewer symptoms of mental stress. Study author Oliver Witard, PhD, says amino acids from protein might reduce levels of perceived exertion and increase availability of carbs.

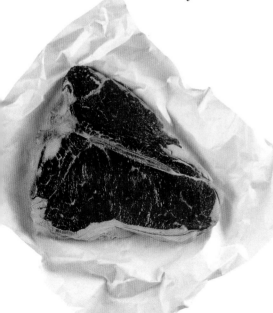

TRY THIS MAGIC POWDER

Baking soda can sharpen your late-match skills on the tennis court, a new Taiwanese study reports. Tennis players who drank water with baking soda before and during a simulated match showed less of a performance decline than players in a placebo group. Bicarbonate might alleviate the fatigue-induced slowdown of nerve signals to muscles, scientists say. Try half a tablespoon in 3 to 4 ounces of water and sip during practice to see if it helps.

BE A SPIN DOCTOR

Science finds the perfect racket—and you can make it yourself!

An effective ground stroke in tennis requires topspin, producing a ball that dive-bombs as it crosses the net and then skips forward low and fast. British researchers who tested several racket designs found that a heavier racket with a higher center of mass increases both ball speed and topspin.

"You can hit the ball harder and it will still land inbounds," says Tom Allen, PhD, lead author of the study, which appeared in the *Journal of Sports Sciences*. The problem is, a heavier racket can slow your stroke. Allen suggests adding lead tape to the top of the racket, on the outside of the rim. Start with 5 grams. Test it, and if your swing feels normal, add another layer of lead. Keep adding lead as long as you don't notice a difference in your swing.

GRUNT WORKS

Annoying, maybe. Effective? Probably. Grunting during a tennis match may throw off your opponent's game. According to a new University of British Columbia study, people watching video clips of matches reacted more slowly and predicted the ball's direction less accurately if players grunted. Grunts blocked the sound of the ball hitting the racket, so speed and spin were harder to gauge. The effect may also work in on-court competition, says study coauthor Scott Sinnett, PhD.

Can you identify the tennis player by his game face? (Answers below.)

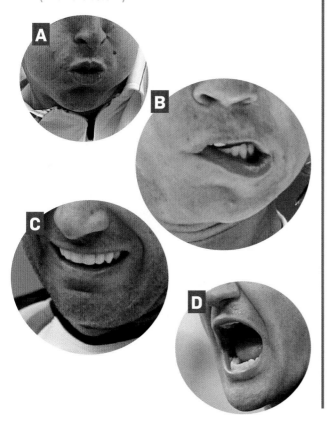

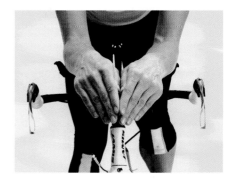

SMOOTH IT OVER

For better aerodynamics, triathletes use "aerobars" on their bikes instead of drop handlebars. A recent New Zealand study found that forming a wedge with your fingers is the most aero dynamic aerobar position. The unfamiliar grip can reduce your power and stability, though, so practice in this position until your output normalizes, suggests study author Lindsey Underwood, PhDc.

DON'T GO FISH

Swimmers who take fish-oil supplements are 2.6 times more likely to accumulate fluid in their lungs than swimmers who don't, a recent study from Texas Tech University reveals. Fish oil may thin the blood, making it easier for fluid to pass into your lungs, says study author Charles Miller, PhD. Less than 2 percent of swimmers suffer the full-blown condition, but partial symptoms might be more prevalent. Lay off the pills for 3 or 4 days before an event, particularly if you have high blood pressure.

Answers: A Igor Andreev, B Rafael Nadal, C Andre Agassi, D Roger Federer

YOU ASKED

Q: Are those new water bottles with the built-in filters worth trying?

A: It depends on whether or not you want to take any chances with what you're chugging. See, these bottles employ miniaturized versions of the carbon technology found in home pitcher and faucet filters, says Robert D. Morris, MD, PhD, an epidemiologist with the University of Washington school of public health.

"The filters meet the National Sanitation Foundation's Standard 42, which certifies an improvement in the aesthetic quality of the water. They will also remove a portion of tap

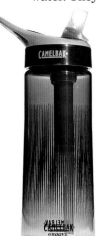

water's potentially toxic volatile organic compounds, including chlorine by-products," says Morris. Because filters reduce the concentration of contaminants by only 50 to 60 percent, they will not ensure the purity of water that started out as unsafe.

The only way to know for certain what's in your water is to request a Consumer Confidence Report from the local water utility, and that isn't exactly practical when you're filling up at a public water fountain. Still, you're better off using these filters than drinking straight tap water.

***MH* PICK:** look for a bottle that meets nsf standards and is bpa-free, such as the camelbak groove ($25, camelbak.com) and the stainless steel watergeeks pure blue ($17, watergeeks.com).

Q: My boss raised an eyebrow when I mentioned a Kinect session. Is 35 too old for gaming?

A: No, but what a 35-year-old man shouldn't do is tell his boss he plays video games. Of course he gave you the evil eye: Most people don't realize that gaming at any age is actually beneficial.

"Games help kids understand different perspectives," says John W. Hagen, PhD, a professor of developmental psychology at the University of Michigan. "It's often assumed that once we mature, we no longer need them, but in reality, we just need more-complex ones that challenge us in new ways."

By trying different games, you can sharpen your problem-solving skills and improve your hand-eye coordination. See our picks for games with proven health benefits.

Shooting: Games like Call of Duty 2 may help you blow off steam, and might increase your tolerance to stress in the real world, report Texas A&M researchers.

Strategy: In a University of Illinois study, Rise of Nations improved the mental performance of older adults. (And the benefits likely extend to younger brains too.)

Active: You could burn 37 calories in 15 minutes of Wii Boxing, a Mayo Clinic study reports. Any game that makes you think and move is good.

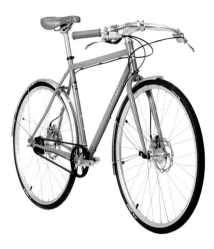

Q: I want a bike I can use for my commute. What should I look for?

A: Here's your checklist: Lightweight yet burly frame, powerful brakes, and stay-clean features to ensure that you arrive sans splatters and grease stains, says Bill Strickland, *Bicycling* magazine's editor at large.

"We're seeing a new breed of commuter bikes. They still have fenders and chain guards, but they're more rakish than dorky."

Use this guide to find a ride that's comfortable, efficient, and safe.

Gearing: Go for three to eight gears. The hottest innovation is the Gates Carbon Drive, a lube-free belt that replaces the chain—and with it the possibility of black marks on your new trousers.

Lock: Always make sure both wheels and the frame are secure. Remove your front wheel and then lock it, the back wheel, and the frame to a post using the Kryptonite Evolution Series 4 LS ($50, kryptonitelock.com).

Fenders: Make sure your frame has fenders—or eyelets to attach them. They'll prevent puddle water from turning your back into a Jackson Pollock abstract and keep you from spattering other riders ($45, planetbike.com).

Cargo: If you need more than a messenger bag, opt for a rack with waterproof panniers that can hold a laptop or a change of clothes. Try the Linus Office Bag ($75, shop.linusbike.com).

Lights: The Planet Bike SuperFlash set ($70, planetbike.com) includes a three-LED red blinking light, visible up to a mile away, and a ½-watt headlight. Make like a Volvo driver and turn them on to boost visibility in daylight.

Brands: Spot's hybrid bikes, like the 8-gear Sprawl, use the carbon drive (from $1,100, spotbrand.com). Two other rigs with it: Raleigh's Alley Way ($1,475, raleighusa.com) and Trek's District ($1,150, trekbikes.com).

Q: How long does it take to earn a black belt in MMA?

A: It's taken Cain Velasquez, the current UFC heavyweight champion, 4 years of training every day to reach brown belt (one below black) in Brazilian jujitsu, the king of mixed martial arts. Derived from judo, it combines grappling and ground-based submissions.

It also has a strong self-defense component, says David Camarillo, a black belt in Brazilian jujitsu and Velasquez's trainer at the American Kickboxing Academy in San Jose, California. "If you train three times a week, you can learn the basics in about 6 months; a black belt typically takes 8 years." During that time you will sculpt a lean, strong physique and possibly sharpen your mind: Training in martial arts can help you develop the area of your brain responsible for concentration and memory, according to a study in the *Journal of Science and Medicine in Sport*. To find a Brazilian jujitsu dojo near you, visit dojolocator.com.

CREDITS

INDEX

Boldface page references indicate photographs. <u>Underscored</u> references indicate boxed text.